**OSCEs for
Medical Finals**

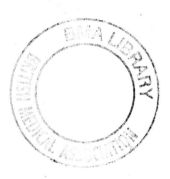

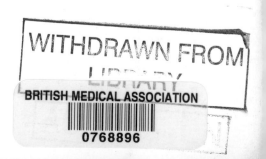

OSCEs for Medical Finals

Hamed Khan

MBBS DGM MRCGP MRCP (London)
GP Principal and Undergraduate Tutor
Oxted, Surrey

Iqbal Khan

BSc MBBS
FY2 Doctor
Homerton University Hospital NHS Foundation Trust

Akhil Gupta

BSc MBBS
Specialist Registrar in Anaesthetics
London Deanery

Nazmul Hussain

MBBS MRPharmS
GP ST3
Newham GP Vocational Training Scheme

Sathiji Nageshwaran

BSc MBBS
FY2 Doctor
Royal Free London NHS Foundation Trust

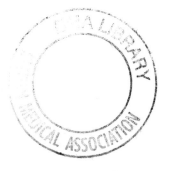

WILEY-BLACKWELL

A John Wiley & Sons, Ltd., Publication

Library of Congress Cataloging-in-Publication Data
OSCEs for medical finals / Hamed Khan ... [et al.].
      p. ; cm.
   Objective structured clinical examinations for medical finals
   Includes bibliographical references and index.
   ISBN 978-0-470-65941-0 (pbk. : alk. paper) – ISBN 978-1-118-44190-9 (eMobi) –
ISBN 978-1-118-44191-6 (ePDF/ebook) – ISBN 978-1-118-44192-3 (ePub)
   I. Khan, Hamed.   II. Title: Objective structured clinical examinations for medical finals.
   [DNLM: 1. Clinical Medicine–Examination Questions.   2. Clinical Competence–
Examination Questions.   3. Communication–Examination Questions.   4. Medical
History Taking–Examination Questions.   5. Physical Examination–Examination
Questions.   WB 18.2]

   616.0076–dc23

                              2012024677

A catalogue record for this book is available from the British Library.

Wiley also publishes its books in a variety of electronic formats. Some content that appears in print may not be available in electronic books.

Cover design by Sarah Dickinson

Set in 8.75/11 Minion pt by Toppan Best-set Premedia Limited
Printed and bound in Malaysia by Vivar Printing Sdn Bhd

1   2013

Contents

Part 4: Procedures

Companion website

This book is accompanied by a companion website:

www.wiley.com/go/khan/osces

featuring:
- Downloadable checklists from the book
- Survey showing which OSCE stations have a high chance of appearing in finals

Contributors

We are grateful to the following doctors and medical students for their contributions to this book.

Contributors to the chapters
Shifa Rahman
Manpreet Sahamey
Ruth-Mary deSouza
Gillian Landymore
Ravi Naik

Contributors to the medical school tables
Saba Ali
Ali Alidina
Nina Arnesen
Svitlana Austin
James Best
Kerry Bosworth
Lisa Burton
Sangeetha Chandragopal
Emily Clark
Laura Clarke
Rebecca Critchley
Nicola Davis
Ruth-Mary deSouza
Pippa Dwan
Matthew Everson
Martin Fawcett
Clare Fernandes

Lyndsey Forbes
Rachel Friel
Ushma Gadhvi
Harminder Gill
Catherine Hatzantonis
Elizabeth Hockley
Laura Hopkins
Towhid Imam
Zara Jaulim
Michelle Kameda
Jennifer Kelly
Pamini Ledchumykanthan
Almas Malik
Sathiji Nageshwaran
Ravi Naik
Sania Naqvi

Siva Nathan
Allan Nghiem
Gary Nicholson
Clarissa Perks
Anna Rebowska
Elissa Scotland
Charly Sengheiser
Nadir Sohail
Charlotte Spilsbury
Sarah Thompson
Elizabeth Khadija Tissingh
Christine Wahba
John Wahba
Siobhan Wild
Anna Willcock
Ahila Yogendra

Acknowledgements

We are immensely grateful to the multitude of friends and colleagues who helped us with various aspects of this book. They include the following:
- All of the patients who kindly permitted us to use their photos in this book
- All the staff at Eversley Medical Centre who assisted us with finding patients with signs that could be photographed – specifically Dr John Chan, Dr Colette Boateng and practice nurses Pauline Kearney and Cheryl Mirador
- Dr Vivek Chayya and Dr Alison Barbour for their advice on gastroenterology
- Dr Sara Khan, Dr Kartik Modha, Dr Nazia Khan and Dr Siva Nathan for their help in recruiting contributors
- Saiji Nageshwaran and Vaitehi Nageshwaran for reviewing several of the chapters
- Mr Ian Skipper for his unparalleled IT expertise and assistance
- Dr Khalid Khan for helping us develop the idea from which this book was derived, and for reviewing, proofreading and critiquing the final manuscript
- All of our parents and families, without whose patience and support this project would never have succeeded

We are also grateful to the Medical Womens Federation, Tiko's GP Group and the Muslim Doctors Association for helping us recruit contributors through their organisations.

Preface

The student begins with the patient, continues with the patient, and ends his studies with the patient, using books and lectures as tools, as means to an end.

Sir William Osler

Few will disagree that the recent overhauls in medical training, together with higher numbers of medical students being trained, has made medicine far more competitive than before. Medical students today have to make definitive career choices much earlier on than they would have had in years gone by, and to start building a portfolio of achievements such as audits and publications very early on at medical school. Time has become even more precious than it was before, and it is understandable that medical students today will opt for concise focused textbooks rather than sprawling prosaic texts, some of which have been used over many generations and gained an almost legendary status.

This book is perhaps unique in that it has been written by a group of doctors who range from those in career-grade posts who have completed postgraduate training and have been OSCE examiners themselves, to those who have very recently sat their finals. We have collated our experiences to create a textbook that we have made as focused, easy to read and, above all, as exam-orientated as possible. While doing this, we have worked hard to ensure that we include everything necessary not only to pass finals, but also to achieve excellent marks and hopefully merits and distinctions.

The structure is based on four sections – clinical examinations, histories, communication skills and procedures. At the beginning of each of these sections, there is a 'Top Tips' page that has generic advice for any OSCE station of that section which would help you boost your marks and performance regardless of what the station is.

Each section is divided into chapters based on the stations we feel are most likely to appear in OSCEs at medical schools. Practice makes perfect – and more so in OSCEs than in any other form of assessment. That is why we have started each chapter with a checklist of items reflecting the areas you are likely to be marked on. You should use these to perfect and consolidate your routines, and also when practising OSCEs with friends and on patients. You should ideally do this in a pair or a group of three, with one student doing the station as a candidate and one allocating mock 'marks' using the checklists to assess the candidate's performance.

Following this in each section, we have included tables that summarise the most common conditions that are likely to present in finals OSCEs. We have ensured that the information on the conditions in these tables is as focused and exam-oriented as possible. There is also a 'Hints and tips for the exam' section in which we have summarised key advice and common pitfalls that finalists tend to make.

We hope that this book will make your revision not only thorough and focused, but also enjoyable. We have spent a lot of time working with our publishers to make the text as vibrant, colourful and easy to read as possible, with a plethora of tables, illustrations and photos that will not only make it easy to remember key ideas and principles, but also make the topic more interesting.

We wish you the very best of luck with your finals OSCEs, and hope that you find this book both enjoyable and useful.

Hamed Khan

Part 1: Examinations

Top tips

Do:

• **Memorise the steps:** The most important thing that OSCE examiners are looking for is an ability to carry out a full examination with reasonable technique and speed. At finals level, you will be forgiven for missing a few signs, and the vast majority of the marks on the mark schemes are allocated for going through the motions and doing all the 'steps'. In contrast, at postgraduate level, for example for the MRCP exam, you would be expected to pick up all the major signs, and be penalised heavily for missing them.

• **Always suggest a number of possible differential diagnoses:** Very few doctors will be able conclusively to put their finger on a diagnosis after examining a patient for 10 minutes without a history. Offering a number of differentials means that you have a higher chance of at least mentioning the correct one, even if it is not at the top of your list. It will also show a healthy awareness of your own limitations.

• **Practise, practise and practise:** The best way to do this is by seeing patients, having a friend to assess you using our checklists and then getting critical (but constructive) feedback from them. Swapping roles and watching colleagues examine is more useful than most students think, as it will reinforce the steps of the examination, and you may see them use techniques and skills that you would not otherwise have thought of. Doing all the major examinations should become such a normal routine for you that you can do it without thinking about what the next step will be – just like riding a bicycle or driving a car.

Don't:

• **Don't be nervous:** Most people have problems in OSCEs not because of poor technique or knowledge, but because of anxiety and nervousness. Don't be overwhelmed by the occasion, and don't be intimated by an examiner's grilling. You will find it much easier to focus on your technique and findings if you are relaxed, and most examiners only grill students who are doing well, as they do not waste their breath on those whom they have decided are a lost cause!

• **Don't worry about minutiae:** Medicine is not an exact science, and different doctors have different ways of examining patients, most of which yield the right conclusions. At undergraduate level, all the examiners are looking for is a decent, fluent technique that appears to be well practised. Don't spend ages trying to figure out exactly how much the chest should expand, or whether the cricoid–sternal notch distance is three finger breadths or four.

• **Don't hurt the patient:** This is the only unforgivable sin in the OSCE. Its always a good idea to start your examination by asking if the patient is in pain anywhere, and reassuring them that if you unintentionally cause pain during the examination, you will be happy to stop. Students often have a tendency to ignore patients saying 'Ouch!' and pretending that they have not heard it, but this is definitely the worst thing you can do. If you do cause pain, acknowledge it immediately, apologise unreservedly and offer to stop – both examiners and patients will appreciate your honesty and professionalism.

Generic points for all examination stations

HELP:

H: 'Hello' (introduction and gains consent)

E: Exposure (nipples to knees/down to groins)

L: Lighting

P: Positions correctly (supine), asks if patient is in any pain

Washes hands

Inspects from end of bed for paraphernalia

Inspects patient (scars, etc.)

Thanks patient

Offers to help patient get dressed

Washes hands

Presents findings

Offers appropriate differential diagnosis

Suggests appropriate further investigations and management

For joints only: Look → Feel → Move → Active/passive/resisted

---

OSCEs for Medical Finals, First Edition. Hamed Khan, Iqbal Khan, Akhil Gupta, Nazmul Hussain, and Sathiji Nageshwaran.
© 2013 John Wiley & Sons, Ltd. Published 2013 by John Wiley & Sons, Ltd.

1 Cardiovascular

Checklist	P	MP	F
HELP:			
H: 'Hello' (introduction and gains consent)			
E: Exposure			
L: Lighting			
P: Positions at 45 degrees, asks if patient is in any pain			
Washes hands			
Inspection:			
• From end of bed: ECG, GTN spray			
• Scars: thoracotomy, mitral valvotomy			
• Pacemaker			
Hands:			
• Clubbing (infective endocarditis, cyanotic heart disease, atrial myxoma)			
• Signs of infective endocarditis (splinter haemorrhages, Janeway lesions, Osler's nodes)			
Radial pulse:			
• Rate			
• Rhythm (regular or irregular)			
• Character (collapsing, slow rising)			
• Radial–radial delay			
Requests blood pressure			
Eyes:			
• Xanthelasma			
• Corneal arcus			
• Anaemia			
Face:			
• Malar flush			
Mouth			
• 'CDD' (central cyanosis, dental hygiene, dehydration)			

Neck:			
• Jugular venous pressure (raised >4 cm)			
• Palpates carotid pulse (character)			
Palpates apex beat			
Checks if apex beat is displaced in axilla			
Palpates sternal edges and subclavicular areas for thrills			
Auscultates chest:			
• Mitral area/apex beat (5th intercostal space [ICS], midclavicular line) • Tricuspid area (4th ICS, right sternal edge) • Pulmonary area (2nd ICS, right sternal edge) • Aortic area (2nd ICS, left sternal edge) • Palpate carotid or brachial pulse simultaneously to time murmur			
Cardiac manoeuvres:			
• Auscultates mitral area with patient lying on left side and in expiration for murmur of mitral stenosis			
• Auscultates aortic area with patient sitting forward and in expiration for murmur of aortic regurgitation			
Auscultates lung bases for pulmonary oedema			
Palpates shins or ankles for peripheral oedema			
Thanks patient			
Offers to help patient get dressed			
Washes hands			
Presents findings			
Offers appropriate differential diagnosis			
Suggests appropriate further investigations and management			
OVERALL IMPRESSION:			

Summary of common conditions seen in OSCEs

	Aortic stenosis	Aortic regurgitation	Mitral stenosis	Mitral regurgitation	Tricuspid regurgitation
Location of murmur (loudest heard)	Aortic area	Aortic area	Mitral area	Mitral area	Tricuspid area
Type of murmur	Ejection **systolic** Radiating to carotids	End-**diastolic**	Mid-**diastolic**	Pan-**systolic** Radiating to axilla	**Systolic**
Manoeuvres to enhance murmur	None	Sit forward and expirate	Roll on left side and expirate	None	None
Pulse	Slow rising	Collapsing Carotid pulsations	Irregular if atrial fibrillation	Normal	Normal
Peripheral features	Narrow pulse pressure Commonly have CABG scar	Quincke's sign Corrigan's pulsation De Musset's sign	Atrial fibrillation on auscultation Right-sided heart failure	None	JVP increased to earlobes
Key management points	Aortic valve replacement if severe Beta-blockers Diuretics Treat heart failure Antibiotic prophylaxis for gastrointestinal/ genitourinary/dental procedures	Aortic valve replacement Treat any heart failure Antibiotic prophylaxis for gastrointestinal/ genitourinary/ dental procedures	Mitral valvotomy Treat atrial fibrillation and heart failure Antibiotic prophylaxis for gastrointestinal/ genitourinary/ dental procedures Anticoagulate (with warfarin)	Mitral valve replacement Treat any heart failure Antibiotic prophylaxis for gastrointestinal/ genitourinary/ dental procedures	Tricuspid valvotomy Treat right heart failure

Hints and tips for the exam

Identifying valvular lesions

Trying to learn all the murmurs and all the conditions associated with them is futile and only really necessary if you are a cardiologist. Trying to correctly differentiate whether murmurs are ejection systolic or pansystolic, end-diastolic rather than mid-diastolic, is also difficult and is not necessary for finals and perhaps even PACES.

The easiest and most logical way of diagnosing the correct valvular lesion from the murmur is by answering the following two questions:

1. Where is the murmur?
Murmurs can frequently be heard throughout the chest, but the area where a murmur is loudest is usually where the murmur is – so a murmur heard loudest in the aortic area will probably be aortic regurgitation (AR) or aortic stenosis (AS), and a murmur heard loudest in the mitral area will probably be mitral regurgitation (MR) or mitral stenosis (MS). Exceptions to this include Gallavardin's phenomenon, in which an AR murmur is heard loudest in the tricuspid area; however,

from the perspective of passing an exam, you would not be penalised for missing that, and in any case it is extremely rare.

2. Is it systolic or diastolic?
In other words, does the murmur correspond with the pulse (systolic) or not (diastolic)?

Murmurs will only be produced if the natural flow of the blood is opposed. In the case of valves through which the blood leaves the heart (such as the aortic valve), systolic murmurs will only be produced when the outflow of blood is hindered, which can only happen in AS (as opposed to AR, which would not hinder the outflow of blood).

In the case of valves where the blood flows into the heart in diastole, the natural flow of blood in diastole is against the aortic valve, as the purpose of the aortic valve is to stop blood flowing into the aorta during diastole. Hence blood hits the aortic valves and stops there when the cardiac muscles relax in diastole. This natural flow would be impaired by AR as the blood flows into the aorta when it should not, which is why a diastolic murmur in the aortic area can only be AR.

If this seems too complex, remember that diastolic murmurs are usually 'ARMS' (AR or MS), and the area where it is loudest is probably where the murmur is.

Right versus left
• LEFT-sided murmurs are louder in EXPIRATION.
• RIGHT-sided murmurs are louder in INSPIRATION. This is because more blood flows into the intrathoracic cavity and lungs on inspiration, and hence more blood flows through the right-sided heart valves as these supply the lungs. The converse is true for left-sided murmurs.

It is vital to ask patients to hold their breath when using this test, but you must not ask them to do this for too long as this can cause the patient pain and you will fail the exam. Its often a good idea to hold your own breath at the same time so that you will know when it is getting too long to allow your patient to breath normally.

Timing the murmur
Timing murmurs is something that both students and experienced doctors have difficulty with. Just remember to palpate the pulse when listening to the heart sound, and see if you hear the murmur at the same time as you feel the pulse.
• If the murmur is WITH the pulse, it is a SYSTOLIC murmur.
• If the murmur if NOT WITH the pulse, it is a DIASTOLIC murmur.
Use a central pulse such as the carotid or brachial to do this, otherwise it will not be accurate.

Diastolic murmurs
A number of conditions can cause diastolic murmurs, but the most common ones are AR and MS – this can be easily memorised using the mnemonic 'ARMS'.

Diastolic murmurs are very difficult to elicit for even the most experienced doctors, and if you can hear a murmur easily, it is most likely to be systolic. However, if you do manage to identify a diastolic murmur, it is handy to remember that MS murmurs are much quieter than AR murmurs, and if you can auscultate a diastolic murmur throughout the chest, it is much more likely to be AR than MS.

Valve replacements
If you see a midline sternotomy scar, you should immediately bring your ear close to the patient's chest and listen carefully for the clicking noise that is indicative of the closing of a metallic valve replacement – this can easily be heard without a stethoscope.

Also remember that you should not hear a murmur with a replaced valve unless it is leaking.

Identifying which valve has been replaced
Remember that the pulse correlates with the first heart sound, which is the mitral valve closing. (The second heart sound is the aortic valve closing.)
• If the loudest sound of the valve closing correlates with the pulse, it is the first heart sound, indicating that the mitral valve has been replaced.
• If the loudest sound of the valve does not correspond with the pulse, it is the second heart sound, indicating that the aortic valve has been replaced.
• The location of the loudest sounds may also be helpful. Bioprosthetic valves sound the same as normal heart valves, so it would be unfair for examiners to expect you to identify them.

Apex beat
The apex beat is palpable in the 5th intercostal space, and is displaced to the apex in MR. Various characters of the apex beat have been described, such as 'heaving' and 'thrusting'; differentiating between them is extremely difficult and probably beyond the scope of a 10-minute OSCE. Other than this, it is more likely to cause confusion than add anything substantive.

The best course of action is to describe where the apex beat it, and whether it is palpable or not. An impalpable apex beat is often caused by obesity, hyperinflation of the lungs, dextrocardia or poor technique.

Scars
Figures 1.1–1.5 show scars and other signs that you will need to note on your examination of the patient.

Questions you could be asked

Q. Which organism causing infective endocarditis is associated with underlying bowel cancer?
A. *Streptococcus bovis* – a colonoscopy should be considered in all patients presenting who are found to have *Streptococcus bovis*.
Q. What is the most common cause of tricuspid regurgitation?
A. Most cases of tricuspid regurgitation are 'functional', due to dilatation of the right ventricle (so that the tricuspid valves flop downwards). This could arise for a number of reasons, such as right heart failure, congestive heart failure and pulmonary hypertension.

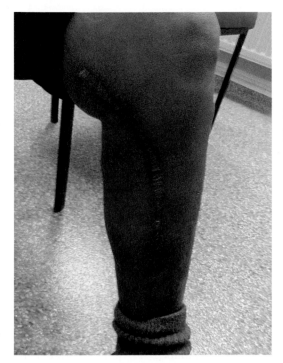

Figure 1.1 Graft scar from leg vein removal in coronary artery bypass grafting

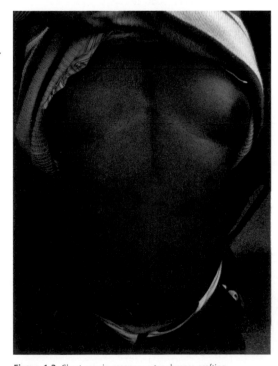

Figure 1.2 Chest scar in coronary artery bypass grafting

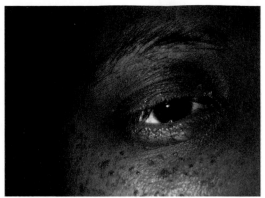

Figure 1.3 Xanthelasma

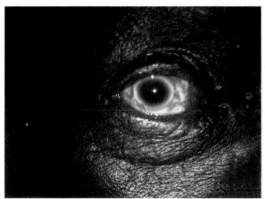

Figure 1.4 Corneal arcus

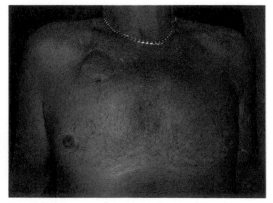

Figure 1.5 Indication of pacemaker insertion

Q. How should a patient with suspected heart failure be investigated in primary care?

A. According to the NICE guidelines (NICE, 2010), the primary investigation of choice is the blood level of brain natriuretic peptide (BNP)– patients with normal results are unlikely to have heart failure, and those with a BNP level >400 pg/mL should be investigated urgently (within 2 weeks).

Reference

National Institute for Health and Clinical Excellence (2010) Chronic heart failure: Management of chronic heart failure in adults in primary and secondary care. Available from http://www.nice.org.uk/nicemedia/live/13099/50526/50526.pdf (accessed June 2012).

2 Respiratory

Checklist	P	MP	F
HELP:			
H: 'Hello' (introduction and gains consent)			
E: Exposure			
L: Lighting			
P: Positions at 45 degrees, asks if the patient is in any pain			
Washes hands			
Inspects from end of bed: • Looks at the front and back for thoracotomy scars • Sputum pots (bronchiectasis, COPD) • Oxygen cylinders (COPD) • Inhalers (COPD, asthma) • Immuosuppressants (pulmonary fibrosis) • Nebulisers (COPD) • Peak flow charts (asthma)			
Hands:			
• Clubbing (suppurative conditions, lung cancer, fibrosis)			
• Tar staining			
• Wasting of small muscles			
Tremor + CO_2 retention flap			
Radial pulse			
Respiratory rate			
Eyes:			
• Horner syndrome (Pancoast syndrome)			
• Anaemia			
Face:			
• Plethora (polycythaemia)			
Mouth:			
• 'CDD' (central cyanosis, dental hygiene, dehydration)			

Neck:			
• JVP (raised >4 cm) in cor pulmonale			
• Palpates lymph nodes			
• Tracheal deviation			
• Cricoid–suprasternal notch distance (<three finger breadths in hyperinflation)			
Palpates:			
• Palpates apex beat			
• Measures chest expansion (6–8 cm is normal) at three places on the anterior and three on the posterior chest			
Percusses:			
• Percusses at three positions on the anterior and three on the posterior chest			
Auscultates:			
• Auscultates at three positions on the anterior and three on the posterior chest			
• Auscultates axillae to listen for right middle lobe signs			
• Auscultates for vocal fremitus			
Palpates shins or ankles for peripheral oedema			
Thanks patient			
Offers to help patient get dressed			
Washes hands			
Presents findings			
Offers appropriate differential diagnosis			
Suggests appropriate further investigations and management			
OVERALL IMPRESSION:			

Summary of common conditions seen in OSCEs

Condition	Key finding	Chest expansion	Percussion	Auscultation	Vocal fremitus
Pulmonary fibrosis	**Fine end-inspiratory crackles**	Decreased bilaterally	Normal/mild decrease at bases	Fine end-inspiratory crepitations	Normal/increased at bases
Pneumothorax	**Increased resonance**	Decreased unilaterally	Increased resonance	Decreased breath sounds at site of pneumothorax	Decreased
Pleural effusion	**Stony dull bases**	Normal	Dull on side of effusion	Dull base(s)	Decreased at base
COPD/asthma	**Wheeze**	Normal	Normal	Wheeze + scattered crepitations in COPD	Normal
Lobectomy	**Scar**	Normal	Dull at site of lobectomy	Normal	Normal
Pneumonectomy	**Scar**	Decreased unilaterally	Dull on side of pneumonectomy	Absent on side of pneumonectomy	Decreased
Bronchiectasis	**Sputum pot, crackles, clubbing**	Normal	Normal	Normal	Normal
Consolidation	**Crackles concentrated in one area**	Normal	Normal	Normal/increased at site of consolidation	Normal/increased at site of consolidation

Hints and tips for the exam

Inspection

Inspection can often provide the diagnosis at the respiratory station. There are some key stereotypical features of a few conditions that can give the case away.

Findings	Condition
Young, thin, short patient with a PEG site near the umbilicus and a tunnelled catheter at the axilla or on the chest	Bronchiectasis secondary to cystic fibrosis
Middle-aged patient with full sputum pot	Bronchiectasis
Cushingoid features (high BMI, bruising, striae) and bruising (from steroid use)	Pulmonary fibrosis
Features of rheumatological disease, e.g. rheumatoid hands (ulnar deviation, swollen metacarpophalangeal joints, swan neck deformity) or scleroderma (beak-shaped nose, small mouth, tight skin, telangiectasia)	Pulmonary fibrosis
Elderly patient with tar-stained fingernails and an oxygen cylinder at the bedside	COPD
Characteristic scars (with pictures)	Lobectomy/ pneumonectomy

Timing

A common problem at the respiratory station is timing as students find it difficult to listen to carefully all the breath sounds in enough places during the 5–10 minutes they have.

Once you have completed your inspection, start examining from the back. Most physicians will agree that it is easier to percuss and auscultate at the back as you have more surface area available. In addition, the position of the heart often makes it difficult to establish findings in the left lower zone of the lung anteriorly.

One of the ways you can minimise collateral time losses is by reducing the time spent in changing the patient's position. When the patient is lying down, palpate, percuss and auscultate the anterior aspect of the chest. When he or she is sitting forwards, palpate, percuss and auscultate the posterior aspect, and examine for lymphadenopathy at the same time.

Lobectomies and pneumonectomies

These are very common in OSCEs as patients are usually stable and ambulant, and the examination findings are obvious. Students are often surprised when they do not hear decreased breath sounds at the site of lobectomy scars, which they may have done during their ward attachments. This is because, after a few months or years, patients with lobectomies develop

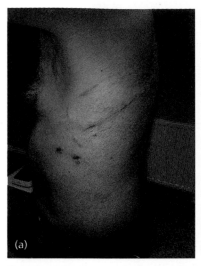
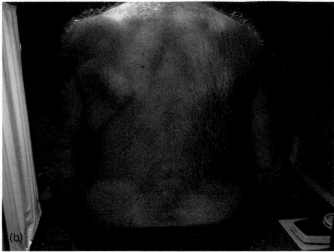

Figure 2.1 Lobectomy scar: side view (a) and back view (b)

compensatory hyperinflation, and lung tissue fills up areas it was removed from. This will not be the case immediately after lobectomy surgery as sufficient time has not surpassed for compensatory hyperinflation to occur.

The scar from a pneumonectomy can be very similar to the scar from a lobectomy (Figure 2.1), although they can immediately be distinguished by the fact that chest expansion and breaths sounds are usually completely absent on the side of a chest that has undergone a pneumonectomy.

'Creps and clubbing'

Remember that bilateral crepitations and clubbing that occur together most commonly present in patients with bronchiectasis or pulmonary fibrosis.

Questions you could be asked

Q. Why are spontaneous pneumothoraces more common in tall men?
A. There are a number of theories for this. One is that the difference between the intrapleural pressure of the apex and the base is greater in taller people, making it easier for a pneumothorax to form spontaneously. Another is that any anatomical defects or blebs will become more stretched if the length if the lung is longer, as is the case in taller individuals.
Q. Why might you hear breath sounds over an area of the lung that has been excised in a lobectomy?
A. See 'Lobectomies and pneumonectomies' above.
Q. Name three causes of bibasal crepitations with clubbing in a patient.
A. See 'Creps and clubbing' above.

3 Abdominal

Checklist	P	MP	F
HELP:			
H: 'Hello' (introduction and gains consent)			
E: Exposure (nipples to knees/down to groins)			
L: Lighting			
P: Positions correctly (supine), asks if patient is in any pain			
Washes hands			
Inspects from end of bed for relevant paraphernalia (e.g. nutritional supplements, CAPD device)			
Inspects patient:			
• Body habitus (BMI, Cushingoid from immunosuppressants following organ transplant)			
• Pallor (anaemia)			
• Jaundice			
• Pigmentation (Addison's disease, Peutz–Jeghers syndrome, 'bronze'/slate grey in haemochromatosis, drugs)			
• Bruising			
• Tattoos			
• Peripheral skin lesions associated with IBD (erythema nodosum, pyoderma gangrenosum)			
Hands:			
• Clubbing (IBD, malignancy, malabsorption states such as coeliac disease, liver cirrhosis)			
• Dupuytren contracture			
• Palmar erythema			
• Leukonychia (iron deficiency)			
• Koilonychia			
• Liver flap			
Arms:			
• Arteriovenous fistula (for dialysis) – auscultate for bruit			
• Tattoos			
Eyes:			
• Jaundice			
• Anaemia			
• Xanthelasmata			
Face:			
• Parotid enlargement (alcohol excess)			
Mouth:			
• Angular stomatitis (iron/vitamin B deficiency)			
• Glossitis (vitamin B deficiency)			
• Peri-oral pigmentation (Peutz–Jeghers syndrome), telangiectasia			
• Ulcers (IBD)			
• Dehydration			
• Dental hygiene			
• Smell of breath (hepatic fetor, uraemia)			
Supraclavicular lymph nodes (Virchow's node/ Troisier's sign for stomach cancer)			
Chest:			
• Gynaecomastia			
• Spider naevi (more than five is significant)			
Inspects abdomen:			
• Scars (see Figure 3.4)			
• Drain insertion sites			
• Peristalsis/pulsations			
• Caput medusae			
• Distension			
• Masses/swellings			
• Stretch marks/striae			
Palpates abdomen (ideally kneeling down):			
• Superficial palpation in nine quadrants for masses and tenderness			
• Deep palpation in nine quadrants for masses and tenderness			
• Hepatomegaly			
• Splenomegaly			
• Ballots kidneys			
• Abdominal aortic aneurysm			
Percusses abdomen:			
• Liver			
• Spleen			
• Ascites with shifting dullness			
• Bladder (dull if full, e.g. in urinary retention)			
Auscultates for bowel sounds, renal bruits, abdominal aortic aneurysm			
Examines for shifting dullness/ascites			
Examines lower legs for oedema			

Tells examiner he would like to complete the examination by examining the following: • Hernial orifices (with cough/sitting up) • Genitalia • Rectum • Lymph nodes • Urine dipstick			
Thanks patient			
Offers to help patient get dressed			

Washes hands			
Presents findings			
Offers appropriate differential diagnosis			
Suggests appropriate further investigations and management			
OVERALL IMPRESSION:			

Summary of common findings seen in OSCEs

- Chronic liver disease
- Hepatomegaly
- Splenomegaly
- Nephrectomy scar/features of end-stage renal failure (ESRF)
- Enlarged kidneys

- Transplanted kidneys
- Ascites
- Hernia
- Stoma
- Surgical scars

Summary of common conditions seen in OSCEs

Common chronic conditions	Chronic liver disease	Inflammatory bowel disease	Renal disease/ESRF
Examination findings			
General inspection	Malnourished Bruising (impaired clotting)	Cushingoid appearance (from steroids)	Cushingoid appearance (from steroids) CAPD paraphernalia
Hands/arms	Clubbing Palmar erythema Dupuytren contracture Liver flap (in hepatic encephalopathy) Leukonychia (due to hypoalbuminaemia)	Clubbing Tubing for total parenteral nutrition Leukonychia/ koilonychia	Arteriovenous fistula (listen to bruit) Elevated blood pressure Renal osteodystrophy
Face	Jaundiced sclera (if decompensated) Parotid enlargement (if liver failure caused by excess alcohol intake)	Mouth ulcers Temporalis muscle wasting	Gum hypertrophy (ciclosporin) Anaemia Collapsed nasal bridge (Wegener's granulomatosis) Molluscum (immunosuppression) Viral skin warts/skin cancers Butterfly rash (if SLE) Hearing aid (if Alport syndrome)
Neck	Raised JVP (if fluid overload secondary to hypoalbuminaemia)		Parathyroidectomy scar (after tertiary hyperparathyroidism) Raised JVP Cushingoid neck

(Continued)

Common chronic conditions	Chronic liver disease	Inflammatory bowel disease	Renal disease/ESRF
Chest	Reduced hair Gynaecomastia Spider naevi		Right internal jugular/subclavian tunnelled intravenous line/scar CABG scar (may indicate atherosclerosis causing renovascular disease)
Abdomen	Jaundice (if decompensated) Ascites (if portal hypertension) Hepatomegaly Splenomegaly (in portal hypertension) Caput medusae	Surgical scars Liver transplant scar (from primary sclerosing cholangitis) Fistulas Stomas	Nephrectomy scars (if renal transplant/dialysis) Enlarged kidneys (if adult polycystic kidney disease) Transplanted kidney palpable in iliac fossa/near groin CAPD scars Injection sites (from subcutaneous insulin) Cushingoid features (if immunosuppression with steroids)
Legs	Peripheral oedema (hypoalbuminaemia)	Pyoderma gangrenosum Erythema nodosum	Peripheral oedema
Key investigations	Liver function tests Clotting and albumin (for synthetic liver function) Alcohol screen Abdominal ultrasound Viral hepatitis screen Autoimmune hepatitis screen Viral serology screen Liver biopsy Oesophago-gastro-duodenoscopy (to look for varices if portal hypertension suspected)	Inflammatory markers Colonoscopy Stool microscopy, culture and sensitivity	Urinalysis (including albumin creatinine ratio) Us+Es and glomerular filtration rate Nephritic/vasculitic screen Renal ultrasound IVU/CT kidneys, ureter and bladder Renal biopsy
Key management principles	Treat underlying cause Stop all hepatotoxic medications Nutritional support Salt restriction Monitor fluid status and input/output Vitamin B/folate supplements Lactulose Monitor blood glucose Monitor Glasgow Coma Scale score Treat clotting abnormalities Assess for portal hypertension (splenomegaly/ascites/caput medusae) → if present do oesophago-gastro-duodenoscopy for varices	Steroids (topical/enema/oral) Mesalazine/ azathioprine/ anti-TNF Assess for toxic megacolon Monitor inflammatory markers Metronidazole for perianal disease Nutritional support/ elemental diet Surgery	Treat underlying cause Stop all nephrotoxic medications Nutritional support Salt restriction Monitor fluid status and input/output Calcium supplements (if hypocalcaemic) Phosphate binders (if high phosphate) Monitor parathyroid hormone level (consider parathyroidectomy if tertiary hyperparathyroidism) Monitor blood gases and treat acidosis Monitor Hb (consider erythropoietin/iron if anaemic) Optimise blood pressure (ACE inhibitor) and cholesterol

Common conditions leading to chronic liver disease

To make things easier, we have summarised here the key clinical features and investigations of chronic liver disease that you can use in the viva/questions part at the end of the OSCE generically, regardless of what the cause of the liver disease is. Table 3.1 outlines common conditions leading to chronic liver disease – the most common ones are marked with an asterisk. This will be especially useful for students aiming for a merit or distinction, as it helps to diagnose not only chronic liver disease, but also the underlying cause.

Hints and tips for the exam

Hepatomegaly and splenomegaly

Hepatomegaly and splenomegaly are also very common findings at this station in finals. We have discussed various key tips below to help you in both the diagnosis and the discussion.

Examining large livers and spleens
• Start low in the right iliac fossa, so that you do not miss giant organomegaly.

Table 3.1 Common conditions leading to chronic liver disease

Common causes of chronic liver disease	Key points in history	Collateral 'clues'	Specific investigations to identify cause
*Alcohol	Alcohol intake CAGE	Rib fractures on chest X-ray	High AST:ALT ratio High MCV
*Hepatitis B and C	Sexual history Intravenous drug abuse Blood transfusions Travel abroad	Tattoos Scars from intravenous access	Hepatitis serology
Primary biliary cirrhosis	Xanthelasmata Pigmentation Clubbing Excoriation marks	Female (>90%) Middle-aged Features of autoimmune/connective tissue/rheumatological diseases Features of immunosuppression (Cushing's disease, molluscum contagiosum)	↑ IgM Antimitochondrial antibodies Cholestatic liver profile (↑ ALP) Liver biopsy
Autoimmune hepatitis	Musculoskeletal pain	Features of autoimmune/connective tissue/rheumatological diseases Features of immunosuppression (Cushing's disease, molluscum)	↑ IgG Antinuclear antibodies Anti-smooth muscle antibodies Liver biopsy
Primary sclerosing cholangitis	Past medical history of or active IBD	Features of IBD (usually ulcerative colitis) Bowel surgery scars Stoma	pANCA ERCP/MRCP Liver biopsy Cholestatic liver profile (↑ ALP)
Wilson's disease	Family history (autosomal recessive inheritance)	'Bronze' skin pigmentation Marked tremor Kayser–Fleischer rings in iris Dysarthria/cognitive impairment	Serum copper 24-hour urinary copper excretion
Haemochromatosis	Family history (autosomal recessive inheritance) Diabetes Arthritis Hypopituitarism	'Slate grey' pigmentation 'Bronzing' of the skin Gonadal atrophy Gynaecomastia	Serum iron studies Liver biopsy
Fatty liver/non-alcoholic steatohepatitis)	Xanthelasmata	Hypertension CABG scar	Ultrasound Lipids
Heart failure	Past medical history of heart disease/hypercholesterolaemia	Signs of heart failure	Echo

• Use the radial aspect of your index finger – but if that doesn't work, use your finger with your hands pointing up towards the patient's head.
• Keep your fingers absolutely still as the patient breathes in and out.
• Make sure that you move your hand upwards superiorly by no more than 2 cm as the patient breathes in and out. If you leave too large a distance as you move up, there is a risk that you may miss the edge of the liver or spleen.
• For the liver, percussion is almost as discriminatory as palpation. It is also useful to differentiate between lung hyperinflation pushing the liver down, and true hepatomegaly. The superior aspect of the liver usually lies between the 4th and 6th ribs, and continues down to the last rib at the inferior border of the rib cage; hence, there should be dullness in all of this area. Hyperinflation pushing down the liver is confirmed if percussion is resonant significantly below the 6th rib.
• For the spleen, use your left hand to stabilise the left ribs in order to prevent them from being pushed towards the left as you palpate the spleen with your right hand. If you still have difficulty, roll the patient on to the right side and repeat this.
• When you do find an enlarged liver or spleen, estimate the size of hepatomegaly in centimeters rather than 'finger breadths', which vary from person to person (depending on how big their fingers are!).
• Avoid the business of trying to identify the liver characteristics (e.g. whether it 'firm', 'hard' or 'soft', or pulsatile, or nodular or smooth). Doing this in an exam will make the patient uncomfortable and use up your valuable time without achieving very much. Once a large liver or spleen has been identified, the most logical way of defining its characteristics would be to carry out some sort of imaging – usually an ultrasound of the abdomen.

Systematic differentiation of the underlying causes of hepatomegaly and splenomegaly

• A large liver and/or spleen is a very common finding at finals OSCE stations. Make sure that you have a generic system for categorising the causes, so that you can reel off a list of differential diagnoses quickly, confidently and systematically.
• Always try to use all the signs to help you devise a differential diagnosis. However, if you find an enlarged spleen or liver and have no clue what the cause is, go for conditions that can cause hepatomegaly and splenomegaly either individually or together – the first column of Table 3.2 summarises these.

• Don't be too pedantic when distinguishing between gigantic, moderate and mild splenomegaly. Identifying splenomegaly and giving a reasonable list of differential diagnoses and investigations will usually be enough to score a decent pass. Distinguishing between mild/ moderate and gigantic splenomegaly will help to get you into the merit/distinction range. Remember that the spleen has to be at least double or triple its normal size to be palpable.
• Remember to piece the other parts of your examination together to complete the diagnostic jigsaw. All the conditions that cause hepatomegaly or splenomegaly have several peripheral signs so look out for these and use them to support your differential diagnosis.

Renal cases

Although students often worry about getting a 'renal case' in finals, it can often be a blessing in disguise. The differential diagnosis is relatively straightforward, and the signs are easy to elicit.

Fundamentally, there are only two findings in renal cases – those of ESRF, and ballotable enlarged kidneys.

End-stage renal failure

There are potentially three findings that are all attributable to ESRF:
• **Nephrectomy scar** (Figure 3.2): Inspect carefully for this, making sure that you look all the way around the lumbar/flank regions through to the back. Finding a nephrectomy scar is alone sufficient to devise a full list of differential diagnoses and a management plan.
• **Palpable transplanted kidney:** This is usually near the groin/iliac fossa with a small scar at the site.
• **Signs of dialysis use** (arteriovenous fistula, right internal jugular vein line, CAPD scars; Figure 3.3): A slicker way of describing this is 'renal replacement therapy', which covers them all – and also sounds more impressive!

Whichever of these signs the patient has, the underlying condition is always ESRF.

The four most common causes of ESRF are as follows:
1) Diabetes
2) Hypertension
3) Adult polycystic kidney disease (APKD)
4) Glomerulonephritis

Once you have got to this stage, your investigations and management should be guided by your differential diagnosis. However, if you are still struggling, merely discuss the generic investigations and management strategies for patients with ESRF, as discussed in the summary table above.

Table 3.2 Causes of hepatomegaly and splenomegaly

	Hepatosplenomegaly	Hepatomegaly only (without splenomegaly)	Splenomegaly only (without hepatomegaly)			Peripheral signs
			Gigantic splenomegaly (palpable in right lower quadrant)	Moderate splenomegaly (5–10 cm)	Mild splenomegaly (2–5 cm)	
Malignancy	All haematological malignancies (myeloproliferative and lymphoproliferative)	Hepatocellular carcinoma Secondary metastases	Chronic myelogenous leukaemia Myelofibrosis	All haematological malignancies (myeloproliferative and lymphoproliferative)	All haematological malignancies (myeloproliferative and lymphoproliferative)	Lymphadenopathy Cachexia Anaemia Bruising and purpura
Infective	Viral hepatitis CMV Toxoplasmosis Malaria Schistosomiasis Histoplasmosis Brucellosis Leptospirosis Kala-azar Weils disease Hydatid disease	Viral hepatitis	Chronic malaria Visceral leishmaniasis	All infectious causes of hepatosplenomegaly	Glandular fever Brucellosis Viral hepatitis Early sickle cell disease HIV	Pyrexia Recent foreign travel Tattoos/intravenous drug abuse scars (viral hepatitis)
Infiltrative	Sarcoidosis Amyloidosis Gaucher's disease	Fatty liver/NASH Haemochromatosis	Gaucher's disease	Gaucher's disease	Sarcoidosis Amyloidosis Gaucher's disease	Sarcoid skin disease
Inflammatory	–	–	–	Felty's syndrome (rheumatoid arthritis, neutropenia, splenomegaly)	Rheumatoid arthritis SLE	Arthropathy Butterfly rash of SLE
Liver disease	Liver disease with portal hypertension	Any cause of chronic liver disease (as above)	–	Portal hypertension	Liver cirrhosis with portal hypertension	Signs of chronic liver disease (as above)
Cardiovascular	–	Right heart failure Tricuspid regurgitation	–	–	Infective endocarditis Constrictive pericarditis	Ankle oedema, raised JVP Haematuria and peripheral signs of endocarditis
Miscellaneous	–	Polycystic kidney disease (causing liver cysts)	–	–	Haemolytic anaemias (autoimmune, hereditary spherocytosis) Thalassaemia	Ballotable kidneys/ nephrectomy scar Jaundice (from haemolysis)

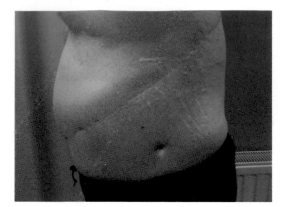

Figure 3.1 Scar from splenectomy after a road traffic accident, also showing the drain insertion site

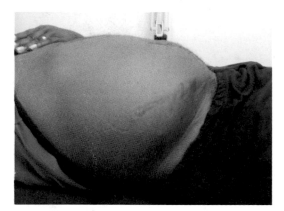

Figure 3.2 Nephrectomy scar

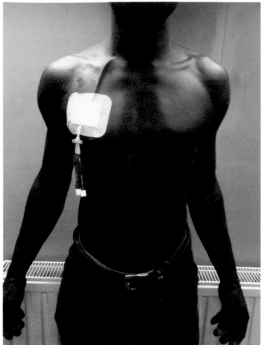

Figure 3.3 Right internal jugular tunnelled catheter (for dialysis)

Ballotable/ enlarged kidneys

Ballotable enlarged kidneys can be palpated in the lateral lumbar regions. As with ESRF, you only need to remember a short list of differential diagnosis:
- APKD
- Renal cell carcinoma
- Bilateral hydronephrosis (secondary to obstruction, e.g. by an external mass, prostate enlargement, etc.)
- Amyloidosis (primary or secondary)

The key investigations with all of these are imaging (CT of the kidney, ureter and bladder/IVU) and renal biopsy, with the management depending on the underlying cause.

Rare findings

- **Clubbing versus pseudoclubbing:** Although these conditions look similar on examination, the underlying causes are fundamentally different. Pseudoclubbing occurs because of tertiary hyperparathyroidism and although it looks like clubbing, with prominence of the distal phalanges, what actually happens is that the proximal phalanges become narrow, and this makes the distal phalanges look prominent despite being normal.

Pseudoclubbing is common after renal replacement therapy – patients with long-standing secondary hyperparathyroidism (due to low calcium levels) develop parathyroid hyperplasia, leading to increased parathyroid hormone production that becomes autonomous of the negative feedback system. Once a patient is undergoing renal replacement therapy and their calcium levels normalise, the parathyroid continues producing excess parathyroid hormone, which results in hypercalcaemia and resorption of bone from the proximal phalanges, causing them to narrow.

- **Chronic liver disease and features of ESRF in the same patient:** This is rare, but don't let it put you off. The most likely cause is hepatitis C (leading to chronic liver disease), which also causes membranous glomerulonephritis (leading to ESRF).
- **Spleen versus kidney:** When palpating the left side of the abdomen, it can sometimes be difficult to distinguish a ballotable kidney from a spleen. Table 3.3 below summarises the key differences.

Theoretically, the spleen should be dull while the kidney has traditionally been documented in most texts to be 'resonant'. This is, however, more theoretical than realistic as in practice both kidneys and spleens feel dull on percussion.

Abdominal scars

As with all OSCEs, the key findings in abdominal examination are often established on inspection (Figure 3.4):

1) Rooftop scar
   - Partial hepatectomy
   - Pancreatic surgery
   - Accessing aorta
2) Kocher incision
   - Cholecystectomy
3) 'Mercedes-Benz' scar
   - Liver transplant
   - Gastric surgery
   - Oesophageal surgery
4) Midline laparotomy
   - Colon surgery
   - Aortic abdominal aneurysm surgery

Table 3.3 Spleen or kidney?

Spleen	Kidney
Cannot get above the spleen	Should be able to get above the kidney
Moves downwards and medially with inspiration	No movement with breathing
Not ballotable	Ballotable
Palpable notch (medial aspect)	No notch

5) Nephrectomy scar (r
   1. Classic caesarea'
   2. Appendicector
   3. Caesarean sec
   4. Inguinal hernia sca.
   5. Femoral hernia scar

Abdominal masses

If you find a mass, try to answer two questions in mind.

1. Where is the mass?

First identify the quadrant where the mass is located, and then think of the organs in that quadrant from which the mass might originate (Figure 3.5).

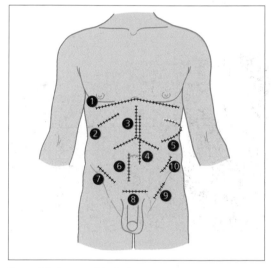

Figure 3.4 Common abdominal scars

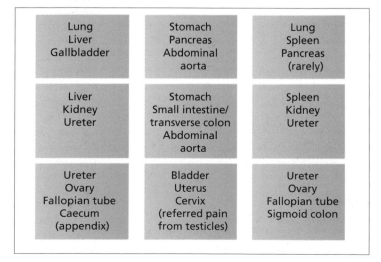

Lung Liver Gallbladder	Stomach Pancreas Abdominal aorta	Lung Spleen Pancreas (rarely)
Liver Kidney Ureter	Stomach Small intestine/ transverse colon Abdominal aorta	Spleen Kidney Ureter
Ureter Ovary Fallopian tube Caecum (appendix)	Bladder Uterus Cervix (referred pain from testicles)	Ureter Ovary Fallopian tube Sigmoid colon

Figure 3.5 Location of organs in the abdomen

mber to describe the mass accurately and logi-
see Chapter 10 on breast examination for a table
aracteristics that you should aim to describe.

What is the lesion?

As with everything in OSCEs, the key is to have a
generic method of categorising potential differential
diagnoses. The categories below can be used to devise
a differential diagnosis for a mass in almost any of the
nine quadrants:

- Tumour
  - Benign
    - **i.** Cyst (liver, renal)
    - **ii.** Fibroids (in the pelvic area in women)
    - **iii.** Vascular (abdominal aortic aneurysm)
  - Malignant
    - **i.** Primary
    - **ii.** Secondary
    - **iii.** Lymphoma
- Infection
  - Abscess
  - Tuberculosis (usually ileocaecal)
- Inflammatory bowel disease
  - Crohn's disease (in right iliac fossa)
  - Diverticular disease (left iliac fossa)

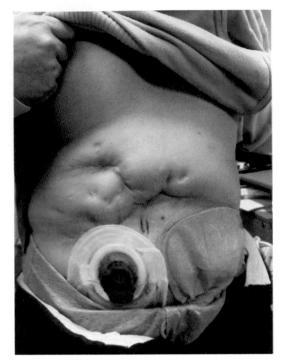

Figure 3.6 Stoma

Key investigations

The crux of investigating a mass is to visualise it and to
get a tissue sample from it. Hence the following investigations are most important:

- **Imaging:** CT/MRI scan
- **Endoscopy:** colonoscopy for colon, oesophago-
gastro-duodenoscopy for oesophagus/stomach, cystos-
copy for bladder
- **Biopsy:** for any non-vascular mass

Stomas

Stomas (Figures 3.6 and 3.7) feature more commonly
in finals than most students think, and they are actually
quite easy to examine and talk about. The most
common stomas are ileostomies and colostomies, and
the key feature that distinguishes them is their location.
Table 3.4 summarises the key features.

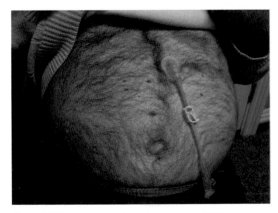

Figure 3.7 Percutaneous endoscopic gastrostomy (PEG)

Questions you could be asked

Q. What is the one investigation you would do in a
patient with known portal hypertension in order to
reduce mortality?

A. The key features of portal hypertension are:
- Splenomegaly
- Ascites
- Caput medusae
- Oesophageal varices

Although the answer to this is debatable, the most
important investigation would be an oesophago-
gastro-duodenoscopy to identify varices, and more
importantly to band them and prevent torrential acute
severe gastrointestinal bleeding.

Q. How big does the spleen have to be before it is
palpable?

A. About twice its normal size.

Table 3.4 Stomas

	Ileostomy	Colostomy	Nephrostomy	Urostomy
Location	Right iliac fossa/lower quadrant	Left iliac fossa	Flank	Right side of umbilicus
Reasons for use	Colon cancer (proximal) IBD Familial adenomatous polyposis	Colon cancer (more distal) Diverticulitis	Any cause of renal tract obstruction	Any cause of renal tract obstruction
Consistency of products	Watery (as there is no colonic absorption of water)	Hard and dry (after colonic absorption of water)	Urine	Urine (often has tiny amounts of mucus produced by the small intestinal conduit)
Mucosal appearance	Mucosa protrudes 3–4 cm as a 'spout'	No protrusion of mucosa	Usually no significant mucosal protrusion	Usually no significant mucosal protrusion
Permanent or temporary	End-ileostomy (most common): permanent Loop ileostomy (rare): temporary	End-colostomy: permanent Loop colostomy: temporary	Usually temporary	Temporary or permanent

Q. Name some causes of a palpable liver without hepatomegaly.

A.

- Lung hyperinflation (e.g. COPD) pushing it down
- Riedel's lobe (on the left lateral side of liver)
- Gallbladder pathology

Q. What are 'Terry's nails'?

A. Terry's nails signify chronic liver disease. They have a characteristic appearance, being white proximally but dark red distally, often in a concave shape.

4 Peripheral nervous system

Upper limbs

Checklist	P	MP	F
HELP:			
H: 'Hello' (introduction and gains consent)			
E: Exposure and explains he or she wants to examine the nerves of the arms			
L: Lighting			
P: Have the patient in a position that they find comfortable and in which the examination can easily be undertaken			
Washes hands			
Inspects from end of bed: • Relevant paraphernalia: walking stick, crutches, foot supports, wheelchair, special glasses, hearing aid			
Inspects patient's arms:			
• Asymmetry			
• Scars			
• Skin changes			
• Deformities			
• Claw hand			
• Wrist drop			
• Fasciculations			
• Wasting of small muscles of hands			
• Scars			
• Contractures			

• Signs of denervation, such as:
    • Injuries
    • Neuropathic ulcers/Charcot joints			

Inspects patient's back:			
• Spinal scars (back or side of neck)			
• Kyphosis			
Abnormal movements:			
• Abnormal movements			
• Tremor			
• Dyskinesia			
• Chorea			

Scars and skin changes + signs of denervation: • Injuries • Neuropathic ulcers • Charcot joints			
Inspects patient's neck:			
• Spinal scars – these can be at the back or on the side of the neck			
• Kyphosis			
Motor examination			
Screening test: Asks patient to raise both arms forwards when in a supine position			
Pronator drift: Asks patient to sit up and close their eyes. Ask them to stretch their arms out with the palms up at the level of their shoulders. Looks for drift into pronation			
Tone: Checks at each joint in flexion, extension, pronation and supination			
Power:			
• Shoulder abduction: C5			
• Shoulder adduction: C6, C7, C8			
• Elbow flexion: C5, C6			
• Elbow extension: C7			
• Wrist flexion: C8			
• Wrist extension: C7			
• Fingers: T1			
Fingers: flexion, extension, abduction, adduction, opposition, grip strength			
Thumb: abduction, adduction, extension			
Reflexes:			
• Reinforces if absent (clench teeth or apply Jendrassik* manoeuvre)			
• Biceps: C5/C6			
• Triceps: C6/C7			
• Supinator: C5/C6			

Hoffman's sign: • Flexes and then suddenly releases distal phalanx of middle finger • Looks for abnormal flexion of other fingers • This indicates an upper motor neuron lesion			
Coordination: • Finger–nose testing bilaterally • Dysdiadochokinesis bilaterally • Looks for intention tremor and past-pointing • Tests for rebound by pushing down on the outstretched arms and looking for rebound past the original position			
Sensory examination			
Explains examination to patient and checks their sensation on a part of the body known to have normal sensation (such as forehead or sternum)			

Examines the following modalities on all dermatomes:
• Dermatomes of the upper limbs:
  • C3: lateral neck
  • C4: lateral shoulder
  • C5: lateral upper arm
  • C6: thumb
  • C7: middle finger
  • C8: little finger
  • T1: medial lower arm
  • T2: medial upper arm
  • T3: axilla
• Dermatomes of the lower limbs:
  • L1: just below groin
  • L2: medial aspect of mid-thigh
  • L3: knee
  • L4: medial lower leg
  • L5: big toe
  • S1: little toe
  • S2: medial aspect of back of knee			

Pin-prick (spinothalamic tract): uses a Neurotip			

Vibration(dorsal column): uses a 128 Hz tuning fork on most distal phalanx, and only proceeds proximally if a deficit is identified			
Joint proprioception(dorsal column): • Only proceeds proximally if a deficit is identified • Holds terminal phalanx of thumb. Shows patient that 'up' means extension and 'down' means flexion. Asks them to close their eyes. Moves phalanx and ask them to say if it is 'up' or 'down'. Only proceeds proximally to the wrists and elbows if a deficit is identified. Offers to perform two-point discrimination using calipers			
Light touch (dorsal column): uses a wisp of cotton wool			
Temperature (spinothalamic tract): offers to use syringes of hot and cold water			
Identifies pattern of sensory loss: • Identifies if the pattern is dermatomal or 'glove and stocking' • Identifies level if it is dermatomal			
Special tests: performs these based on the likely diagnosis from the examination. Common ones to know are Phalen's, Tinel's and Froment's			
Thanks patient			
Offers to help patient get dressed			
Washes hands			
Presents findings			
Offers appropriate differential diagnosis			
Suggests appropriate further investigations and management			
OVERALL IMPRESSION:			

*If the reflexes are difficult to elicit, reinforce them by asking the patient to interlock their fingers and pull them in opposite directions (Jendrassik manoeuvre).

Lower limbs

Checklist	P	MP	F
HELP:			
H: 'Hello' (introduction and gains consent)			
E: Exposure (shorts or underwear) + explains he or she wants to examine the nerves of the legs			
L: Lighting			
P: Have the patient in a position that they find comfortable and in which the examination can easily be undertaken. Ensure privacy and dignity			
Washes hands			
Inspects from the end of the bed for paraphernalia: walking stick, crutches, foot supports, wheelchair, special glasses, hearing aid			
Inspects patient's legs:			
• Fasciculations			
• Wasting of proximal and distal lower limb muscles			
• Scars			
• Skin changes			
• Signs of denervation (injuries, neuropathic ulcers, Charcot joints)			
• Contractures			
• Pes cavus			
• Foot drop			
• Deformities			
• Abnormal movements			
Inspects patient's back:			
• Spinal scars			
• Kyphosis, scoliosis			
MOTOR EXAMINATION			
Gait: Asks patient to walk and turn, and observes gait carefully and any walking aids the patient uses. Assesses heel–toe gait and patient's ability to stand on tiptoes			
Romberg's test:			
• Asks patient to stand with both feet together and their arms to their sides, first with their eyes open and then with their eyes closed			
• Positive if patient appears to be falling (indicates dorsal column or sensory nerve pathology) – **ensure that patient does not fall!**			

Tone:			
1) Lifts the knees quickly off the ground			
2) 'Rolls' both hips gently			
3) Checks for clonus (using ankle dorsiflexion)			
Power:			
Hip flexion: L1, L2			
Hip extension: L5, S1			
Knee flexion: L5, S1			
Knee extension: L3, L4			
Ankle dorsiflexion: L4, L5			
Ankle plantarflexion: S1, S2			
Foot inversion: L4, L5			
Foot eversion: L5, S1			
Toe movements: L5, S1			
Reflexes:			
Reinforces if absent (clench teeth or Jendrassik* manoeuvre)			
Knee: L3/4			
Ankle: L5/S1			
Plantar: Up (upper motor neurone lesion) or down (lower motor neurone lesion/normal)			
Coordination: Heel–shin testing bilaterally, gait			
SENSORY EXAMINATION			
Explains examination to patient and checks their sensation on a part of the body known to have normal sensation (such as forehead or sternum)			
Examines following modalities on all dermatomes:			
• **Pin-prick** (spinothalamic tract): uses a Neurotip			
• **Vibration** (dorsal column): uses a 128 Hz tuning fork on most distal phalanx, and only proceeds proximally if a deficit is identified			
• **Joint proprioception** (dorsal column): • Holds great toe and shows patient that 'up' means extension and 'down' means flexion. Then asks them to close their eyes, and moves the toe, asking patient to say if it is moving 'up' or 'down' • Only proceeds proximally if a deficit is identified • Offers to perform two-point discrimination using calipers			

• **Light touch** (dorsal column): uses a wisp of cotton wool			
• **Temperature** (spinothalamic tract): offers to use syringes of hot and cold water			
• **Identifies pattern of sensory loss:** • Identifies if the pattern is dermatomal or 'glove and stocking' • Identifies level if it is dermatomal			
Thanks patient			

Offers to help patient get dressed			
Washes hands			
Presents findings			
Offers appropriate differential diagnosis			
Suggests appropriate further investigations and management			
OVERALL IMPRESSION:			

*If the reflexes are difficult to elicit, reinforce them by asking the patient to interlock their fingers and pull them in opposite directions (Jendrassik manoeuvre).

Summary of common conditions seen in OSCEs

List of common cases

Lower limb	Upper limb
Foot drop	Carpal tunnel syndrome
Post stroke	Ulnar nerve palsy
Cerebellar degeneration	Wrist drop
Sensory neuropathy	Axillary nerve palsy
Radiculopathy secondary to spinal pathology	Volkmann's contracture
Cerebral palsy	Cervical rib
Muscular dystrophy	Cerebellar degeneration
Pes cavus	Tremor – Parkinson's disease, essential tremor
Old cauda equina syndrome	Post stroke
Old polio	Motor neurone disease
Brown–Sequard syndrome	Erb's or Klumpke's palsy

Common patterns of weakness, and common causes for them

Pattern of weakness	Common causes
Proximal muscle weakness	Myopathy
Distal weakness	Inherited myopathies
Hemiparesis	Cerebral pathology
Paraparesis	Thoracic or lumbar cord lesion Cauda equina syndrome
Tetraparesis	Cervical cord lesion
Monoparesis	Plexus lesion

Summary of common conditions and findings in the peripheral nervous system

Upper motor neurone (UMN) conditions	Lower motor neurone (LMN) conditions	Combined UMN and LMN lesions

Stroke:
• Unilateral hemiplegia
• Patient is commonly elderly
	Peripheral neuropathy: secondary to:
	• Common causes:
	  • Diabetes (most common)
	  • Alcohol
	  • Vitamin B/B12 deficiency
	  • Excess toxins (e.g. from liver or renal failure)
	  • Malignancy
	  • Inflammatory disease (such as vasculitis)
	• Rarer causes:
	  • HIV
	  • Guillain–Barré syndrome
	  • Chronic inflammatory demyelinating polyneuropathy
	  • Lead poisoning
		Motor neurone disease:
		• Elderly
		• Dysarthria
		• Fasciculations
		• Weakness
		• Hypertonia

Multiple sclerosis: • UMN signs • Cerebellar signs • Often a young woman in a wheelchair	**Nerve root lesion:** • Specific dermatome/myotomal signs • Sensory level	**Subacute combined degeneration of spinal cord:** • Features of pernicious anaemia or vitamin B12 deficiency
Spinal cord lesion/damage: • Spastic paraplegia	**Proximal myopathy:** • Secondary to endocrine causes (Cushing's disease, Addison's disease) • Polymyalgia rheumatica	**Friedreich's ataxia:** • Upgoing plantars and weak ankle reflexes • Kyphoscoliosis • Pes cavus • High-arched palate
	Hereditary neuropathies: • e.g. Charcot–Marie–Tooth disease	
	Mononeuritis multiplex: • Secondary to anything that damages the nerve intrinsically, e.g. diabetes, excess toxins	

UMN vs LMN signs

	UMN (brain and spinal cord)	LMN (distal to anterior horn cells)
Inspection	Spastic gait	Muscle wasting Fasciculations
Tone	Increased tone (spastic – pyramidal, or rigid – extrapyramidal)	Reduced/normal tone
Power	Weakness	Weakness
Reflexes	Brisk reflexes	Hyporeflexia
Plantars	Upgoing plantars	Downgoing plantars

Gait in examination of the peripheral nervous system

Type of gait	Findings
Spastic gait	Both legs affected
Hemiplegic gait	Circumduction, usually post stroke
Waddling gait	Proximal myopathy
Festinant gait with freezing and no arm movements	Parkinson's disease
Broad-based ataxic gait	Cerebellar dysfunction
Antalgic gait	Joint or back pain in which the patient takes their weight off the affected side
High-stepping gait	Sensory neuropathy, and in foot drop
Scissor gait	Cerebral palsy and multiple sclerosis
Stamping gait	Sensory neuropathy
Apraxic gait	Diffuse cerebral disease and dementia

Hints and tips for the exam

Before going any further, it is important to remove from your mind the myth that neurology is difficult, and ingrain some structures that will simplify your examination findings and help you come to the right conclusions.

First of all, always ask yourself the following two questions when encountering neurological cases:

1. **Where is the lesion?**

If the findings relate to an UMN, the lesion is affecting the brain or the spinal cord. If it is an LMN lesion, it is affecting the peripheral nerves.

In UMN lesions, tone and power are increased, whereas in LMN lesions they are decreased.

2. **What is the lesion?**

Once you have localised the lesion, you need to have a list of causes that you systematically go through.

UMN

- **Neoplastic:** primary, secondary, benign
- **Vascular:** ischaemic stroke, haemorrhage
- **Trauma**
- **Demyelination:** multiple sclerosis
- **Inflammation:** vasculitis, post-infectious inflammation

These causes could affect the brain or spinal cord, and could all be considered and presented in an OSCE as potential differential diagnoses for a UMN lesion.

LMN

With LMN lesions, the pattern of the clinical findings often helps to distinguish the diagnosis. The most common patterns of presentation are as follows.

Asymmetrical weakness

For a structured answer that will demonstrate a robust understanding of the pathological processes of the peripheral nervous system, consider where the lesion could be, working your way from the proximal area of the CNS near the spinal cord, to the distal part areas the peripheries:

- **Anterior horn cell:** This lies at the border of the spinal cord and peripheral nerves, and hence lesions will exhibit both UMN and LMN signs, for example in motor neurone disease, syringomyelia or cervical myelopathy.
- **Nerve root lesion:** Commonly due to prolapsed spinal cord discs, these lesions usually cause a mixed motor and sensory neuropathy, and the level of the lesion can be localised.
- **Plexus lesion (brachial plexus in the upper limbs, sacral plexus in the lower limbs):** These lesions usually cause problems in a diffuse group of multiple nerves, so would not be easily defined to a spinal cord level or a specific nerve.
- **Mononeuritis multiplex:** If you are grilled in your viva after the OSCE on any asymmetrical LMN lesion, an easy 'one-size-fits-all' answer is mononeuritis multiplex. This basically describes a group of nerves being affected and could result from a huge variety of metabolic and structural causes.
- **Neuromuscular junction:** This includes conditions such as Guillain–Barré syndrome and Eaton–Lambert syndrome. There would usually be a global affect on all the nerves of an upper or lower limb, or there would be a clear pattern, as there is in both of the above-mentioned conditions.

Proximal symmetrical weakness/proximal myopathy

- **Inflammatory/rheumatological:** polymyositis, dermatomyositis, vasculitis, rheumatoid arthritis
- **Endocrine:** Cushing's disease, Addison's disease, diabetes, hypothyroidism
- **Paraneoplastic**
- **Muscular dystrophy:**
  - Duchenne muscular atrophy
  - Becker's muscular dystrophy
  - Fascio-scapulo-humeral dystrophy
- **Drugs:** such as statins and insulin
- **Metabolic:** osteomalacia

Distal symmetrical weakness

• **Peripheral neuropathy:** This is by far the most common neurological condition. It is caused by a vast number of pathologies that affect the intrinsic nerve, usually metabolically, but sometimes physically compressing it. Common causes to remember for OSCEs are given above. Most peripheral neuropathies affect both sensory and motor modalities in the distal limbs.

• **Mononeuritis multiplex:** Again, there is a vast list of pathologies that can cause this, most of which overlap with those of peripheral neuropathy. However, the nerve distribution is not necessarily distal and symmetrical, which makes this a useful differential diagnosis, as virtually any LMN condition can potentially be due to mononeuritis multiplex.

Grading power using the Medical Research Council scale

As a finalist, you would pass if you described power subjectively as normal, weak or absent. But if you are aiming for a merit, you should use the Medical Research Council's (MRC) grading scale, which is more specific – and actually very easy to remember and use (Table 4.1).

Plegia versus paresis

If you are going to use the terms 'paresis' and 'plegia', make sure you know the difference: 'plegia' refers to when there is absolutely no ability to move the limb, whereas 'paresis' refers to a weakness in which some ability to move is retained.

Grading reflexes

As with power, you could pass by describing reflexes as present, absent or hyperreflexic. However, you will look much more slick if you use the descriptions shown in Table 4.2.

Table 4.1 MRC grading of muscle power

0	No movement at all
1	Flicker of muscle
2	Can move but cannot oppose gravity
3	Can oppose gravity
4*	Can perform resisted movements but weak
5	Normal power

*Grade 4 is sometimes broken into 4+ and 4− to further quantify the degree of resistance. This is not much use other than in serial examinations to show the change from one examination to the next.

Table 4.2 Grading of reflexes

+	Present
++	Brisk
+++	Pathologically brisk
+/−	Present with reinforcement
−	Absent

Know your tracts

This is important when diagnosing the cause of a specific sensory deficit. In summary:

• **Spinothalamic tract:** temperature, sharp pain sensory

• **Dorsal column:** vibration, proprioception, fine touch

Increased tone in UMN lesions

Remember that it takes a good few weeks for tone to become increased following an UMN lesion – so don't be surprised if you elicit UMN signs in a patient but find that he or she has normal tone. If you are aiming for a merit or distinction, use this knowledge to diagnose whether an UMN lesion is acute or chronic.

What is pronator drift?

Pronator drift is a sign of an UMN lesion. It is present when there is spasticity from a pyramidal lesion and occurs due to an imbalance between pronation and supination of the forearms. Upwards drift may represent cerebellar dysfunction.

Remember the pain factor

Movement can sometimes be limited by pain, so try to distinguish whether a muscle weakness is neurological or the result of pain. At the very least, if the patient is in pain, state during your presentation that the patient was in pain, and that this made it difficult to accurately assess power.

Bladder, bowel and sexual function

Patients with lower limb neurology as a result of spinal pathology may also have bladder, bowel and sexual dysfunction. Although it is not appropriate to check these in an OSCE, it is worth mentioning that you would consider a rectal examination and would check the residual bladder volume in cases where leg neurology was caused by spinal pathology.

Questions you could be asked

Q. Name some Parkinson-plus syndromes and their salient signs.

A. • **Multisystem atrophy:** autonomic dysfunction, postural hypotension, bladder dysfunction

• **Progressive supranuclear palsy:** loss of vertical gaze, then loss of horizontal gaze (causing frequent falls), pseudobulbar palsy, proximal rigidity, dementia later on

Q. What is the difference between 'plegia' and 'paresis' (e.g. hemiplegia and hemiparesis)?

A. As described in the text above, plegia = paralysis, paresis = weakness.

Q. How do you elicit Hoffman's test?

A. See the upper limb checklist at the start of the chapter.

Q. What is the pronator drift test used to assess?

A. See the section on pronator drift above.

Q. How long does it take for tone to become increased after a UMN lesion?

A. A few weeks, as described in the text.

5 Central nervous system

Checklist	P	MP	F
HELP:			
H: 'Hello' (introduction and gains consent) Explains that needs to examine the nerves of the face			
E: Exposure of head and eyes – sits opposite the patient at eye level			
L: Lighting			
P: Positions correctly (sits opposite patient at eye level), asks if patient is in any pain			
Washes hands			
Inspection:			
• Facial asymmetry (stroke, parotid gland tumour)			
• Ptosis (complete – cranial nerve III palsy, or partial – Horner's syndrome)			
• Convergent or divergent squint (congenital or muscle/nerve pathology)			
• Medical aids – glasses, eye patch, hearing aids, pen and paper for communication			
• Hearing aids (deafness – peripheral or central cause)			
• Fasciculations (LMN)			
• Dyskinesia			
• Wasting (LMN, UMN, disuse atrophy)			
• Abnormal movements (tremor, chorea, myoclonus)			
• Speech defects (see Chapter 8 on speech)			
• Scars (back of ear – acoustic neuroma, craniotomy; in front of ear – parotid gland tumour, and may have associated ipsilateral facial nerve palsy)			
• Tracheostomy, nasogastric or PEG tubes (lower cranial nerve dysfunction leading to breathing difficulties and unsafe swallow)			
Cranial nerve I: olfactory nerve (sensory): • Sense of smell can be tested with smelling salts • Any change/loss of smell? • Most likely cause of abnormal sense of smell is conductive/mechanical (e.g. due to obstruction)			

Cranial nerve II: optic nerve (sensory): • Any change in vision? • 'AFRO-C': • **A**cuity: With glasses (if worn), gets to the patient to identify how many fingers are held up, and then tests with a Snellen chart • **F**ields: • Confrontation (can the patient see the student's face? – central vision) • Asks them to cover their right eye with their right hand. Student covers their own left eye with the left hand, and asks patient to keep looking into their eye. Using free hand, student tests fields, and then swaps hands and repeats on other side • During this part of the exam, maps the blind spot (the area where the patient's view of the finger temporarily disappears) • Tests each eye separately: brings in fingers from outside the field of vision. Does this match the student's field (peripheral vision)? • Pupillary **R**eflexes: • Comments on whether the pupils are the same size • Direct and consensual • Accommodation (pupils constrict on convergence) • Considers testing for relative afferent pupillary defect (RAPD) – damage to optic nerve on one side results in a delay in constriction when swinging a light between the eyes. Pupil appears to dilate when the light is swung to the eye with the damaged optic nerve • Red pins for colour desaturation • Fundi: See Chapter 6 on **O**phthalmoscopy • **C**olour vision: Ishihara plates • Uses a pinhole to correct refractive error			

Cranial nerves III, IV and VI: oculomotor, trochlear, abducens (all motor):
- Tests nerves individually:
  - IV: superior oblique
    - Damage means eye is unable to look down when abducted
  - VI: lateral rectus
    - Damage means eye is unable to abduct
  - III: Other movements: Examine smooth pursuit and nystagmus with a hat pin moved in a 'H' pattern
    - Damage causes dilated pupil, ptosis and restricted eye movements
  - Look for exophthalmos
- Double vision
  - Whether it is going across/up/down and in which direction
- Nystagmus

Cranial nerve V: trigeminal nerve (motor and sensory):
- Tests sensation in three areas supplied by branches V1, V2 and V3 (light touch and pin-prick)
- States intent to elicit a corneal reflex (wisp of cotton on the sclera of the eye – both eyes should blink)
- Opens the patient's mouth against resistance and moves it from side to side (pterygoids)
- Feels the temporalis and masseter muscles while the patient clenches their teeth
- Jaw jerk

Cranial nerve VII: facial nerve (motor and sensory):
- Asymmetry – look for a Bell's palsy
- Is the forehead spared?
- Asks the patient to raise their eyebrows and shut their eyes tight against resistance
- Asks them to show their teeth
- Asks them to puff out their cheeks
- Taste in anterior two-thirds of the tongue

Cranial nerve VIII: vestibulocochlear (sensory):
- Simple test of hearing – whispers a number into each of patient's ears while rubbing the fingers next to the other ear (to prevent the whisper being heard in that ear)
- Rinne and Weber tests (256 Hz tuning fork) – see 'Hints and tips for the exam' below
- States intent to perform caloric testing

Cranial nerves IX and X: glossopharyngeal and vagus (both motor and sensory):
- Assesses cough ('bovine' cough if Xth nerve lesion)
- Listens and identifies hoarseness of voice
- Asks patient to say 'Ah' (uses a torch to see if the palate rises uniformly bilaterally and the uvula is central)
- Taste: posterior third of tongue
- Offers to test gag reflex (using a tongue depressor, carefully touches the back of the throat. Patient should gag. Positive reflex shows intact afferent cranial nerve IX and efferent cranial nerve X)

Cranial nerve XI: accessory (motor):
- Asymmetry of muscles
- Asks patient to shrug shoulders against resistance – trapezius
- Asks patient to turn head to left and right against resistance – sternocleidomastoid

Cranial nerve XII: hypoglossal (motor):
- Visualises tongue at rest (fasciculation)
- Asks patient to protrude tongue (deviation)
- Asks patient to moves tongue to left and right

Thanks patient

Offers to help patient get dressed

Washes hands

Presents findings

Offers appropriate differential diagnosis

Suggests appropriate further investigations and management

OVERALL IMPRESSION:

Summary of common conditions seen in OSCEs

Condition	Cranial nerves involved	Symptoms and signs	Causes
Bulbar palsy	IX, X, XI, XII	**Lower motor neurone** Fasciculating tongue Normal or absent jaw jerk Quiet/nasal speech	Motor neurone disease Guillain–Barré syndrome Myasthenia gravis Brainstem tumour Central pontine myelinolysis
Pseudobulbar palsy	V, VII, X, XI, XII	**Upper motor neurone** Expressionless face Cannot protrude tongue Increased jaw jerk Emotional instability	Disease of corticobulbar tracts Motor neurone disease (UMN and LMN signs) Multiple sclerosis Stroke Central pontine myelinolysis associated with progressive supranuclear palsy
Cerebellopontine angle tumour	V, VII, VIII	Scar behind ear Unilateral hearing loss Vertigo Signs of nerve palsy	Acoustic neuroma • Neurofibromatosis type 2
Oculomotor nerve palsy	III	Down and out Large pupil (surgical) Complete ptosis	Surgical or medical Surgical (unlikely in finals – result of posterior communicating artery aneurysm) Medical – diabetes (pupil spared)

Facial nerve palsy	VII	Contralateral facial weakness (UMN)
		Loss of nasolabial fold
		Inability to wrinkle forehead **only in LMN** (in UMN forehead is spared due to dual cortical representation)
		Hyperacusis
		Scar in front of ear – tumour resection (involving nerve = malignant)
			UMN:
			• Multiple sclerosis
			• Stroke
			• Space-occupying lesion
			LMN:
			• Neuromuscular:
			  • Myotonic dystrophy
			  • Myasthenia gravis
			  • Guillain–Barré syndrome
			  • Bilateral Bell's palsy
			• Compressive:
			  • Sarcoidosis
			  • Cerebellopontine lesion
			  • Parotid tumour
			• Mononeuritis multiplex:
			  • Diabetes
			  • Lyme disease

Vagus nerve palsy	X	Uvula **pulled away** from side of lesion	
Hypoglossal nerve palsy	XII	Tongue **pushed towards** side of lesion	
Cavernous sinus	III, IV, VI, V1		
Jugular foramen	IX, X, XI		
Horner's syndrome – damage to sympathetic ganglion		Ipsilateral: • Partial ptosis • Miosis (small pupil) • Anhydrosis • Enophthalmos	See below Apical lung tumour: Pancoast tumour – invades sympathetic plexus. If invades brachial plexus: arm pain. If invades recurrent laryngeal nerve: hoarse voice
Myasthenia gravis		Fatigability Sternotomy scar	Antibodies to acetylcholine receptor Thymoma

Cranial nerves

Write in your mnemonic and tick whether you think the nerve is motor/sensory or both. (Refer to the examination mark sheet for the answers).

Number	Name	Mnemonic	Motor	Sensory
I	Olfactory			
II	Optic			
III	Oculomotor			
IV	Trochlear			
V	Trigeminal			
VI	Abducens			
VII	Facial			
VIII	Vestibulocochlear			
IX	Glossopharyngeal			
X	Vagus			
XI	Accessory			
XII	Hypoglossal			

Where is the lesion?
Upper motor neurone

Cranial nerves	Site of pathology	Investigation
I–IV	Above (cranial nerves I and II) and within the midbrain	CT or MRI
V–VIII	Pons	
IX–XII	Medulla	

Lower motor neurone

Cause	Investigation
Compression	Nerve conduction studies
Trauma	
Mononeuritis multiplex	

Common eye signs

Pupillary defects commonly turn up in finals, so know your differential diagnoses well.

Large pupil	Small pupil
Palsy of cranial nerve III	Horner's syndrome
Holmes–Adie syndrome (young women, absent ankle and knee reflexes)	Argyll Robertson pupil – neurosyphilis: accommodates (on convergence) but does not react to light
Traumatic (may be irregular)	Age-related miosis
Drugs (dilating eye drops – tropicamide, atropine, illicit drugs (cocaine, ecstasy)	Drugs (opiates)
	Anisocoria (difference in pupil sizes)

Horner's syndrome

Identifying Horner's syndrome is easy, but diagnosing the cause is much more difficult. The table below shows how you do it systematically according to the site of the lesion.

Central lesion	Preganglionic lesion	Postganglionic lesion
Stroke	Pancoast tumour	Carotid artery dissection
Syringomyelia	Thyroidectomy	Carotid aneurysm
Multiple sclerosis	Trauma	Cavernous sinus thrombosis
Tumour	Cervical rib	Cluster headache
Infection		

Visual field defects

You should know the following information inside out by the time you sit finals.

Field defect	Visual fields	Site
Monocular blindness	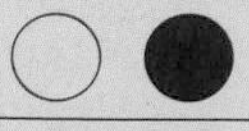	Lesion in front of nerve (vitreous, retina) Ipsilateral optic nerve lesion
Homonymous hemianopia	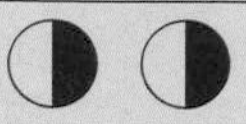	Contralateral optic radiation Contralateral occipital lobe
Bitemporal hemianopia	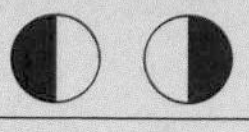	Optic chiasm
Left/right superior quadrantanopia	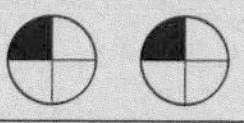	Contralateral temporal optic radiation
Left/right inferior quadrantanopia	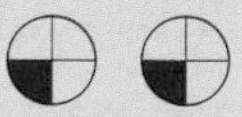	Contralateral parietal optic radiation
Left/right homonymous hemianopia with macular sparing	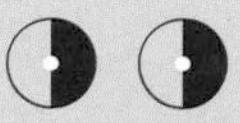	Contralateral occipital lobe infarct due to posterior cerebral artery infarct (the middle cerebral artery also supplies the occipital pole – the area representing the macula)
Arcuate scotoma	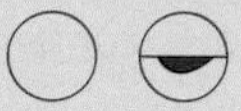	Glaucoma
Central scotoma	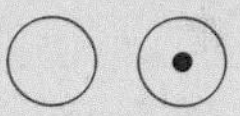	Macular degeneration Macular oedema

Figure 5.1 Visual field defects

Hearing

Air conduction (AC) should be louder than bone conduction (BC), i.e. AC > BC.

Start with a simple test by covering one of the patient's ears with your finger and whispering a number into the other. Ask the patient to repeat what you have said.

Rinne test

Use a 256 Hz tuning fork. Place it near the ear (air conduction). Tell the patient that this is sound 1.

Then place the tuning fork behind the ear (bone conduction). Tell the patient this is sound 2

Ask which was louder. Repeat it if necessary, and remember to test both ears.

Weber test

Place a 256 Hz tuning fork on the centre of the patient's forehead. Ask whether the sound is heard in the middle of the head or towards one side.

Interpreting the Rinne and Weber tests

Rinne test	Result	Findings
Normal	Rinne positive	Air > bone
Conductive	Rinne negative	Bone > air
Sensorineural	Rinne positive	Air > bone

Weber test	Findings
Normal	Heard in centre of head
Conductive	Lateralises to same side
Sensorineural	Lateralises to opposite side

Hints and tips for the exam

Examination of the cranial nerves is testing to say the least. It is feared among students, and most students take longer to prepare for it than for examination of any other area. Yet doing it well will definitely distinguish you from other candidates.

Know the names of the cranial nerves

The first step to learning this examination is to know the names of the 12 cranial nerves.

It is unlikely that you will have to examine the entire 12 nerves at one station, and you will most likely be directed by the blurb outside your station (e.g. 'Examine this patient's lower cranial nerves: V and VII–XII' or 'Examine this patient's eyes' – therefore implying nerves II–IV and VI).

But you don't have to examine in that order

It is not necessary to examine the cranial nerves in the order I–XII. An alternative way to examine all the cranial nerves is to examine each part of the head separately in an orderly manner that covers all the cranial nerves (but not necessarily in numerical order). A possible order could be:

1. Inspection: face, eyelids, symmetry of the pupils, back of the ears for an acoustic neuroma scar

2. Simple test of fields and acuity: 'Can you see my face?' 'Is any part of my face missing?'

3. Eyes:
  • AFRO-C (II, III, IV, VI)
  • Corneal reflex

4. Face:
  • Sensation (V)
  • Facial expression/muscles (VII)
  • Jaw muscles

5. Ears (VIII):
  • Hearing
  • Weber/Rinne tests

6. Tongue and throat (IX, X, XII):
  • Tongue movement
  • Gag
  • Taste
  • Cough
  • Voice

7. Shoulders and neck (XI):
  • Power

See some pathology – real or otherwise

In preparation for this station, include pathology into your practice once you have mastered the slick routine. Have people pretend to have cranial nerve lesions such as of III (ptosis with a down and out eye) or a pseudo-bulbar palsy (difficult but possible to mimic!). This topic can really put you off in the OSCE so it's worth preparing for it.

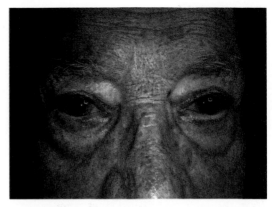

Figure 5.3 Mydriasis of the left pupil

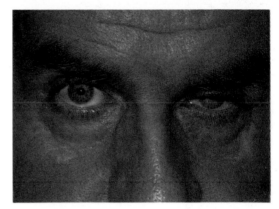

Figure 5.4 Ptosis

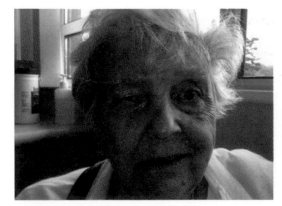

Figure 5.2 Right facial nerve palsy

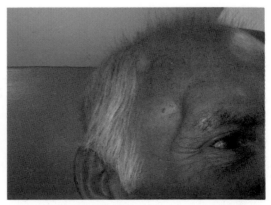

Figure 5.5 Surgical clipping of a berry aneurysm following a subarachnoid haemorrhage

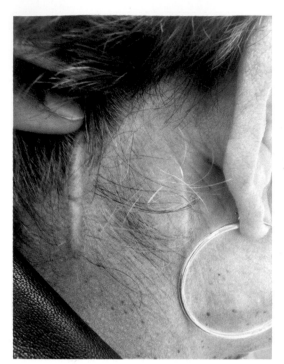

Figure 5.6   Scar from resection of an acoustic neuroma

Diplopia could be myogenic or neurogenic

Diplopia can be caused by either myogenic/myopathic (muscle) or neurogenic (CNS) dysfunction. Myopathic causes result in diplopia being greatest when looking in the direction of the affected muscle.

- Neurogenic:
  - UMN:
    - Brainstem
  - LMN:
    - Mononeuritis multiplex
    - Nerve compression/trauma
- Myogenic:
  - Myasthenia gravis
  - Hypothyroidism
  - Myositis
  - Myotonic dystrophy
  - Lambert–Eaton syndrome

The 'outer image' is produced by the abnormal eye

Of the two images seen, that furthest away is the false image caused by the damaged muscle. Ask the patient to cover each eye and tell you when the outer image disappears – **the eye producing the outer image is the defective eye.**

Simple versus complex ophthalmoplegia

To further understand eye movement disorders (ophthalmoplegias), you can classify them as **simple** or as **complex**.

Simple ophthalmoplegias refer to disorders of movement in one direction. These are most often due to the neurogenic causes. Complex ophthalmoplegias most often arise from disorders related to muscles and neuromuscular junctions (the myogenic causes).

Complex ophthalmoplegias are:
- Myopathies (examine muscle fatigability)
- Graves' disease (check thyroid function tests and MRI of the orbits)
- Retro-orbital tumour

Internuclear ophthalmoplegia

A CNS cause of eye movement disorder that is rather rare but often finds its way into finals, either physically or on questioning from your examiner, is internuclear ophthalmoplegia (INO).

INO describes the phenomenon in which there is failure of adduction of an eye when the other eye is abducting. The neuroanatomy of this eye movement disorder is covered in the questions at the end of this chapter. INO is often associated with infarction or multiple sclerosis. WEBINO (wall-eyed bilateral INO) is very rare (Figure 5.7).

Master the technique from a neurologist

The real finesse of cranial nerve examination cannot be brought to life by reading, and I would advise those with a passion for neurology to have a neurologist show them the examination on the wards.

Know your neuroanatomy

Those who really want to shine at this station should have a good grasp of neuroanatomy. Some medical schools have been known to ask the path of various nerves in the head. Two of the more common ones are outlined below:
- **Abducens nerve (VI):**
  - Leaves the brainstem at the pontomedullary junction.
  - Ascends on the front of the brainstem and then turns sharply forwards over the petrous temporal bone (where it is stretched and damaged, giving rise to the 'false localising sign').
  - It then runs forwards into the carotid sinus to enter the orbit via the superior orbital fissure.
  - Finally, it runs laterally to supply the lateral rectus.

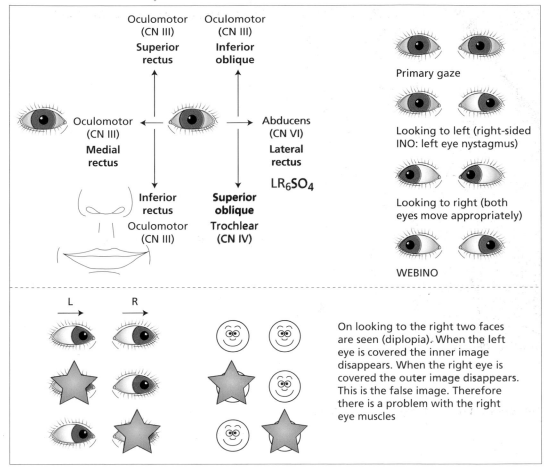

Figure 5.7 Cranial nerves with their corresponding eye muscles

- **Facial nerve (VII):**
  - The motor part arises from within the pons.
  - The sensory part arises from the naevus intermedius.
  - It enters the petrous temporal bone and then the internal auditory meatus.
  - It then forms the geniculate ganglion.
  - It runs through facial canal and the then stylomastoid foramen.
  - Branches within the skull are:
    - Greater petrosal nerve
    - Nerve to stapedius
    - Chorda tympani
  - Finally, the nerve passes through parotid gland and divides into give branches:
    - Temporal
    - Zygomatic
    - Buccal
    - Marginal mandibular
    - Cervical

If you have managed to be asked and answer these questions, you have more than likely gained a distinction.

Possible variations at this station

You could be asked to examine a patient with a possible subarachnoid haemorrhage (SAH). This would be a rather shorter station than the CNS and might involve an actor who is visually in distress.
- Before starting the examination, tell the examiner you would resuscitate the patient with regard to ABC.
- Acknowledge the patient's distress early on, ask them to tell you if anything you do is painful, and say that they can tell you to stop at any point.

• Comment on their state at rest and on any signs of (head) trauma.

• You may try to perform a brief Glasgow Coma Scale assessment – this is, however, optional.

• Your examination should aim to elicit the signs of raised intracranial pressure (ICP) and meningism.

• Comment on pupil size. (You may have to ask the patient to open their eyes first.)

• Tell the patient before you shine a light in their eyes. Test for photophobia and for direct and consensual light reflexes.

• Test the eye movements. Comment on any palsies such as of the lateral rectus (possibly a false localising sign in raised ICP).

• Ask about diplopia.

• State that you would like to look at the back of the eye with a fundoscope (SAH/raised ICP: papilloedema).

• State that you would like to test visual acuity (may be reduced).

• Test for Kernig's sign – flexing the patient's knee to 90 degrees and then extending it causes pain.

• Test for Brudzinski's sign: ask patient to flex their neck – this causes flexion at the hips.

  • Note that Kernig's and Brudzinski's signs are signs of meningism.

  • Other signs of a raised ICP that may feature include Cushing's reflex – hypertension and bradycardia. This is a late sign.

• How would you investigate the likely diagnosis?

  • 15–30-minute neurology observations (Glasgow Coma Scale, pupils, heart rate, blood pressure, respiratory rate, temperature)

• CT followed by lumbar puncture.

  • Early: red blood cells appear in each bottle.

  • Late: xanthochromia (a yellow colour) appears after 12 hours.

Questions you could be asked

Q. What is the difference between a medical and surgical IIIrd cranial nerve palsy?

A. • A medical IIIrd nerve palsy is due to ischemia of the IIIrd nerve. As the parasympathetic fibres travel peripherally, they are not affected. Hence the patient's pupil is 'down and out' but not dilated.

  • Cause: Diabetes mellitus

  • In a surgical IIIrd nerve palsy, the parasympathetic fibres are damaged so the pupil is also dilated.

  • Cause: Posterior communicating artery aneurysm

Q. What symptoms might lead you to consider the presence of an acoustic neuroma (vestibular schwannoma)?

A. • Sensorineural hearing loss

  • Tinnitus

  • Loss of sensation of the ipsilateral face

Q. What are the features of internuclear ophthalmoplegia and where is the lesion?

A. • A lesion in the ipsilateral medial longitudinal fasciculus will result in failure of adduction of the ipsilateral eye (IIIrd cranial nerve) and nystagmus of the contralateral eye during abduction.

  • The medial longitudinal fasciculus connects the ipsilateral IIIrd cranial nerve nucleus to the contralateral VIth nerve nucleus.

6 Ophthalmoscopy

Checklist	P	MP	F
HELP:			
H: 'Hello' (introduction and gains consent)			
E: Exposure			
L: Lighting			
P: Positions correctly (sitting in a chair), asks if the patient is in any pain			
Washes hands			
Explains need to darken the room and to use dilating eye drops			
Explains and consents need to use drops to dilate pupils			
Asks patient if they use glasses/contact lenses (asks patient to remove any glasses)			
Inspection:			
• Around the room: glasses, visual aids, Braille charts			
• Facial asymmetry			
• Scars (edges of lids and cornea)			
• Strabismus (convergent or divergent squint)			
• Ptosis			
• Pupil size and asymmetry			
• Red eyes			
Checks the ophthalmoscope light is 'bright and white'			
Asks patient to fixate their eye on a distant object			
Fixates patient's upper eyelid with a thumb			
Uses right eye to examine patient's right eye, and left eye to examine patient's left eye			
Approaches eye from an angle of 30 degrees			
Checks red reflex in both eyes (sets the ophthalmoscope to '0') • This is lost if any opacity is present (e.g. cataract, vitreous haemorrhage)			
Examines fundus (sets the ophthalmoscope to own refractive error to focus):			

• Examines the anterior chamber (between the iris and cornea – starts by focusing on iris or sclera)
  • Cataracts
  • Hyphaema			

Checklist	P	MP	F
• Colour of the retina			
• Disc (colour, contour, cupping, pigmentation, new vessels, haemorrhages, laser photocoagulation scars)			
• Examines the retina and blood vessels systematically in anatomical quadrants			
• Superior temporal arcade + retina (vessel tortuosity, haemorrhages, exudates, hypertensive changes, colour of retina)			
• Inferior temporal arcade + retina (as above)			
• Inferior nasal arcade + retina (as above)			
• Superior nasal arcade + retina (as above)			
• Fovea (light reflex)			

• Macula (fovea is at the centre of the macula)
  • Asks patient to look directly at the light, or angles ophthalmoscope temporally
  • Macula appears as a slightly darker/dense area on temporal aspect of fundus			

Repeats with other eye			
Tells examiner he or she would like to complete the examination by doing the following:			
• Assess visual acuity			
• Assess visual fields			
• Assess light reflexes			
• Assess range of eye movements			

• Undertake further examinations based on the diagnosis:
  • Urine dipstick/blood glucose for suspected diabetic retinopathy
  • Blood pressure in suspected hypertensive retinopathy			

Thanks patient			
Washes hands			
Presents findings			
Offers appropriate differential diagnosis			
Suggests appropriate further investigations and management			
OVERALL IMPRESSION:			

Summary of common conditions seen in OSCEs

Condition	Findings on examination	Management
Diabetic retinopathy	Background retinopathy: blot haemorrhages, microaneurysms, hard exudates Pre-proliferative: cotton wool spots, intraretinal microvascular abnormalities (IRMAs), venous loops Proliferative: new vessels at disc or elsewhere Maculopathy: exudates at macula	Regular referral to ophthalmology if background retinopathy All other findings require urgent referral Tighter control of diabetes: conservative and medical management
Hypertensive retinopathy	Grade 1: Silver wiring Grade 2: Arteriovenous nipping Grade 3: Flame haemorrhages, cotton wool spots Grade 4: Papilloedema Macular star	Antihypertensive (oral and intravenous) Grades 3 and 4 are regarded as medical emergencies If hypertension is refractive to treatment, look for rarer causes: • Phaeochromocytoma • Conn's syndrome
Optic atrophy	Pale optic disc	Investigate for a cause and treat accordingly: • Ischaemic optic neuropathy • Optic neuritis • Toxins: tobacco
Papilloedema	Raised disc Blurred disc margin	Treat cause: hypertension, raised intracranial pressure
Age-related macular degeneration (AMD)	Elderly patient Drusen at macula New vessels (neovascularisation) – wet AMD	Urgent ophthalmology referral Dry AMD: No treatment. Smoking may be a risk factor Wet AMD: Intravitreal anti-VEGF
Retinitis pigmentosa	Black specks following retinal veins Optic atrophy Cataract	Urgent ophthalmology referral No treatment is available Genetic counselling may be appropriate for inherited forms
Central retinal artery occlusion	Pale retina Cherry red spot on macula	Urgent ophthalmology referral No treatment is available Look for a cause: • Atherosclerosis • Embolic: carotid, cardiac • Vasculitis: giant cell arteritis
Central retinal vein occlusion	Haemorrhages along venous distribution Partial areas may be affected from retinal vein branch occlusion 'Stormy sunset'	Urgent ophthalmology referral Treat cause: • Compression by atherosclerotic retinal artery • Chronic glaucoma • Hyperviscosity, e.g. hyperlipidaemia, myeloma
Cataract	Absence (partial or complete) of red reflex	If early onset, investigate for a cause: congenital infection, hyperparathyroidism, corticosteroids Treatment: Cataract removal and implantation of intraocular lens

Hints and tips for the exam

Ophthalmoscopy is a difficult technique to master. Under the pressure of an OSCE, those who have neglected to practise this station sufficiently are likely to unravel.

Communication, communication, communication . . .

As with many of the stations, your opening communication with the patient is absolutely fundamental, and that starts with your introduction and explanation of the examination. You can avoid making them anxious by explaining that you will be getting very close to them, resting your thumb on their eyebrow, and shining a very bright light in their eye. Add that they should look at a point on the wall and try to keep still; if they become uncomfortable at any point, the examination can be stopped.

Get your technique right

Try to familiarise yourself with the ophthalmoscope used at your medical school. First test the light from the ophthalmoscope by shining it onto the back of your hand. Then assess for a red reflex by looking through the scope at the patient's eyes while standing at approximately 15 degrees from the midline. At this point, the lens on the scope should be set to zero. You should only start to focus the lens as you move in towards the patient.

Remember to use your right hand with your right eye to look into the patient's right eye (and vice versa). A common mistake is to stand too far from the midline.

Be clear and systematic when describing your findings

You will probably have to examine a model in which various retinal slides have been placed. Be sure to look carefully into both eyes as different pathologies might be presented. To maximise your marks, give your description in the following order:

1. **Optic disc:** If you cannot see this straight away, follow the blood vessels medially to the disc. Then comment on the '3 Cs' – colour, contour and cupping.

2. **Retinal vessels:** Examine these by quadrant.
3. **Macula and peripheral retina.**

Pathological signs may be seen at any of these points, and these should also be commented upon. This will usually be followed by the examiner asking for your differential diagnosis and management options.

A simple statement at the end of your examination mentioning the importance of examining the posterior chamber and using a slit lamp will guide you towards the marks earmarked for merit students. The posterior chamber is not to be confused with the vitreous area behind the lens: it is the area in front of the lens and behind the iris, and is important in the pathology of glaucoma.

Questions you could be asked

Q. What are the causes of an absent red reflex?
A. • Cataract (acquired or congenital)
   • Retinoblastoma
   • Coloboma
   • Ocular toxocariasis
Q. What are the causes of optic atrophy?
A. • Multiple sclerosis
   • Compression of the optic nerve: tumour/glaucoma
   • Central retinal artery occlusion
Q. What is normal intraocular pressure?
A. 11–21 mmHg.
Q. What drugs dilate/constrict the pupil?
A.

Dilate/mydriatic	Constrict/miotic
Antimuscarinic:	Pilocarpine
• Tropicamide	
• Cyclopentolate	
• Atropine	
Sympathomimetic:	
• Phenylephrine	

7 Cerebellar

Checklist	P	MP	F
HELP:			
H: 'Hello' (introduction and gains consent)			
E: Exposure			
L: Lighting			
P: Positions correctly (supine), asks if the patient is in any pain			
Washes hands			
Asks patient which hand is dominant			
Inspection:			
• Posture (truncal instability, titubation of the head)			
• Walking aids			
• Catheter			
Assesses eye movements for nystagmus:			
• Asks patient to keep their head still while they follow student's finger from side to side and then up and down. A few beats of nystagmus can occur at the extremes of gaze – this is normal			
Assesses articulation (dysarthria):			
• 'Baby hippopotamus'/'British Constitution'			
Tests for cerebellar drift in the arms:			
• Asks patient to hold their arms out in front of them with the palms facing up – 'like holding a plate'. (The ipsilateral arm will drift upwards and hyperpronate – Riddoch's sign – due to hypotonia)			
Tests for cerebellar rebound:			
• Patient holds arms out in front of them but now with palms facing down. Student briskly pushes down on each hand. (Positive rebound will result in the arm bouncing up higher than its neutral position)			
Finger–nose test (intention tremor and past-pointing – dysmetria)			

Assesses for dysdiadochokinesis. (Asks patient to clap quickly while turning top hand back and forth – test is positive if patient is unable to smoothly perform rapidly alternating movements)			
Assesses precision movements of the fingers (patient touches each finger to their thumb and 'plays the piano')			
Heel–shin test (coordination – can be done while in seated position)			
• Asks patient to place one heel on the opposite knee, then run it down the front of the shin, lift it off and then place it back on the knee. Asks them to do this three times quickly and then repeat on the other side. (Movement will not be smooth in cerebellar disease)			
Assesses tone in the limbs (for hypotonia)			
Assesses reflexes in limbs (for hyporeflexia): • Knee reflex. (Pendular reflex In cerebellar disease – the lower leg swings back and forth like a pendulum)			
Assesses gait:			
• With a walking aid if required • Asks patient to walk to end of the room, turn around and walk back • Asks the examiner to walk alongside patient ready to support them if required, or offers to do this themself • Notes which direction patient deviates towards (falls towards side of lesion in cerebellar disease) • A wide stance (base) may signify ataxia (hence widening the feet for stability)			
Assesses heel–toe (tandem) gait:			
• Demonstrates heel–toe gait while explaining the test – 'walking on a tightrope' • By lowering the base, tandem gait will reveal finer ataxia that would otherwise be missed			

Romberg's test:			
• Asks patient to stand with feet together and arms by their sides, and then to close their eyes			
• Test will help to differentiate between sensory ataxia and cerebellar ataxia			
• Positive result occurs when patient is more unstable with the eyes closed – sensory ataxia due to dorsal column damage. (Patients are unable to use visual feedback to steady themselves)			
• Negative result signifies cerebellar disease (unstable with the eyes open)			
States intent to complete the examination with the following:			

• Full examination of central and peripheral nervous systems			
• Examination of the fundus for signs of optic atrophy in cases of multiple sclerosis			
• Examination of speech			
Thanks patient			
Washes hands			
Presents findings			
Offers appropriate differential diagnosis			
Suggests appropriate further investigations and management			
OVERALL IMPRESSION:			

Summary of common conditions seen in OSCEs

Causes of cerebellar symptoms
Multiple sclerosis
Stroke
Posterior fossa tumour
Degenerative: alcohol, Friedreich's ataxia
Iatrogenic (anticonvulsants: carbamazepine, phenytoin)
Hypothyroidism
Paraneoplastic syndrome (lung cancer)

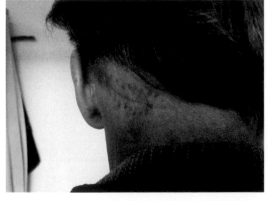

Figure 7.1 Scar from resection of a cerebellar tumour. This patient presented with classical cerebellar symptoms. He was found to have a cerebellar haemangioblastoma that was successfully resected surgically

Hints and tips for the exam

The mnemonics in the table below will make it easier to remember the signs and causes of cerebellar disease.

D	Dysmetria & dysdiadochokinesis
A	Ataxia
N	Nystagmus
I	Intention tremor
S	Slurred/staccato speech
H	Hypotonia
P	Posterior fossa tumour
A	Alcohol
S	Multiple sclerosis
T	Trauma
R	Rare
I	Inherited (e.g. Friedreich's ataxia)
E	Epilepsy medication (carbamazepine, phenytoin toxicity)
S	Stroke

Describing gait

In the cerebellar examination, the gait can point to a set of diagnoses, so it is important to get this right. It may be valuable to start with the gait assessment to localise the side of the cerebellar damage, which you can confirm with the rest of your examination. In cerebellar disease, the patient will deviate (or fall!) to the side of the lesion.

A wide-based gait is classic in cerebellar disease, with patients choosing to place their feet wide apart to improve their stability. This may not be very obvious and is the reason for subsequently performing a tandem (heel–toe or tightrope) gait assessment.

Things to note when assessing gait
Use of walking aids
Stance-phase symmetry (how long the patient spends on each foot)
Heel strike
Toe-off
Stride length
Arm swing (symmetrical, reduced, absent)
Time to turn and smoothness of turn (turn slowly, en bloc – Parkinson's disease)

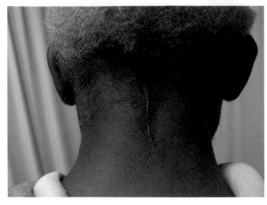

Figure 7.2 Scar after posterior craniotomy and resection of an infarcted cerebellar mass

Types of gait

Type	Description	Cause
Ataxic	Wide base (feet apart for greater stability) Unable to walk heel-to-toe Falls to side of lesion	Cerebellar disease
Antalgic	Decreased stance phase on one leg (patient spends less time on the painful leg)	Pain
Festinant	Difficulty starting, turning and stopping Small hurried steps 'Forever in front of one's centre of gravity'	Parkinson's disease
Stomping	Broad base Slams feet down Patient looks at feet Romberg's text positive	Peripheral neuropathy Dorsal column loss (proprioception) • Freidreich's ataxia
High stepping	Patient steps high to avoid foot scraping the floor Inability to dorsiflex (foot drop)	Common peroneal palsy (e.g. trauma) Sciatic nerve palsy L4 or L5 root lesion Peripheral motor neuropathy (e.g. alcoholic) Distal myopathy Motor neurone disease
Waddling	Unable to stand from sitting or climb stairs	Muscular dystrophy Proximal myopathy
Spastic/scissoring	Stiff Circumduction movements (patient moves leg out and up as unable to flex knee to prevent scuffing foot)	Stroke Multiple sclerosis

Looking for an intention tremor

A common mistake students make when assessing this aspect is to have their finger too close to the patient. The sign can be very faint so make sure the patient's arm is fully extended when reaching to touch your finger. This gives you the best chance of revealing an intention tremor.

Neuroanatomy

The cerebellum can be separated for the purpose of OSCEs into the midline and the cerebellar hemispheres.

With midline damage, the patient will exhibit imbalance and ataxia. He or she may also have titubation (bobbing) of the head. Eye movements may also be affected with nystagmus.

Damage to the cerebellar hemispheres will result in incoordination of movement such as dysdiadochokinesis and intention tremor.

The key investigation for these conditions is an **MRI scan** of the brain.

When in doubt, think cerebellum

Within the finals OSCE, it is likely that any sign of incoordination is due to cerebellar pathology. So if you are stuck for a diagnosis, mention a cerebellar syndrome within your differential diagnosis.

Questions you could be asked

Q. Name some causes of a cerebellar syndrome.
Q. List possible cerebellar signs.
Q. Where is the lesion in this patient?
A. The answers can all be found in the text above.

8 Speech

Checklist	P	MP	F
HELP			
H: 'Hello' (introduction and gains consent)			
E: Exposure			
L: Lighting			
P: Positions correctly (sitting in chair), ask if patient is in any pain			
Washes hands			
Inspection:			
• Any signs of stroke: facial asymmetry, arm flexed across chest			
• Hearing aids			
• Scars on neck (e.g. thyroid surgery, carotid endarterectomy)			
Identifies dominant side (is patient right- or left-handed?)			
Assesses orientation:			
• Time			
• Place			
• Person			
Simple questions for general initial assessment of speech ('How did you get here today?'):			
• Fluency (are words used correctly?)			
• Volume			
• Coherence			
• Quality			
Assess articulation for dysarthria (patient repeats words with increasing difficulty; if wrong, student asks once more):			
• Brown			
• Butter			
• Artillery			
• British constitution			
• Baby hippopotamus			
Assess language for dysphasia (expression, comprehension and repetition):			
• Expression (naming with increasing difficulty, allows time and prompts):			
• Watch			
• Strap			
• Winder			
If incorrect responses, asks 'Is it a watch?', etc.:			
• Comprehension (one-, two- and three-step commands, no visual prompts):			
• Asks patient to point to ceiling			
• Asks patient to point to ceiling and floor			
• Asks patient to point to ceiling, floor and window			
• Repetition (asks patient to repeat):			
• 'No ifs, ands or buts' or 'Today is Tuesday'			
Assesses phonation for dysphonia:			
• Lips: 'Ma ma ma'			
• Tongue: 'La la la'			
• Palate: 'Ka ka ka'			
• Vocal cords: asks patient to cough			
States intent to complete the examination by assessing the following:			
• Reading			
• Writing (assessing dysgraphia, hand dominance, other neurological signs such as tremor)			
• Swallow			
• Abbreviated Mental Test Score			
• CNS – 'Nerves in head and neck'			
Thanks patient			
Washes hands			
Presents findings			
Offers appropriate differential diagnosis			
Suggests appropriate further investigations and management			
OVERALL IMPRESSION:			

Summary of common conditions seen in OSCEs

Dysphasia: language problem

Conditions	Specific signs	Lesion
Broca's expressive dysphasia (BED)	Non-fluent speech Can understand Cannot answer appropriately and is aware of this (naming objects) – may become frustrated Word-finding difficulty Reading and writing affected	Inferolateral dominant **frontal** lobe
Wernicke's receptive dysphasia	Fluent speech Confident in responses Paraphasias (incorrect words) Neologisms (made-up words) Does not understand questions Reading and writing affected	Posterior superior dominant **temporal** lobe
Global aphasia	Unable to speak or understand	Dominant lobe infarction
Conduction aphasia	Repetition affected	Connecting fibres (arcuate fasciculus) between Wernicke's and Broca's areas
Nominal dysphasia	Only naming objects is affected	Posterior dominant temporoparietal lesion

Dysarthria: articulation (difficulty coordinating muscles of speech)

Conditions	Specific signs	Cause
Cerebellar disease	Slow and deliberate speech Slurring Scanning/'staccato' speech	Multiple sclerosis Stroke
Pseudobulbar palsy (UMN)	'Donald Duck' speech Slow Indistinct Jaw jerk increased	Tongue cannot protrude, is 'stuck' at base of mouth Tongue is 'spastic' Disease of corticobulbar tracts Motor neurone disease (UMN and LMN signs) Multiple sclerosis Stroke
Bulbar palsy (LMN)	Nasal quality Quiet Slurred Jaw jerk decreased/normal	Tongue hangs out Motor neurone disease Guillain–Barré syndrome Myasthenia gravis Brainstem tumour
Myogenic (muscular) defect	Features of underlying condition	Hypothyroidism Any myopathy

Dysphonia: speech volume (weak respiratory muscles and vocal cords)

Conditions	Specific signs	Cause
Myasthenia gravis	Fatigability (ask patient to say letters of alphabet/count to 100) Nasal quality Poor swallow Sternotomy scar	Antibodies to acetylcholine receptor Thymoma
Guillain–Barré syndrome	History of infection (gastroenteritis) Ascending weakness	Various infections Autoimmune Idiopathic
Vagal nerve palsy	Dysphonia Uvula dropping away from side of lesion	Trauma Compression Medullary pathology
Vocal cord weakness/paralysis		Recurrent laryngeal nerve damage: • Tumour • Surgery
Hypothyroidism	Signs of hypothyroidism	Causes of hypothyroidism

Hints and tips for the exam

The speech station is can be tricky. Having a speedy system that covers all possible causes is key. The algorithm outlined in Figure 8.1 will allow you to diagnose any defect.

Look around for clues

On entering the station, you should inspect carefully for clues to what is going on with the patient. They may be sitting in a chair with their right arm across their lap, imitating a left hemisphere stroke (i.e. one that may result in a speech deficit). Most people are left-side dominant, even those who are left-handed.

Remember the three components of speech

• Articulation – mechanical action to produce speech (**dysarthria**)

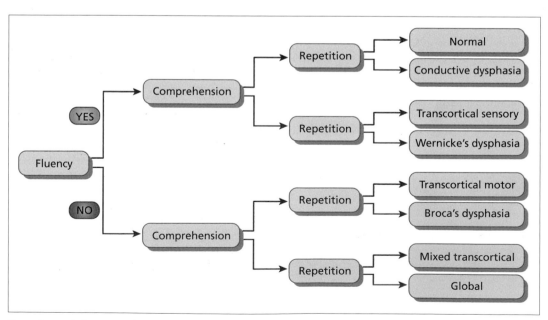

Figure 8.1 Quick algorithm to identify where a lesion is located

- Phonation – the act of producing voice sounds (**dysphonia**)
- Language – the content of what is said (**dysphasia**)

Confusion versus speech defect

If you suspect that the patient is exhibiting signs of confusion or dementia *and* you have time to complete the station comfortably, quickly run through the AMTS at the end of your speech examination. **RATY2B2MH20** is an easy acronym (see below) to remember for the Abbreviated Mental Score Test – a score of <7 suggests cognitive impairment. Having a shot at this is (if cognitive impairment is a possibility) may push you into the realms of distinction – even if you don't quite complete it.

R	Give the patient an address to **R**ECALL at the end: 42 West Register Street
A	**A**GE
T	**T**IME
Y	**Y**EAR
2	Recognise **2** people
B	Date of **B**IRTH
2	Dates of the **2**nd World War
M	Name of current **M**ONARCH
H	Name of **H**OSPITAL
20	Count backwards from **20**

Finding the right words

A skilful trick to use is to ask directly 'Are you able to understand me but are just having difficulty finding the right words?' In patients with a Broca's dysphasia, you may be greeted with a reassuring nod. This will show the examiner that you are both acknowledging the patient's frustration and exploring the diagnosis.

Make sure the patient is orientated and can hear you

This will show the examiner that you have learnt this examination not just for an OSCE but for real life, where such questions can guide whether or not it is appropriate to conduct a speech examination.

Be calm, professional and empathetic

Maintaining a professional manner at this station can be difficult but is important. There are marks at this station for assessing your professionalism when faced with disability. Marks are awarded at this station for maintaining an open body posture and active listening.

The patient may say things that are both unexpected and random. If patients are exhibiting a Broca's dysphasia, they may also become visibly frustrated at their inability to answer your questions appropriately. Be empathetic towards the patient's situation and stay calm. And try not let it put you off what you are doing (although this is easier said than done!)

Take your time and listen carefully

Continue with your examination and make sure you give the patient an appropriate time to answer your question without interruption. Rushing the patient is likely to lose you communication marks. A mark will be awarded for active listening. If you suspect that the patient has not understood your question, try to rephrase it once (do this for only one question during the examination for sake of time). If you are unsure about a response, do not be afraid to ask the patient to repeat the answer.

Multidisciplinary team

The multidisciplinary team is instrumental to the management of speech problems:
- Speech and language therapist (SALT) (who will also test for a safe swallow)
- Counsellor for psychological support
- Physiotherapist for associated stroke rehabilitation
Remember that dysphasia following stroke is associated with a poor prognosis, and that ongoing multidisciplinary team interventions may be needed by specific stroke therapists.

Questions you could be asked

Q. What speech defect is this patient exhibiting?
Q. Where is the lesion?
Q. What other symptoms and signs could they have?
Q. What are the causes?
Q. How would you treat this patient?
Q. What are the different components of speech?
A. The answers to these can all be found in the text above, although the answer to the first question obviously depends on your specific case.

9 Thyroid

Checklist	P	MP	F
HELP:			
H: 'Hello' (introduction and gains consent)			
E: Exposure (neck)			
L: Lighting			
P: Positions correctly (supine), asks if the patient is in any pain			
Washes hands			
Inspects from end of bed:			
• Relevant paraphernalia (e.g. drugs: levothyroxine, propranolol, amiodarone)			
• Body habitus			
• Clothing (e.g. suggestion of heat or cold intolerance)			
Examination of thyroid gland:			
• Identifies neck swelling			
• Examines for JVP, distended neck veins			
• Palpates lobes of thyroid:			
• At rest			
• During swallowing			
• During tongue protrusion			
• Appropriate technique for palpating thyroid gland (e.g. stabilises ipsilateral lobe while palpating contralateral lobe)			
• Assesses tracheal deviation			
• Palpates carotid pulses			
• Palpates cervical lymph nodes			
• Percusses downwards from sternal notch to detect retrosternal extension of goitre			
• Auscultates for bruits over thyroid lobes			

• Auscultates over aortic area to rule out radiated aortic stenosis murmur			
• Attempts/states intension to examine for Pemberton's sign			
Examination of peripheral signs of thyroid disease:			
• Examines hands:			
• Inspects for palmar erythema, warmth, tar staining and acropachy			
• Checks pulse for rate and rhythm			
• Examines for a tremor			
• Examines legs:			
• Inspects for pretibial myxoedema			
• Correctly tests for proximal myopathy			
• Examines for slow-relaxing knee reflex			
• Examines eyes:			
• Inspects from front, sides and above for proptosis, lid retraction and exophthalmos			
• Ensures patient is able to shut eyes completely (if appropriate)			
• Correctly tests for lid lag			
• Correctly tests for ophthalmoplegia			
Thanks patient			
Offers to help patient get dressed			
Washes hands			
Presents findings			
Offers appropriate differential diagnosis			
Suggests appropriate further investigations and management			
OVERALL IMPRESSION:			

Summary of common conditions in OSCEs

Pathology	General inspection	Neck	Hands	Legs	Eyes	Additional information
Hyperthyroidism	Agitated, restless patient Sweating Clothing suggesting heat intolerance Thin hair Underweight	Goitre (Figure 9.1) Impalpable thyroid gland	Thyroid acropachy Warm, excess sweating Tremor Palmar erythema Tar staining	Pretibial myxoedema Proximal myopathy	Exophthalmos Proptosis Ophthalmoplegia (worst on upward gaze) Conjunctival oedema Corneal ulcers Normal	If you see a patient with clinical features of hypothyroidism with Graves eye disease, this may be due to overtreatment If patient has marked scoliosis with clinical features of hyperthyroidism, this may be due to a predisposition to osteoporosis
Hypothyroidism	Pallor Hair loss Lack of facial expression Loss of outer third of eyebrows Obese	Goitre Normal	Cool *Low pulse rate Irregular pulse due to heart block	Ankle swelling Slow-relaxing reflexes Proximal myopathy	Puffy eye lids	Other signs include ataxia, ascites and pleural effusions
Post-thyroidectomy hypothyroidism	May be signs of Graves eye disease	Thyroidectomy scar (Figure 9.2) Impalpable thyroid gland			Signs of Graves eye disease possible	
Thyroglossal cyst	Spherical neck lump in midline	Small spherical lump that moves upwards on tongue protrusion				

The three main pathologies likely to appear in the examination are as follows:

- Thyroglossal cyst
- Hyperthyroidism
- Hypothyroidism

Patients with hyper- or hypothyroidism may be brought to the examination, but it is equally likely that these conditions will be simulated by actors (particularly in short-station OSCEs). Simulating the signs of hyperthyroidism (e.g. tremor, irritability/fidgeting, ophthalmoplegias, heat intolerance) is particularly easy for well-trained actors. Therefore it is very important to inspect for subtle signs such as restlessness, frequent yawning, over- or underweight body habitus and tremor from the end of the bed as these signs can instantly give away the diagnosis.

Key investigations

- **Thyroid function tests:** Free thyroxine and triiodothyronine levels are more useful than total levels.
- **Thyroid autoantibodies:** Anti-thyroid peroxidase may be increased in Hashimoto's and Graves diseases. Its presence in Graves disease signifies an increased likelihood of post-treatment hypothyroidism.
- **Thyroid-stimulating hormone receptor antibody:** Increased in Graves disease.
- **Blood lipids and glucose:** Patients with hypothyroidism are at risk of cardiovascular disease and diabetes.
- **Ultrasound scan:** Useful to distinguish cystic from solid lumps (which are more likely to be malignant).
- **Isotope scan:** Can be used to differentiate different causes of a goitre and identify ectopic thyroid tissue and hot and cold nodules. Note that cold nodules are much more likely to be malignant than hot nodules.

Key treatment modalities for thyroid disease

Hyperthyroidism

- **Drugs:**
  - Symptom control: beta-blockers, e.g. propranolol.
  - Disease modification: carbimazole + thyroxine (simultaneously) for 12–18 months. (NB. Agranulocytosis is a serious complication of carbimazole therapy.)
- **Radioiodine:** This is contraindicated in active hyperthyroidism (due to an increased risk of thyrotoxic storm), pregnancy and breast-feeding.
- **Complete or partial thyroidectomy:** This is reserved for cases refractory to medical treatment, compression of important structures, and patient preference for cosmetic reasons. (NB. Damage to local structures, including the recurrent laryngeal nerve and parathyroid glands, is a serious complication.)

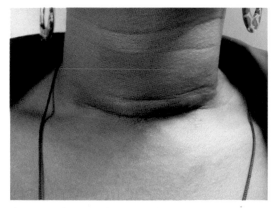

Figure 9.2 After successful resection of the goitre

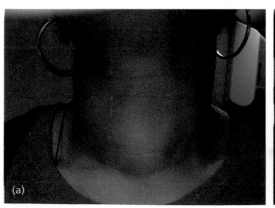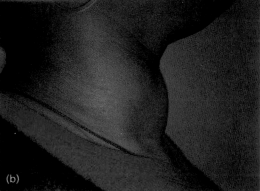

Figure 9.1 Multinodular goitre: (a) frontal and (b) lateral view. Remember that patients with a goitre may have hyperthyroidism or hypothyroidism, or may be euthyroid. This patient was euthyroid

Hypothyroidism

Treatment is with **levothyroxine** – but remember that:
• Enzyme-inducing drugs increase the breakdown of levothyroxine
• Thyroxine can increase the risk of a myocardial infarction in patients with ischaemic heart disease.

Hints and tips for the exam

Examination of the thyroid gland and thyroid function are very commonly tested in short- and long-station finals. Beware as there is a lot to do, especially in just 5 or 10 minutes. There is no 'right' or 'wrong' order in which to perform the examination, but it would be wise to dedicate most of your time examining the thyroid gland itself (as opposed to peripheral stigmata), especially if it appears abnormal in any way upon general inspection.

Performing a slick examination

• **Inspection from the end of the bed:** Be quick! Have a system. For example, start with the bedside paraphernalia, then move on to the general body habitus and then on to the face.
• **Examining the thyroid gland:** Do not forget to ask about pain and check for scars (even underneath necklaces and collars!). To palpate the gland, stabilise one lobe with one hand and palpate the other lobe with the other hand using the flat of your fingers. Once you have started palpating, try not to lift your hand off the neck until you finish palpating that lobe so that you do not miss small lumps. If you detect a lump, use the same protocol to describe it as you would for any other lump – comment on **site, size, surface, texture, temperature, tenderness, consistency, pulsatility and adherence** to any underlying or overlying structures. Specifically for thyroid lumps, you must also comment on whether they **move with swallowing or tongue protrusion**. It is extremely important to palpate the cervical lymph nodes. If you notice a lump, it may be wise to examine Pemberton's sign.
• **Examining the hands:** Again, be quick because this is probably the easiest part of the examination and could give you vital clues to the diagnosis. Look for tar staining because Graves eye disease is much more common in smokers.
• **Examining the legs:** Expose the shins to look for pretibial myxoedema (Figure 9.3). When testing for proximal myopathy, sit the patient on the edge of the couch, and instruct them to fold their arms and then stand from the sitting position without using their hands. Remember that reflexes are slow-relaxing in

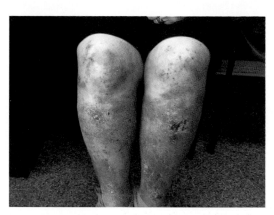

Figure 9.3 Pretibial myxoedema caused by hypothyroidism

hypothyroidism – the twitch is normal but relaxation back to the resting position afterwards is delayed.
• **Examining the eyes:** If there is proptosis or exophthalmos, you should check that the eyes can be shut because inability to shut the eyes can result in corneal damage. To test lid lag, instruct the patient to keep their head still and follow your rapidly downwards-moving horizontal finger with the eyes only. It is sometimes necessary to place your other hand gently on the patient's forehead to prevent head movements. To test for, test eye movements in an 'H' pattern (see Chapter 5 on the central nervous system) and on vertical upwards and downwards gaze. Ophthalmoplegia in hyperthyroidism is typically most marked on upwards gaze.

Potential variations at this station

• **Focused history followed by examination of thyroid function:**
  Ask about:
  • Changes in weight and appetite
  • Changes in mood and energy level
  • Changes in bowel habit
  • Changes in menses (in females)
  • Heat/cold intolerance
  • Palpitations
  • Previous history of thyroid disease
  • Past medical history of other autoimmune disease
  • Drug history (e.g. amiodarone)
  • Family history of thyroid disease
  • Smoking
• **Thyroid examination followed by interpretation of thyroid function tests.**
• **Thyroid examination followed by focused examination for other autoimmune disease:**

- Examine skin for depigmented patches of vitiligo.
- Examine fingertips for evidence of regular blood glucose testing suggestive of diabetes mellitus.
- Examine skin folds/creases in the palms and axillae, and examine any old scars for increased pigmentation – its presence suggests Addison's disease.

Questions you could be asked

Q. What are the causes of goitre?
A. Physiological, autoimmune thyroid disease, multinodular goitre, solitary adenoma, malignancy, pregnancy-induced.

Q. How would you manage Graves eye disease?
A. • Treat underlying hyperthyroidism
  • Advise/assist patient with smoking cessation
  • Conservative measures: artificial tears, taping the eyelids together at night, use of a Fresnel prism to reduce diplopia
  • Medical measures: high-dose intravenous methylprednisolone
  • Surgery: surgical decompression

10 Breast

Checklist	P	MP	F
HELP			
H: 'Hello' (introduction and gains consent)			
E: Exposure			
L: Lighting			
P: Position – asks patient to lie down or sit up			
Washes hands			
Asks for a CHAPERONE			
Inspects the breasts with patient in the positions below for asymmetry, lumps, dimples, scars, skin changes, peau d'orange:			
• With her hands by her sides			
• With her arms raised above her head (for masses tethered to the skin)			
• Underneath the breasts			
Palpates the breasts with patient lying flat or at 45 degrees:			
• Asks about pain and lumps felt by patient – starts examining away from these areas			
• All four quadrants (see below)			
• Nipple, including for discharge and underlying lumps			
Palpates axillary lymph nodes:			

• Supports the patient's arm with their non-dominant arm and palpates following areas:
  • Superior aspect
  • Inferior aspect
  • Anterior aspect
  • Posterior aspect
  • Apex			

Covers patient and offers to help her get dressed			
Tells the examiner that they would like to do the following to look for secondary metastasis: • Palpate for cervical lymphadenopathy • Palpate for hepatomegaly • Auscultate the lung bases for effusions • Percuss the spine for tenderness			
Advises the patient to sign up to breast screening			
Suggests a mammogram for greater diagnostic certainty			
Thanks patient			
Washes hands			
Presents findings			
Offers appropriate differential diagnosis			
Suggests appropriate further investigations and management			
OVERALL IMPRESSION:			

Summary of common conditions seen in OSCEs

	Breast malignancy	Fibroadenosis	Fibroadenoma	Abscess	Mammary duct ectasia	Fat necrosis
Borders	Irregular	Well-circumscribed	Well-circumscribed	Regular, symmetrical	Usually peri-areolar	Irregular
Skin changes	Often tethered to underlying skin	None	None	None	None	May be tethered to skin
Changes with menstruation	None	Pain and size often vary during menstruation	None	None	None	None
Age group	Rare under 30 years\n\nCommonly 50–70 years old	<30 years	Middle-aged	Often lactating women	Around menopause	Any age, often post-trauma
Pain	Painless	Painful	Painless	Very painful, tender	Painful, tender	Painful
Consistency	Hard	Firm	Firm	Firm, fluctuant	Firm	Hard

Hints and tips for the exam

Patient welfare and dignity

This is arguably the most intimate clinical examination of all, and it requires a specific and deliberate emphasis on showing respect for the patient and her dignity. If you appear to make the patient uncomfortable or treat her without adequate respect, the examiners will almost certainly fail you, even if your technique is clinically sound. Remember the following points:

• **Chaperone, chaperone, chaperone:** You will definitively fail if you do not ask the examiner for a chaperone, even if the patient says that she does not mind you examining without one.

• **Explain what you will be doing:** Be clear in your wording, and ensure that the patient understands that you will be feeling her breasts for lumps or any other abnormalities.

• **Don't leave the patient naked while you present the findings:** Although your patient will be a person dressed normally with a breast manikin, it is essential that you treat the patient as if she were undressed. So make sure that you cover the patient with a blanket (if one is available), and offer to help her get dressed – you will never be asked to do this, but it will show that you

have a robust grounding in basic professional medical etiquette.

Techniques for palpation

Students often find it difficult to decide which technique to use when palpating the breasts. Ultimately it does not matter how you do it, as long as you cover all four quadrants using a technique that minimises the chances of missing lumps. It is also vital that you complete the examination in the time frame given, so keep an eye on the watch. Use the pulp of the fingers and move them in a rotatory manner in each area being palpated. We have described a number of techniques below (see also Figure 10.1)– use whichever you feel most comfortable with.

Lawnmower technique

This describes 'up and down' movements in parallel lines on a breast as for a lawnmower in a garden. You could start from the superior medial aspect of the breast and then palpate down that aspect of the breast in a straight line. Once you reach the inferior aspect of the breast, move your fingers 2 or 3 cm laterally, and then go up in a straight line. Carry on up and down the breast in lines until you reach the most lateral aspect,

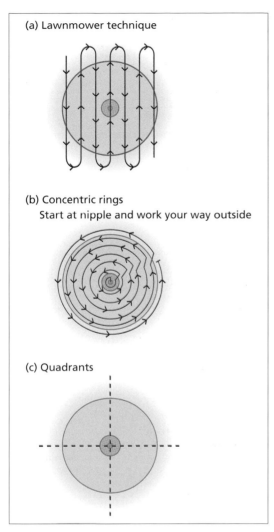

(a) Lawnmower technique

(b) Concentric rings
Start at nipple and work your way outside

(c) Quadrants

Figure 10.1 Breast examination techniques

where you can finish. This is a very thorough technique, but often time-consuming (Figure 10.1a).

Concentric rings

Here, you palpate the breast in concentric rings, each ring moving closer and closer to the centre of the breast and the nipple. So you would start at the outermost border of the breast, palpating in a clockwise or anti-clockwise direction until you reached the point at which you started. You would then move your fingers about 2 cm closer to the centre, and palpate the 'next' concentric ring. And carry on doing that until you reached the nipple (Figure 10.1b).

Quadrant by quadrant

This is where you palpate each of the four quadrants of the breast in turn, ensuring that you cover the whole area of each quadrant. The area around the nipple is usually done separately at the end (Figure 10.1c).

Describing the lump

A clear and logical description of a breast lump is the icing on the cake of any post-examination presentation. Use the parameters in the table to describe any lumps.

Parameter	Description
Number of lumps	
Location within the breast	There are five areas: • Superior-medial • Inferior-medial • Superior-lateral • Inferior-lateral • Nipple region
Shape	Round, circular, oval
Borders	Regular, well-circumscribed, irregular
Consistency	• Soft (like your lips feel) • Firm (like your nose feels) • Hard (like your forehead feels)
Size	In millimeters or centimetres
Tenderness	Tender or non-tender
Tethering	Tethered to skin/underlying structures

An easy way to remember this is to use the '4Ss/4Cs/4Ts' – see Chapter 13 on testicular examination.

Breast screening

This can be done quickly and always impresses examiners as it demonstrates a consideration for wider health promotion and prevention issues.
• Advise the patient to self-examine on a regular basis, and to see her GP immediately if she feels any lumps.
• Ensure that the patient is under the National Breast Screening Programme. All women aged 50–70 years old receive regular mammograms every 3 years, and any suspicious lumps are biopsied.

Questions you could be asked

Q. How would you distinguish between a benign and a malignant lump on examination?
Q. What age group does the NHS Breast Screening programme cover, and how frequently is screening offered?
A. The answers appear in the text above.

11 Rectal

Checklist	P	MP	F
HELP			
H: 'Hello' (introduction and gains consent)			
E: Exposure			
L: Lighting			
P: Positions correctly (lying on side, fetal position with hips and knees flexed), asks if the patient is in any pain			
Washes hands			
Explains purpose and routine of examination in a sensitive manner			
Explicitly asks for consent before proceeding			
Explains that having a CHAPERONE is essential for the examination, and requests one from examiner			
Explains repositioning on couch (e.g. 'Please remove your trousers and undergarments down to your knees, and lie on your left hand side on the couch with your knees tucked in to your chest and your bottom close to the edge')			
States intention to draw the curtain/step outside to allow privacy to undress			
Gathers appropriate equipment: tray, gloves, tissues, lubricating gel			
States intention to optimise lighting			
Wears gloves			
Parts buttocks and inspects for: skin tags, ulcers, abnormal growth, warts, fissures, fistulas			
Tells patient before inserting finger			
Inserts one lubricated finger into anus			
Examines sensation of the perianal skin			
Instructs patient to 'bear down' and squeeze on finger to examine anal tone			

Checklist			
States intention to feel for:			

• Entire wall of rectum by moving finger 180 degrees in either direction:
  • Polyps
  • Lumps
  • Faecal impaction/hard stool			

• Prostate: Comments on:			
• Size			
• Symmetry			
• Midline sulcus			
• Texture			
Tells patient before removing finger			
Inspects glove of finger for melaena, mucus, fresh blood			
Removes gloves and disposes of them appropriately in clinical waste			
Thanks patient, says examination is complete and allows patient to re-dress with dignity and privacy			
States intention to complete examination by examining abdomen			
States intention to perform neurological examination of lower limbs (if told by examiner that anal tone was reduced)			
Washes hands			
Presents findings			
Offers appropriate differential diagnosis			
Suggests appropriate further investigations and management			
OVERALL IMPRESSION:			

Summary of common conditions seen in OSCEs

Condition	Appearance on manikin	Investigations	Treatment
Melaena	Black tarry stool Characteristic foul smell	Full blood count Oesophago-gastro-duodenoscopy Colonoscopy	Blood transfusion Identify and treat cause
Cauda equina syndrome	Impaired perianal and anal sensation Anal atony LMN weakness below L1 Reduced sensation below L1	Urgent MRI of whole spine Transfer to neurosurgical centre	Urgent neurosurgical intervention
Benign prostatic hypertrophy	Symmetrical increase in firmness, size and 'knobbly' texture compared with the model of the normal prostate Palpable midline sulcus	Prostate-specific antigen Transrectal ultrasound scan Biopsy	Conservative: bladder training exercises, avoidance of caffeine, alcohol and anticholinergic drugs Medical: first line are alpha-blockers (e.g. tamsulosin), second line are 5-alpha-reductase inhibitors (e.g. finasteride) Surgical: TURP, TUIP, prostatectomy
Prostate carcinoma	Localised area of the prostate that will be harder and more 'knobbly' than the remainder Also, the midline sulcus may be impalpable	Prostate-specific antigen Transrectal biopsy Bone X-ray or bone scans MRI for staging	Symptom control: TURP (to relieve obstruction), NSAIDs/bisphosphonates/radiotherapy for relief of pain from bony metastases Management: • Prostatectomy • Radiotherapy + hormone therapy
Rectal tumour	Palpable irregular mass high up on wall of internal anal canal	Full blood count Liver function tests Sigmoidoscopy Colonoscopy CT, MRI, liver ultrasound for staging	Abdominoperineal resection if distal
Perianal haematoma	Visible blue lump when buttocks are parted	(Clinical diagnosis)	Drain under local anaesthetic
Perianal abscess	Visible white/green lump when buttocks are parted	Microscopy, culture and sensitivity of drained pus	Incision + drainage + antibiotics Rule out underlying causes (diabetes mellitus, Crohn's disease, malignancy)
Haemorrhoids	Protruding tissue from the anus Alternatively you may be able to palpate them when you insert your finger in to the anal canal of the manikin	Proctoscopy	Conservative: increase dietary fibre and fluid intake Medical: topical anaesthetic, band ligation Surgery NB. Treatment of acutely thrombosed external piles is conservative if patient presents after 72 hours. With presentation within 72 hours, treatment of choice is surgical excision
Anal fissure	Crack in lining of external anal canal exuding blood	Examination under anaesthesia if required	Classified as acute if present <6 weeks: • Conservative: dietary advice • Medical: bulk-forming laxatives, lubricants prior to defecation, topical anaesthetic Classified as chronic if present >6 weeks. In addition to treatment for acute fissure: • Topical GTN • Refer for surgery if GTN ineffective after 6–8 weeks of treatment

Summary of relevant investigations and management

• Proctoscopy (to visualise anus)
• Sigmoidoscopy (to visualise rectum)
• Colonoscopy (to visualise colon)
• Haemoglobin and iron studies (to check if the patient has iron deficiency anaemia)
• Tumour markers (carcinoembryonic antigen for bowel cancer)
• Prostate-specific antigen (if prostate is enlarged)
• MRI of the spine (if cauda equina suspected)

Hints and tips for the exam

This is a relatively easy OSCE station. You may get opportunities to practise on actual patients during colorectal surgery and gastroenterology outpatient clinics. However, it is highly likely that you will be asked to perform the examination on a manikin in the OSCE. Therefore it is important to go to the clinical skills centre at your medical school and practise this examination before the OSCE. There are several important things to remember for this station.

Do NOT forget to request a chaperone

This is vitally important for any intimate examination, and could easily make the difference between a fail and a pass.

Cauda equina syndrome

This is exceedingly rare, but is an acute neurosurgical emergency that requires immediate neurosurgical intervention. The spinal cord ends at L1/L2, below which the spinal cord branches into smaller roots – similar to how a horsetail roots out into smaller branches at the end; these branches are called the 'cauda equina' (cauda meaning tail, equina relating to horse). Anything that causes compression of these roots will result in cauda equina syndrome. Symptoms can very quickly become irreversible, resulting in permanent disability, which necessitates urgent neurosurgical intervention and decompression.

Communicate clearly when explaining how the examination will be carried out

One suggestion is to say something like:
> Hello Mr Jones. I'm —, one of the junior doctors. I understand you have recently noticed some bleeding from your back passage so is it OK if I examine your back passage to try and find out what may be causing the bleeding? You will need to undress down to your knees and lie down on your left side on the couch with your knees tucked in to

> your chest. I will examine your back passage with a gloved, lubricated index finger. It may be slightly uncomfortable, but if it hurts don't hesitate to stop me. It should take no more than 5 minutes. If you are happy with my explanation, do you give consent for me to examine you?

Although this may take up a few seconds of your precious time in the exam, it is extremely important to demonstrate clear communication before performing any intimate examination. There are certain to be a sizeable proportion of marks for good communication in this station.

Ask if the patient is in any pain

This is specifically important in the PR station because anal fissures (which can be simulated on the manikin) are exquisitely painful.

Tell the patient before you insert or remove your finger from the back passage, and say what you are doing as you proceed through the examination

This is important because the examiner will not be able to see what you are doing when your finger is in the rectum. There are five important things to comment on:
• External abnormalities around the anus
• Abnormalities palpated on the walls of the anal canal
• Prostate (size, symmetry, sulcus, texture/hardness)
• Anal tone
• Presence of blood, melaena or mucus on the glove

Inform the patient clearly when the examination is complete

This is an intimate examination, and often a very uncomfortable one, especially if there is a significant pathological abnormality. Therefore it is very important that you tell the patient when you have finished.

Potential variations at this station

• **Examine the abdomen (on an actor patient) and perform a PR examination (on a manikin)** (5–10 minutes)
• **Examine this patient's rectum and then explain to the patient what you have found. Answer the patient's questions regarding further management** (10 minutes). This is perhaps the most difficult possible variation at this station. Remember to stick to your generic management template. For example, if the examination reveals benign prostatic hypertrophy, talk about conservative measures (e.g. avoiding anticholin-

ergic drugs), medical measures (e.g. alpha-blockers) and surgery as the last line (TURP).

Questions you could be asked

Q. How many hours does it take for cauda equina symptoms to become irreversible?
A. Potentially within 4–6 hours.
Q. Above which point in the gastrointestinal tract does bleeding cause melaena (as opposed to fresh red bleeding)?

A. Although there is no specific point immediately after which fresh red blood suddenly becomes melaena, generally speaking bleeding from an area **proximal to the terminal ileum is more likely to be melaena**, as there is scope for significant 'digestion' in that part of the gastrointestinal tract.

12 Hernia

Checklist	P	MP	F
HELP			
H: 'Hello' (introduction and gains consent)			
E: Exposure (ideally waist downwards)			
L: Lighting			
P: Positions correctly (initially standing, then lying supine), asks if the patient is in any pain			
Washes hands			
Inspects from end of bed for any relevant paraphernalia			
Requests CHAPERONE			
Asks patient to stand			
Inspection:			
• Inspects patient with them in a standing position: • Scars • Swellings • Lumps			
• Inspects scrotum			
• Inspects groin			
• Inspects abdomen			
• Asks patient to cough to exaggerate the hernia, observing for any impulse around groin and scrotum			
Palpation:			
• Identifies relevant anatomical landmarks: • Pubic tubercle • Anterior superior iliac spine • Mid-inguinal point • External (superficial) ring • Internal (deep) ring			

• Attempts to palpate external ring through scrotum (or states intent to do so)			
• Identifies any swelling/lump			
• Examines swelling/lump thoroughly: • 4 Ss • 4 Cs • 4 Ts			
• Attempts to get 'above' swelling			
• Attempts to manually reduce the hernia			
• Asks patient to cough to exaggerate the hernia and feel a 'cough impulse'			
• Uses finger to obstruct internal ring (at the mid-inguinal point) and asks patient to cough • Direct hernia appears • Indirect hernia does not appear			
Auscultates swelling for bowel sounds			
Examines both sides for comparison			
Tells examiner he or she would like to complete the examination by examining the scrotum			
Thanks patient			
Offers to help patient get dressed			
Washes hands			
Presents findings			
Offers appropriate differential diagnosis			
Suggests appropriate further investigations and management			
OVERALL IMPRESSION:			

Summary of key points for OSCEs

Key anatomical landmarks	
Inguinal ligament	From pubic tubercle to anterior superior iliac spine
Internal (deep) ring	Mid-inguinal point 10–15 mm above femoral artery pulse
External (superficial) ring	Superior and medial to pubic tubercle
Inguinal canal	Starts at internal ring Ends at external ring Contains spermatic cord in men Contains round ligament in women 4–5 cm in length
Femoral canal	Inferior and anterior to inguinal ligament Contains fat and a lymph node Femoral vein, femoral artery and femoral nerve lie lateral to the femoral canal (in that order)
Types of hernia	
Inguinal hernias	Superior and medial to pubic tubercle
Femoral hernias	Lateral and inferior to pubic tubercle Protrude through femoral canal More common in females *Commonly strangulate: as the femoral canal is very narrow*
Direct versus indirect hernias	
Direct inguinal hernias	Protrude through a muscular defect in the transversalis fascia (which is the posterior wall of the inguinal canal) *Rarely strangulate: as the opening is wider*
Indirect inguinal hernia	Protrude after exiting through internal inguinal ring >75% of inguinal hernias are indirect Occur due to existence of processus vaginalis and non-closure of internal inguinal ring after birth) Can protrude down to scrotum *Commonly strangulate: as the internal ring is narrow*

Summary of common groin lumps

Cause of lump	Key diagnostic features
Saphena varix	Soft Disappears when supine Cough impulse present Positive tap test Blue tinge
Femoral aneurysm	Pulsatile Bruit
Lymph node	Firm Round Well-circumscribed Fixated to underlying soft tissue Could be tender (depending on cause)
Lipoma	Soft/firm consistency Well-circumscribed
Testes	Characteristic features

Key features and location of different types of hernia (Figure 12.1)

Inguinal (indirect/direct) ⎫ Most common
Femoral
Umbilical and paraumbilical
Incisional
Epigastric ⎭ Least common

Hints and tips for the exam

Hernia examinations are traditionally neglected by students before they reach their exams, despite hernias being a common and easily examinable clinical finding. Moreover, with a bit of practice, the examination is easy to carry out and interpret.

Standing or supine?

Most hernias are easier to examine with the patient standing, as the hernia is less likely to reduce and more likely to protrude outwards. But do not spend too much time thinking about what to do – you will be fine as long as you do a comprehensive logical examination and devise a reasonable list of differential diagnoses.

Request a chaperone

As with all examinations of an intimate nature, this is vital. It obviously depends on the level of exposure, but you will never lose marks for unnecessarily requesting a chaperone – although you will if you do not request one when one is required.

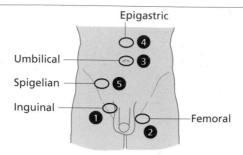

1 Inguinal hernias
Inguinal hernias are the most common type of hernias. The anatomical landmark of the hernia is superior and medial to the pubic tubercle. The majority are indirect, the remaining being direct or a combination of both. Direct hernias pass through the posterior wall of the inguinal canal into the abdominal wall. Inguinal hernias may be congenital or acquired e.g. straining. Do ask about pain radiation as the patient can have referred pain. Do learn about the management options, e.g. conservative or surgical management (use of mesh)

2 Femoral hernias (see above)
Femoral hernias are more common in females (remember 'F' for Femoral and Females) and are acquired. The anatomical landmark is below and lateral to the pubic tubercle. These are more likely to strangulate so early diagnosis is of paramount importance

3 Umbilical hernias
These develop around the umbilicus and are called paraumbilical hernias. There is usually a congenital defect in the umbilical area. In children this hernia may close and surgery can be prevented unless it becomes symptomatic. However, in adults it will require surgical repair if it causes problems

4 Epigastric hernias
Epigastric hernias develop in the upper part of the mid abdomen. These are small in size and can be very uncomfortable especially if pinched

5 Spigelian hernia
These occur due to a defect in the fascia between the external oblique and rectus abdominis. They appear lateral to the umbilicus and medial to the anterior superior iliac spine

Obturator hernia
This will *not* appear in your OSCE. However, you may be asked about it in the viva. It presents with a vague pain in the medial aspect of the thigh. The investigation of choice is an MRI scan. As it occurs in the obturator canal, it may be palpable on a bimanual pelvic examination

Figure 12.1 Types of hernia

Remember that hernias are more common on the right side, and more common in males

This is because the processus vaginalis is more likely to exist in adulthood in males and on the right side (although no one seems to know quite why this is the case). The size of the external ring is also larger in males, so there is a bigger space for the bowel to protrude through.

Investigations and management

This is really simple. The only investigation that helps with diagnosing a hernia is an **ultrasound** – it is sensitive, quick and non-invasive, and does not involve radiation.

The only options for managing hernias are as follows:
• **Emergency surgery** for strangulated or obstructed hernias
• **Elective surgery** for hernias that are either symptomatic or the patient would like resected
• **Conservative management** if the hernia is asymptomatic, if the patient does not want surgery, or if the patient is not fit for surgery. This includes the following measures:
  • Treat any cause of chronic/severe cough
  • Avoid lifting heavy weights

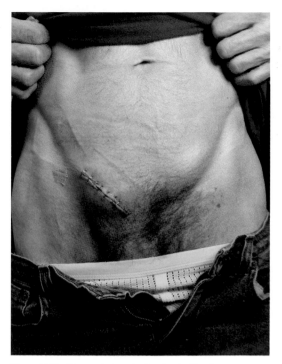

Figure 12.2 After surgical repair of an inguinal hernia

- Avoid/treat constipation
- Use a 'truss' or tight-fitting underwear

Questions you could be asked

Q. On which side are hernias generally more common?

Q. What is the difference between direct and indirect hernias?

Q. What are your differential diagnoses for lumps in the groin?

A. The answers to these three other questions can be found in the text above.

Q. What in the management for a strangulated hernia?

A. The management of a strangulated hernia is urgent surgical repair.

13 Testicular

Checklist	P	MP	F
HELP			
H: 'Hello' (introduction and gains consent)			
E: Exposure			
L: Lighting			
P: Positions correctly (supine), asks if the patient is in any pain			
Washes hands			
Requests CHAPERONE			
Inspection:			
• Comments on patient's general appearance (secondary sexual characteristics, gynaecomastia – if shirt has been removed)			
• Hair distribution (face, axilla, pubis)			
• Skin of pubic region and scrotum (scars, colour, rash, lumps, ulcers)			
• Examines penis from base to shaft			
• Prepuce (if present) is examined and retracted (phimosis, paraphimosis)			
• Asks patient for permission to retract foreskin			
• Meatus (hypospadias, epispadias, discharge)			
• Scrotum (front and back, size, shape, symmetry, height of testes – left usually lower than right)			
• Returns foreskin to normal position			
Palpation:			
• Testicles (number, size, consistency, other masses, epididymis, vas deferens)			

Checklist	P	MP	F
• Epididymis (location, swellings)			
• Spermatic cord			
• Uses correct technique, 'rolling' the testes between finger and thumb, and covering the entire surface area of the testes			
• Examines any swellings if present (size, shape, fluctuance, transilluminable, cough impulse)			
• Tries to palpate 'above' swelling to determine where it originates from (testes, inguinal canal)			
• Examines inguinal lymph nodes			
• Asks patient to stand and comments on any changes (varicocele, hernia)			
Complete examination:			
• Examine abdomen			
• Hernial orifices			
• Rectal examination for prostate			
• If a lump was felt, offers to examine the lungs, liver and spine for bony tenderness			
Thanks patient			
Offers to help patient get dressed			
Washes hands			
Presents findings			
Offers appropriate differential diagnosis			
Suggests appropriate further investigations and management			
OVERALL IMPRESSION:			

Summary of common conditions seen in OSCEs

Testicular mass	How to differentiate
Testicular tumour	Woody hard/firm Smooth or craggy surface Not separate from testicle Not transilluminable Can get above it Patient is young to middle-aged May show signs related to side effects of chemotherapy (e.g. hair loss)
Inguinal hernia (usually indirect)	Cannot get above it Does not transilluminate Above and medial to the pubic tubercle Can be controlled once reduced by pressure on the deep inguinal ring
Epididymal cyst	Separate from testicle Transilluminates
Varicocele	'Bag of worms' consistency Seen when standing and disappears on lying down Left-sided is more common: • Right testicular vein drains directly into inferior vena cava • Left testicular vein drains into left renal vein and then inferior vena cava May be the presenting sign of a renal cell carcinoma that has invaded the renal vein
Penile ulcer	May be on glans (so retract foreskin) Offer to take a swab for microscopy, culture and sensitivity
Hydrocele	Soft, smooth, not separate from testicle Transilluminates Cannot get above it

Making a diagnosis

The algorithm in Figure 13.1 will help you make a diagnosis quickly and systematically.

Look out for an absent vas deferens. This may be the only clue to the patient having cystic fibrosis.

Key investigations

• Bedside: swab discharge for microscopy, culture and sensitivity (? sexually transmitted infection)
• Ultrasound scan: confirm solid or cystic
• Tumour markers (alphafetoprotein – yolk sac tumour; beta-human chorionic gonadotropin – teratomas and seminomas; lactate dehydrogenase)
• Chest X-ray: metastases
• Staging CT: metastatic disease
• Excision biopsy
• Four stages:
  1. No metastases
  2. Infradiaphragmatic nodes (remember para-aortic spread)
  3. Supradiaphragmatic nodes
  4. Haematogenous spread: lung involvement

Hints and tips for the exam

Chaperone

The importance of this cannot be emphasised enough, and could well be the difference between a pass and a fail.

Respect the mannequin

In your OSCE, it is more than likely that a model will be in place of a real patient (for obvious reasons!). This can make the station easier for some, but make sure you conduct yourself as if a patient were in front of you. Take the same care you would if faced with a real patient, and talk to the model as you proceed with the examination. Warn the patient before retracting their foreskin and talk to the patient during the examination, explaining what you are doing.

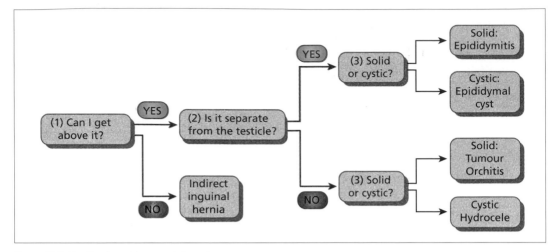

Figure 13.1 Algorithm for making a good diagnosis

Marks will be awarded for trying to maintain the patient's dignity throughout the station. Use appropriate language and, when the examination is complete, cover the patient with a sheet if provided.

When palpating the testes, look at the patient's face and ask about tenderness. Comment on anything you find and attempt to get above it.

Know the basics of the lymphatic system

The lymphatic drainage of the penis and scrotum runs into the inguinal lymph nodes. These can be felt in the inguinal crease. The testicles drain via the para-aortic nodes.

Describing a lump

These are easy marks to remember to famous **4Ss, 4Ts and 4Cs.**

Ss	Ts	Cs
Site	Tender	Colour
Size	Transilluminability	Consistency
Shape	Tethering	Contour
Skin	Temperature	Cough

Questions you could be asked

Q. Which testicular tumours are malignant?

A. • **Seminoma:** peak incidence 30–40 years old, most common, 35–45% of all cases
• **Teratoma:** peak incidence 20–30 years old, about a third of cases

• **Mixed teratoma-seminoma:** 20–40 years old, about 15–20%
• **Lymphoma:** non-Hodgkin's, 60–70 years old, least common

Q. List some risk factors for testicular malignancy.

A. • Cryptorchidism
• History of malignancy in the contralateral testis
• Male infertility
• Family history
• Klinefelter's syndrome
• Infantile hernia
• Testicular microlithiasis

Q. What symptoms may a patient complain of?

A. • A painless lump in the scrotum
• Pain
• A dragging feeling
• Back pain

Q. What is the prognosis of common testicular malignancies?

A. Your answer should begin by stating that this will depend on:
• Staging
• Tumour type
• Tumour marker levels
Seminoma:
• 5-year survival of 90% survival with stage I and II disease
• Radiosensitive
• Spreads late
Non-seminomatous:
• 5-year survival of approximately 90%
• Early haematogenous spread

Q. How is testicular malignancy managed?

A. • Multidisciplinary team approach
  • Exploration and orchidectomy if malignant
  • Radiotherapy
  • Chemotherapy (BEC: bleomycin, etoposide, cisplatin) – used if there is spread beyond the regional lymph nodes

• Monitor treatment success with CT and tumour marker levels
• Before treatment is started, patients should be counselled on the risk of infertility and offered sperm collection

14 Vascular (arterial)

Lower limb

Checklist	P	MP	F
HELP			
H: 'Hello' (introduction and gains consent)			
E: Exposure (entire leg up to groins)			
L: Lighting			
P: Positions correctly (supine), asks if the patient is in any pain			
Washes hands			
Inspection (patient on bed):			
• From end of the bed:			
• Comfortable, cyanosis, pallor			
• Obvious pathology (amputation, stockings, scars)			
• Around the bed (cigarettes, medication [GTN], walking stick)			
• Skin colour (pallor, cyanosis)			
• Trophic changes (hair loss, muscle wasting, shiny skin)			
• Scars (e.g. vein harvesting)			
• Ulceration (heel, tips of toes, in between toes, lateral malleolus, punched-out, painful, over pressure points)			
• Gangrene (dry/wet – infected)			
• Amputation			
• Dressings (states would ideally examine underneath)			
• Stigmata of vascular disease: nicotine staining (smoking), xanthoma, xanthelasmata (hypercholesterolaemia), necrobiosis lipoidica (diabetes)			
Palpation:			
• Examines abdomen for abdominal aortic aneurysm (size)			
• Skin temperature with back of hands			
• Assesses capillary refill in both feet (<2 seconds)			
• Palpates pulses bilaterally: femoral (mid-inguinal point), popliteal, dorsalis pedis (between 1st and 2nd metatarsals) and posterior tibial (half way between tip of heel and medial malleolus)			
• Comments on rhythm (atrial fibrillation – increased risk of embolic disease)			
• If unable to palpate, states intent to use Doppler ultrasonography			
• Measures Buerger's angle and performs Buerger's test, commenting on reactive hyperaemia if present (feet become a dusky red colour)			
• Assess for venous guttering (elevate leg to 15 degrees)			
Auscultates:			
• Bruits (abdominal aorta, femoral pulses)			
States intention to do the following to complete the examination:			
• Examine remainder of peripheral vascular system			
• Examine cardiovascular system			
• Measure ankle–brachial pressure indexes (ABPIs) using Doppler assessment			
• Conduct a neurological assessment of the lower limbs			
• Conduct a musculoskeletal examination			
Thanks patient			
Offers to help patient get dressed			
Washes hands			
Presents findings			
Offers appropriate differential diagnosis			
Suggests appropriate further investigations and management			
OVERALL IMPRESSION:			

Summary of common conditions seen in OSCEs

Condition	Symptoms	Signs
Intermittent claudication	Pain on exercise Relief on rest Location of pain dictates site of narrowing: • Aortoiliac disease – buttock claudication and impotence (Leriche's syndrome) • Weak/absent leg pulses (all) • Iliofemoral – thigh pain , popliteal and foot pulses weak/absent • Femoropopliteal – calf pain, foot pulses absent/weak	ABPI = 0.8–0.06 (falsely high in diabetes mellitus due to calcified arteries)
Critical ischaemia	Intermittent claudication > rest pain > ulceration > gangrene Hangs leg out of bed while sleeping (which improves blood flow) – may sleep sitting up	The '6 Ps' of an acutely ischaemic limb: • Pain • Pallor • Perishingly cold • Pulselessness • Paraesthesia • Paralysis ABPI = <0.5
Diabetic foot	Pain Skin changes Charcot joint: severe joint deformity due to lack of sensation and repetitive trauma	Loss of ankle jerk (autonomic neuropathy) Reduced vibration sense Ulcers
Amputation	Toes, lower leg or entire leg Social impact Buerger's disease: • Young male • Heavy smoker • Severe Raynaud's phenomenon	Above knee Through knee Below knee

Features of arterial and venous lower limb disease

Arterial	Venous
Shiny skin	Brown pigmented skin
Lateral malleolus	Medial malleolus
Deep ulcer	Shallow ulcer
Punched-out	Irregular sloping edge
Little exudate	Lots of exudate
Little/no swelling	Oedematous
Cold skin	Warm skin
No granulation tissue*	Granulation tissue* present
Pulses weak/absent	Pulses normal
Increased capillary refill time (>3 seconds)	Normal capillary refill

*Granular dark red or pink tissue is seen in wound healing.

Important investigations to remember for this station

• **Bedside:** ABPI, ulcer swab, ECG (arrhythmias and ischaemic heart disease), urine dipstick (glycosuria – diabetes mellitus screen)
• **Blood:** Full blood count, Us+Es, lipid profile, glucose
• **Special tests:** Colour duplex ultrasound, angiography

Basic management of peripheral vascular disease

• **Conservative and medical:**
  • Exercise (there is evidence that this may have even better outcomes than surgery)
  • Addressing risk factors (weight, smoking, blood pressure, cholesterol, glucose and aspirin).
  • Other medications that may be used: cilostazol and naftidrofuryl

- **Surgical:**
  - Endovascular: percutaneous transluminal angioplasty
  - Bypass
  - Amputation
- **Outcomes:** approximately one-third improve, one-third stay the same, and one-third deteriorate.

Hints and tips for the exam

The arterial examination is an easy station and can allow you to demonstrate a number of clinical skills. Although you should undoubtedly look for and comment on features of acute conditions (such as acute limb ischaemia), seeing such a patient is almost impossible in the OSCE – if you do, it would be reasonable to stop your examination and get the patient admitted to the nearest surgical ward!

Adequate exposure
When asking the patient to expose appropriately, ensure that you are clear and unambiguous. Ask them to remove their trousers, shoes and socks, leaving their underwear on. Some actors are told to keep their socks on unless specifically asked to remove them – forgetting this can lose you valuable seconds in the OSCE.

It is even more important to treat the patient in a dignified respectful manner, as many patients feel quite anxious when asked to expose their legs and abdomen.

Inspect systemically
Inspection is fundamental in all of the vascular examination, and it is imperative that you are systematic – inspect either from the hips towards the feet or vice versa.

Ulcers
When examining for ulcers, make sure that you inspect all the pressure points and in between the toes (where an ulcer can easily be missed.) Lift each foot up to look at the heel, and use this opportunity to comment on the back of the leg as well. Arterial ulcers are classically 'punched-out'.

When describing an ulcer comment on:
- Site
- Floor
- Size
- Exudate
- Shape
- Surrounding skin
- Edge

Palpating peripheral pulses
When palpating the pulses, it is easiest to start at the femoral arteries. If these pulses cannot be felt, the problem is above this level and the pulses below are unlikely to be felt. Never say that you can feel a pulse when you cannot! Simply add that you would like to have a Doppler scan at the end of the examination to assess the pulses you could not palpate.

The popliteal pulse is best felt with the patient's legs slightly bent and relaxed. Grasp the calf with both hands. Place your thumbs on the tibial tuberosity and use your fingers to feel behind the knee in the popliteal fossa. The popliteal pulses can be difficult to feel so do not waste much time attempting this.

To save time, palpate both pairs of femoral and the foot pulses simultaneously. The abdominal aorta should be felt in the midline **above** the umbilicus (it bifurcates at L4 – below the umbilicus).

Don't forget to check the capillary refill time as this is also a good indicator of perfusion – up to 2 seconds is normal, whereas more than 3 seconds shows that the limb is poorly perfused.

Buerger's test
This has traditionally been one of the most feared parts of the vascular examination – the following bullet point plan should make it easier for you:
- Ask the patient about pain in the hips, and ask whether you can lift their legs up.
- Lift both legs and note the angle at which the sole of the foot goes white.
- Note the angle made between the leg and the bed – this is Buerger's angle (<20 degrees signifies severe ischaemia; normal is >90 degrees).
- Ask the patient to sit up from this position with their legs over the side of the bed:
  - Comment on any change in colour of the legs: bluish (deoxygenated blood) and then red (reactive hyperaemia) if present.

As the station is quite straightforward, it can be incorporated with measuring an ABPI or be followed by questions on management of the common conditions. Knowing the arterial tree of the lower limb can assist you in your examination and impress the examiner when you finally present your findings (Figure 14.1).

How to measure an ABPI
Although it is unlikely that this will appear in the OSCE, you may well be asked to describe the process – especially if you are aiming for a merit or distinction:
- The patient lies on the bed.
- Their legs must be at rest for 20 minutes before the measurement and the patient must be horizontal (remember to state this).

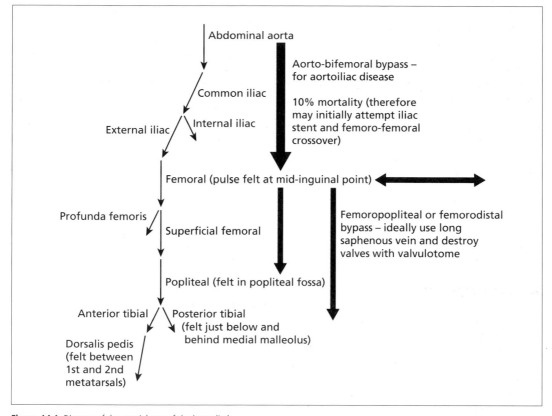

Figure 14.1 Diagram of the arterial tree of the lower limb

• Select an appropriately sized cuff for the patient's arm.
• Measure the systolic blood pressure in the arm.
• Use the appropriate cuff for the calf and place the cuff above the malleoli at mid-calf level.
• Use Doppler scanning at either the dorsalis pedis or posterior tibial pulses (if you are struggling to locate the dorsalis pedis, move to the posterior tibial).
• Inflate above the systolic blood pressure measured in the arm.
• Slowly deflate until the pulse is again heard on the Doppler.
• Use the higher of two readings (although you will only have time to take one in the exam).
• Offer to repeat on the other leg.
• Calculate ABPI = ankle pressure/arm pressure
   • Normal = 1 or more
   • Intermittent claudication = 0.6–0.8
   • Rest pain = 0.3–0.6
   • Ulceration and gangrene = <0.3

• If the result is normal, you should offer to repeat the test after the patient has undertaken a bout of exercise.
• Diabetic patients may have falsely reassuring ABPIs due to calcification of their arteries.

Questions you could be asked

Q. Describe the anatomy of the lower limb arterial tree
A. See Figure 14.1.
Q. Identify and describe common vascular surgical scars.
A. Try to find these on the wards – even if it takes a whole day:
   • Open aneurysm: midline laparotomy
   • Femoro-femoral crossover: bilateral longitudinal groin incisions
   • Femoropopliteal bypass: longitudinal incisions above and below the knee
   • Carotid artery: longitudinal incision in the neck

Q. Discuss the potential complications of vascular surgery.

A. In your answer, classify these as:
- **Intraoperative:** bleeding, infection, thrombosis
- **Early:** compartment syndrome (treat with fasciotomy), reperfusion injury
- **Late:** infection, stenosis, false aneurysm (haematoma outside the arterial wall), amputation

Q. What are the indications for elective abdominal aortic aneurysm repair (placing an endovascular stent through the femoral artery)?

A.
- Size >5 cm
- Expansion rate >1 cm/year
- Symptomatic (back pain, distal emboli, tender abdomen)

15 Vascular (venous)

Lower limb

Checklist	P	MP	F
HELP			
H: 'Hello' (introduction and gains consent)			
E: Exposure (expose legs up to groins)			
L: Lighting			
P: Positions correctly (supine), asks if the patient is in any pain			
Washes hands			
Inspection from end of bed:			
• Comfortable			
• Varicose veins – note which vein			
• Coexistent arterial pathology (amputation, pallor)			
• Relevant paraphernalia (walking aids)			
Inspection of legs: front, side and behind:			
• Trophic changes (venous eczema, haemosiderin deposition, lipodermatosclerosis, thrombophlebitis, atrophie blanche)			
• Scars (e.g. vein harvesting, healed ulcer)			
• Ulceration (gaiter area – medial malleolus)			
• Oedema (around ankles)			
• Dressings (states would ideally examine underneath)			
Palpation:			
• Skin temperature with back of hands, moving up leg from feet in distribution of the long and short saphenous veins			
• Skin thickening (lipodermatosclerosis)			
• Thrombophlebitis (warmth and tenderness over a vein)			

• Locate saphenofemoral junction (SFJ) (4 cm below and lateral to pubic tubercle):
  • Feel for saphena varix
  • Assess for cough impulse			

• Tap test: • Place your hand over varicose vein and tap proximally. Test is positive if pulsation is felt over the varicose vein			

• Oedema			
Auscultates:			
• Bruits (listen over any varicose veins – bruit may signify a vascular malformation)			
Special tests:			

• Trendelenburg test:
  • Lay patient flat
  • Empty varicose veins by lifting leg
  • Place your fingers at SFJ
  • Ask patient to stand up and look for refilling of the veins
  • If veins refill, incompetence is below the SFJ			

• Tourniquet test:
  • Lay patient flat
  • Empty varicose veins by lifting leg
  • Apply a tourniquet at level of the SFJ and tighten it (this acts as an artificial valve)
  • Ask patient to stand up and look for refilling of the veins
  • If they do not refill, incompetence is at the level of the SFJ
  • If they do refill, incompetence is below the SFJ
  • If they refill, work your way down leg by applying tourniquet just above knee, then below it, then at mid-calf region, and look for refilling of vein			

• Perthes test:
  • Lay patient flat
  • Empty varicose veins by lifting leg
  • Apply a tourniquet around mid-thigh area (4–5 cm above knee)
  • Ensure this is not very tight (so that it compresses only the superficial veins and not the deep veins)
  • Ask patient to stand up and tiptoe up and down about 10 times (so that calf muscles contract)
  • If varicose veins remain full of blood, may be a deep vein obstruction (e.g. thrombosis)
  • If varicose veins empty, there is no deep vein obstruction			

• Doppler test:			
• Place Doppler probe over varicose vein. Squeeze distal to vein and listen for double 'whoosh.' This indicates an incompetent valve			
States intent to complete the examination with the following:			
• Examine remainder of the peripheral vascular system			
• Examine abdomen for masses			
• Do a rectal examination for masses			
• Examine external genitalia			

• Carry out brief local neurological examination			
Thanks patient			
Offers to help patient get dressed			
Washes hands			
Presents findings			
Offers appropriate differential diagnosis			
Suggests appropriate further investigations and management			
OVERALL IMPRESSION:			

Summary of common conditions seen in OSCEs

Pathology	Notes
Varicose veins	Abnormal dilatation and tortuosity of superficial venous circulation due to incompetent valves and resulting venous hypertension
Saphena varix	Dilatation of saphenous vein at the SFJ
	May have a cough impulse and can be differentiated from a femoral hernia by its blue colour and the fact that it disappears when the patient lies flat
Chronic venous insufficiency	Presence of valvular dysfunction and chronic venous hypertension will cause a number of trophic changes to occur
	See the above checklist for features of trophic disease
Venous ulcers	See Chapter 14 for notes on arterial examination

Hints and tips for the exam

Venous examination of the lower limb is fairly straightforward and is likely to appear as these patients have a chronic illness and are plentiful in number. To do well at this station, you must first have a sound understanding of the venous anatomy of the legs, and then demonstrate it during the examination. For example, when palpating the vasculature, remember to go from the feet upwards (as the veins take blood towards the heart!).

Inspect thoroughly

Inspect the room carefully for any walking aids. If you manage to complete your examination in good time, you can try to perform a functional assessment to show the examiner you are trying to clarify the level of disability caused by the disease. This can also guide management as painful varicose veins are an indication for surgical treatment.

Figure 15.1 illustrates various features of chronic venous disease, including thread veins, lipodermatosclerosis and haemosiderin deposition.

Examine a varicose as an autonomous entity

If you see a varicose vein, examine it as you would any lump or skin lesion. Do this before proceeding with the rest of the examination. Look carefully for scars from previous vascular surgery as these can often be hard to spot.

Remember that a large proportion of venous pathology coexists with arterial pathology

Mention this in your closing statement. It is an important safety issue as the compression bandaging used to treat venous disease is contraindicated in those with severe arterial disease. Hence an ABPI should be undertaken before compression bandaging is issued.

Questions you could be asked

Q. What are varicose veins?
Q. How are they treated?
Q. What are the trophic skin changes of chronic venous insufficiency?
Q. How do you treat a venous ulcer?
Q. What investigations would you perform for an ulcer?
Q. What is the management of an ulcer?
A. Answers to all these questions can be found in the text above.

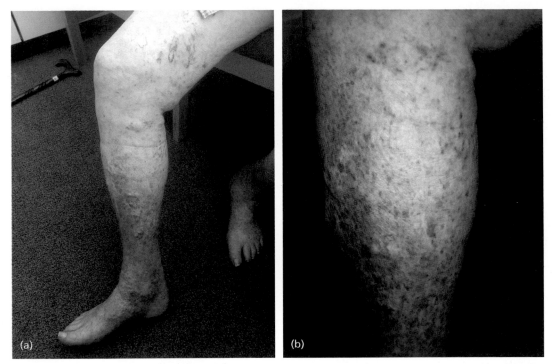

Figure 15.1 (a, b) Features of chronic venous disease

16 Ulcer

Checklist	P	MP	F
HELP			
H: 'Hello' (introduction and gains consent)			
E: Exposure			
L: Lighting			
P: Positions correctly, asks if patient is in any pain			
Washes hands and wears gloves			
Inspects from end of bed:			
• Surgical scars (e.g. bypass grafts for arterial disease, varicose vein stippling)			
• Amputations			
• Diabetes paraphernalia (e.g. insulin pens)			
• Ischaemic heart disease paraphernalia			
Inspection:			
• Number			
• Site/distribution			
• Size (in two dimensions)			
• Shape			
• Surrounding skin			
• Edge			
• Depth			
• Base			
• Colour			
• Discharge (blood, pus, fluid)			
Palpates:			
• Temperature of surrounding skin			
• Tenderness of surrounding skin			
Brief neurovascular examination:			
• Assesses sensation in surrounding dermatomes			
• Assesses power in surrounding myotomes			
• Palpates peripheral pulses			
Examines regional lymph nodes (sign of infection or malignancy)			
Examines for other systemic signs related to cause of ulcer:			
• Necrobiosis lipoidica			
• Corneal arcus, xanthelasmata			
• Signs of chronic venous disease			
• Signs of rheumatological, autoimmune or vasculitic conditions			
States intent to carry out relevant investigations:			
• Microscopy, culture and sensitivity on any fluid/discharge			

• Relevant blood tests to find cause:
  • Cholesterol (ischaemic heart disease)
  • Fasting blood glucose (diabetes)
  • Autoantibody screen (vasculitis)
  • Tumour markers (malignancies)			

• Investigations for arterial and venous disease (see Chapters 14 and 15, respectively)			
• X-ray (to rule out osteomyelitis, if appropriate)			
Thanks patient			
Offers to help patient get dressed			
Washes hands			
Presents findings			
Offers appropriate differential diagnosis			
Suggests appropriate further investigations and management			
OVERALL IMPRESSION:			

Summary of common conditions seen in OSCEs

Type of ulcer	Signs on examination	Management
Arterial	See Chapters 14 and 15	
Venous		
Diabetic/neuropathic	Punched-out ulcer Amputations Charcot joints Scars from bypass surgery Insulin by bedside	Educate patient about the illness Lifestyle modification (diet, exercise and smoking) Medical (optimise monitoring and antihyperglycaemic regimens) Surgical (bypass surgery and amputation)
Pressure	Over pressure points (e.g. sacrum) Walking aids Signs associated with reduced mobility or peripheral neuropathy (altered sensory perception)	Educate patients and carers Encourage movement Frequent repositioning Special mattresses
Basal cell carcinoma (rodent ulcer)	On the face Rolled edge Pearly colour Overlying telangiectasias Necrotic centre Local spread (rarely associated with lymphadenopathy)	Medical (topical 5-fluorouracil) Surgery (resection)
Keratoacanthoma	Central necrosis and horn	Reassure as lesion should resolve spontaneously Surgery may leave a scar that is bigger than the lesion!

Describing the edges of an ulcer

Descriptive term	Pathology	Likely cause	Picture
Punched-out	Full-thickness skin death Relatively quick onset	Arterial Neuropathic Rarely syphilis	
Flat, sloping	Healing ulcer Shallow	Venous	
Undermined	Infection at ulcer site Damages subcutaneous tissue	Infection	
Heaped/everted	Edge is growing quickly	Carcinoma	
Pearly rolled	Slow growth at the edge, telangiectasia in ulcer	Basal cell carcinoma	

Hints and tips for the exam

The ulcer examination station may be encountered as a medical, surgical or dermatology case in finals. It is a short station, and in most cases candidates will have a brief viva or questions to answer.

Find out about function/activities of daily living

Before attending to the ulcer, remember to inspect the patient and the surroundings. A walking aid or wheelchair will aid in your functional assessment and guide your management plan when you come to summarise.

Looking at the patient from a holistic and functional perspective will help you stand out as a candidate for merit or distinction.

Be clear and systematic in your description of the ulcer

The key to this station is in the description of the ulcer, and that is where most of your marks can be gained. The best way to master this is through practice!

When you embark on describing the ulcer, be sure to use the correct terminology, as in most cases it is likely be a spot diagnosis. Use the internet (when not on the wards) to look up and describe pictures of ulcers with a friend. Try not to skip parts of the description because they are 'obvious'. The point is to engrain the method of describing an ulcer, rather than the description itself.

To begin with, comment on the **site** of the ulcer as a distance from a bony landmark or obvious point of reference (e.g. the medial malleolus). The **distribution** of an ulcer may give you a clue to its cause so it is important to mention this too.

You should then attempt to measure the **size** and **shape** of the ulcer. Look around as there may be a ruler to help with this (if not have a guess). The larger an ulcer, the longer it will take to heal and the more likely it will be to become infected. Mentioning this rather obvious fact in your summary will show the examiner you are thinking of both the current clinical picture and the prognosis.

The **edge** of an ulcer is one of its most defining characteristics (at least for finals!). It can allow you to show the examiner you are aware of the diagnosis and also the pathological processes underway within the ulcer (see the table above).

When palpating, use the back of your hand to assess the **temperature** of the surrounding skin.

After thanking the patient, remember to cover them appropriately and complete your examination, tailoring any further examination to your most likely diagnosis, such as an examination of the peripheral nerves if a neuropathic ulcer is found, or a peripheral vascular examination if arterial or venous insufficiency is the suspected aetiology.

Here is one example of describing an ulcer:

> There is a single lesion 1 cm above the left nostril. It is round and approximately 1 cm by 1 cm in size, and 3 mm deep, with a rolled edge. The border is well circumscribed and shiny (opalescent) with several overlying telangiectasias. The base is necrotic. The surrounding skin is not erythematous. There is no associated lymphadenopathy.

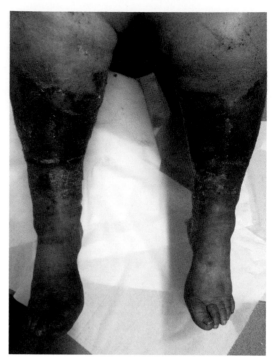

Figure 16.1 Chronic venous ulcers before appropriate dressing

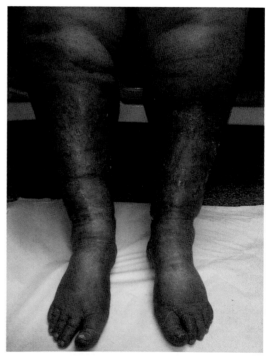

Figure 16.2 Chronic venous ulcers after appropriate dressing has been used

This is the classical description of a basal cell carcinoma (rodent ulcer).

Questions you could be asked

The questions are likely to be specific to the case. Here are a few general questions that you should consider before your OSCE.

Q. What is an ulcer?

A. An ulcer is a breach in the epithelial surface of the skin with **complete** loss of the mucosa.

Q. What is an erosion?

A. An erosion is a breach in the epithelial surface with **partial** loss of the mucosa.

Q. What are the four stages of wound healing?

A. • Haemostasis
  • Inflammation
  • Proliferation
  • Remodelling

Q. What is granulation tissue?

A. This is the pink, soft, granular tissue that is seen after injury. Histologically, new blood vessel formation is seen alongside the proliferation of fibroblasts.

Q. What factors affect wound healing?

A. • Local factors:
    • Blood supply
    • Infection
    • Mechanical stress
  • Systemic factors:
    • Age
    • Anaemia
    • Diabetes
    • Malnutrition

Q. How would you manage an arterial/venous leg ulcer?

A. To answer this question, be sure to include community-based services in your answer in addition to conservative, medical and surgical management. See Chapters 14 and 15 for more information on how to treat these.

17 Shoulder

Checklist	P	MP	F
HELP			
H: 'Hello' (introduction and gains consent)			
E: Exposure (remove top)			
L: Lighting			
P: Positions correctly (supine), asks if patient is in any pain			
Washes hands			
Inspects from end of bed for relevant paraphernalia: • Slings, casts, splints • Walking aids • Zimmer frames			
Inspects patient (patient standing – takes a 360-degree look): • Muscle wasting • Deformities • Scars – arthroscopy portals, surgical scars • Sinuses • Swelling • Erythema • Position of the shoulders – Bryant's sign (lowering of the axillary fold demonstrates dislocation) • Bony deformity (fractures, winging of the scapula)			
Does a quick screening test for all main muscle groups: • Arms raised above head with shoulder fully abducted • Hands raised and placed behind back of head • Hands placed at lower lumbar back			
Palpates shoulder joint: • Temperature • Swelling • Muscle bulk around joint, scapula • Joints: sternoclavicular, acromioclavicular, glenohumeral joints • Scapula			

Assesses movements: • Flexion (0–180 degrees) • Extension (0–50 degrees) • Abduction (0–180 degrees) • Adduction (0–50 degrees) • External rotation (0–90 degrees) • Internal rotation (0–70 degrees) • Assesses passive, active and resisted movements • Assesses degree of passive and active movement • Assesses for pain and crepitus • Stabilises with other hand while assessing movement • Checks for painful arc (70–120 degrees) upon abduction			
Assess for winging of scapula – push against wall			
Special tests: • Rotator cuff tests: • Full can test • Lift-off test • Infraspinatus and teres minor test • Impingement tests: • Neer's impingement test • Hawkins–Kennedy test • Instability test: • Anterior instability test • Sulcus sign • Load shift sign • Yergason's test: • Biceps – resisted supination with long head of the biceps pathology causes pain in the bicipital groove			
Thanks patient Offers to help patient get dressed Washes hands Offers to examine elbow (joint below) and neck (joint above) Offers to examine neurovascular function of lower limbs Presents findings Offers appropriate differential diagnosis Suggests appropriate investigations and management			

Summary of common conditions seen in OSCEs

Condition	History	Symptoms and signs
Most common conditions		
Adhesive capsulitis (frozen shoulder)	Two phases: pain, then stiffness Common in diabetics and middle-aged patients (age around 50 years) Lasts about 18 months Pain often worse at night	Pain in all directions of movement Worse on external rotation
Rotator cuff impingement (supraspinatus tendonitis)	Pain on abduction	Pain on abduction in characteristic 'arc' (70–120 degrees)
Rotator cuff tear	Trauma Cannot lift objects above head	Pain on abduction in characteristic arc (70–120 degrees) Pain worse on resisted abduction Active movements more painful than passive movements
Others – inflammatory/ degenerative		
Biceps tendonitis	Anterior shoulder pain Pain lifting heavy objects	Tenderness at bicipital groove upon palpation
Calcific tendonitis	**Three different presentations:** • Sporadic flares, mild pain, chronic • Obstruction of elevation of shoulder due to calcific deposit • Acute pain with inflammatory symptoms	Stiffness, weakness, crepitus. Radiation of pain from shoulder tip to deltoid insertion Decreased range of movement, painful arc 70–120 degrees Pain on abduction of shoulder or lying on shoulder
Acromioclavicular joint arthritis	Decreased range of movement Pain at tip of shoulder Pain on overhead lifting	Pain with cross-body movements Tenderness upon palpation at the acromioclavicular joint
Rotator cuff tendonitis	Pain over shoulder at night	Painful arc relieved by external rotation, worsens with internal rotation
Others – conditions causing instability		
Acute anterior dislocation	Trauma Decreased range of movement	Humeral head projects anteriorly Axillary nerve palsy Deltoid muscle dysfunction
Acute posterior dislocation	Seizures Elderly Electric shock	Limitation of external rotation
Recurrent shoulder instability	Young Trauma Joint laxity: Ehlers–Danlos syndrome	Examine other joints for laxity, including hands, elbows and knees Sulcus sign Load shift sign

Hints and tips for the exam

Know your scars

Upon inspecting the patient, you may be faced with a multitude of scars, the indications for which may help with your diagnosis.

Scar	Location of incision	Indication
Anterior	Lateral side of clavicle downwards following medial border of deltoid muscle	Shoulder replacement Open reduction/internal fixation of fracture of humerus
Posterior	Along border of scapular spine	Fractures of scapula or glenoid neck Posterior stabilisation surgery
Superior strap	Lateral to the border of the acromion	Rotator cuff surgery
Arthroscopy portals (Figure 17.1)	Through deltoid and posterior lateral edge of acromion	Adhesive capsulitis Loose bodies Chronic synovitis Impingement syndrome: rotator cuff tears and tendonitis Osteoarthritis Shoulder instability

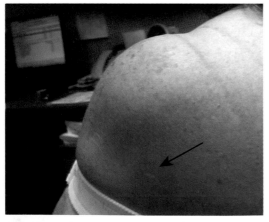

Figure 17.1 Arthroscopy insertion site

Know your muscle groups

The following muscles are responsible for the movements elicited within the shoulder examination.

Movement	Muscle
Flexion	0–60 degrees • Pectoralis major • Biceps brachii • Anterior deltoid • Coracobrachialis 60–120 degrees • Trapezius • Serratus anterior 120–180 degrees • Deltoid plus the all the above muscles
Extension	0–20 degrees • Teres major • Deltoid 20–50 degrees • Rhomboids • Trapezius
Abduction	0–90 degrees • Supraspinatus • Deltoid 90–150 degrees • Serratus anterior • Trapezius 150–180 degrees • Serratus anterior plus all the above muscles
Adduction	0–50 degrees • Coracobrachialis • Teres major • Latissimus dorsi • Pectoralis major
Internal rotation	0–70 degrees • Subscapularis • Teres major • Latissimus dorsi • Pectoralis major • Deltoid
External rotation	0–90 degrees • Teres minor • Deltoid • Infraspinatus
Circumduction	All the muscles listed above as being involved in extension, adduction, flexion and abduction

An easy way to remember the names of the muscles that form the rotator cuff is to use the mnemonic **SSIT**:
- Subscapularis
- Supraspinatus
- Infraspinatus
- Teres minor

Know your special tests
There are many 'special tests' you can do when examining the shoulder, but if time is limited you may have to utlilise them selectively.

Rotator cuff tests
Empty can test
Aim – To assess the supraspinatus.

Patient position – The patient stands with the arms abducted to 90 degrees. The hand imitates holding an empty can for full internal rotation and imitates holding a full can with thumbs up for external rotation.

Clinician position – The clinician stands behind the patient applying downward stress at the mid-forearm while stabilising the patient's shoulder joint.

Clinical significance –
• Positive test: Weakness, pain located in the subacromial region
• Negative test: No pain or weakness

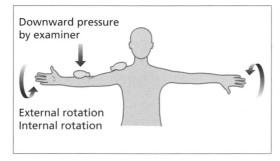

Lift off test
Aim – To test for a subscapularis tear.

Patient position – The patient stands with the shoulder held in a position of internal rotation. The patient's hand gently rests on the lumbar spine.

Clinician position – The clinician passively lifts the hand from the lumbar spine.

Clinical significance –
• Positive test: If the arm extends and the patient is unable to maintain the position of internal rotation, this is evidence of a subscapularis tear.
• Negative test: The arm is maintained in an position of internal rotation.

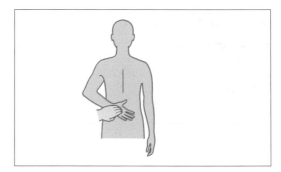

Infraspinatus and teres minor test
Aim – To test for infraspinatus and teres minor weakness.

Patient position – The patient stands with the arm by the side, with the elbow flexed to 90 degrees.

Clinician position – The clinician stands next to the arm, stabilising the elbow and wrist while the patient resists external rotation.

Clinical significance –
• Positive test: Pain and weakness indicate a rotator cuff tear.
• Negative test: Good resistance, no pain or weakness.

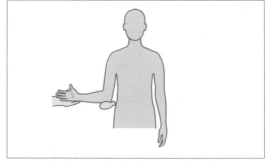

Impingement tests
Hawkins–Kennedy test
Aim – To assess for impingement.

Patient position – The patient stands with the arm flexed to 90 degrees and the elbow flexed to 90 degrees.

Clinician position – The clinician stabilises the elbow and wrist, and swiftly passively internally rotates the arm.

Clinical significance –
• Positive test: Pain upon internal rotation. This action creates impingement of the structures of the greater tuberosity of the humerus against the coracohumeral ligament.
• Negative test: No pain.

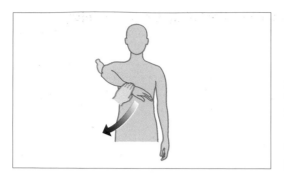

Neer's impingement test

Aim – To assess for subacromial impingement.

Patient position – The patient stands or sits relaxed with the arms in the anatomical position and allows the clinician to carry out the passive movement.

Clinician position – The clinician passively raises the patient's arm in a pronated position while stabilising the scapula to prevent scapulothoracic movement.

Clinical significance –
• Positive test: Pain upon abduction in the subacromial space or anterior edge of the acromion. This demonstrates impingement of the long head of the biceps, supraspinatus or infraspinatus.
• Negative test: No pain upon full flexion.

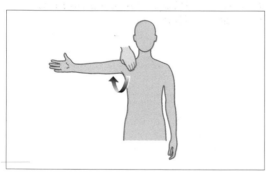

Tests for instability
Anterior instability test

Aim – To assess for anterior instability of the glenohumeral joint.

Patient position – The patient lies supine with the arm abducted to 90 degrees and the elbow flexed to 90 degrees.

Clinician position – The clinician attempts to externally rotate the arm to 90 degrees and gently pushes downwards on the anterior aspect of the humerus, assessing the degree and direction of instability.

Clinical significance –
• Positive test: An anterior fullness can be palpated that denotes subluxation of the glenohumeral joint. Pain is

elicited at the point of full external rotation, extension and abduction, the ideal position from which to dislocate the shoulder.
• Negative test: No pain or fullness at the shoulder joint.

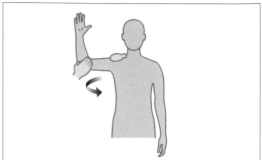

Sulcus sign
The arm is gently pulled downwards, creating an observable enlarged subacromial space and a clear deep skin sulcus.

Load shift sign
Anterior or posterior dislocation can be detected by gripping the humerus with one hand and grasping the scapula with the other hand. The injured shoulder joint will shift more with movement than it does on the normal side.

Test for acromioclavicular joint: Scarf test
Aim – To assess for acromioclavicular joint pathology.

Patient position – The patient sits with the arm abducted to 90 degrees and the elbow flexed to 90 degrees with the palms supinated.

Clinician position – The clinician attempts forcibly to adduct the flexed arm across the chest while supporting the posterior aspect of the shoulder on contralateral side.

Clinical significance –
• Positive test: Pain on the posterior aspect of the affected side.
• Negative test: No pain.

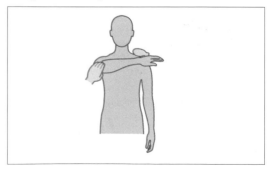

Know your shoulder nerves and how they could be affected by a shoulder injury

Shoulder injuries are common and can often result in nerve injuries producing classical signs that are ideal for OSCE situations. We have summarised the common ones in the table.

	Brachial plexus	Long thoracic nerve injury	Suprascapular nerve injury	Musculocutaneous nerve injury
Aetiology	Fall on shoulder	Traction of arm	Entrapment from backpacking, weightlifting or volleyball	Frontal blows
Symptoms/signs	Paraesthesia Upper limb weakness Does not typically affect motor component	Serratus anterior palsy – winging of scapula medially Spinal accessory nerve palsy – winging of scapula laterally	Supraspinatus and infraspinatus weakness	Muscle – weak elbow flexion and forearm supination Absent biceps tendon reflex Cutaneous – sensory loss over lateral and volar aspects of forearm
Management	Conservative: • Rest • Anti-inflammatories • Physiotherapy	Conservative: • Rest • Anti-inflammatories • Physiotherapy	Conservative: • Rest • Anti-inflammatories • Physiotherapy	Conservative: • Rest • Anti-inflammatories • Physiotherapy

Winging of the scapula

The scapula, also known as the shoulder blade, has a multitude of muscles attached to it in order to create fluid shoulder movement. Dysrhythmia relates to the abnormal movement of these antagonist and agonist muscles when one or many muscles do not function. The result is 'winging of the scapula' – the protrusion of the medial border of the scapula.

The most common cause is paralysis of the serratus anterior muscle, but other causes must not be excluded as follows:

• Trapezius muscle paralysis
• Dislocation of the acromioclavicular joint, causing rupture of the coracoclavicular ligaments
• Secondary to pain – an overcompensation of movement
• Brachial plexus injury
• Recurrent dislocations of the shoulder
• Facioscapulohumeral dystrophy – an inherited bilateral displacement

Referred pain

Shoulder pain is not an exclusive symptom confined to this joint. Other causes not directly related to the shoulder may cause pain, falling under the umbrella of referred pain. These include:

• Cervical spine trauma
• Myocardial ischaemia
• Referred diaphragmatic pain, such as from gallbladder disease
• Malignancy, for example apical lung disease

Therefore, upon examining your patient, ensure you do not forget to examine the other systems if you suspect an alternative cause.

Thoracic outlet syndrome – a rare but serious condition

Thoracic outlet syndrome deserves a special mention. Although it is not a common cause of shoulder pain, it is an important diagnosis that must not be missed.

Anatomy

Thoracic outlet syndrome relates to the compression of the following structures within the small anatomical space of the interscalene triangle:

• Neurology: Brachial plexus (B)
• Venous: Subclavian artery (A)
• Arterial: Subclavian vein (V)

The diagram shows how these structures pass through the interscalene triangle.

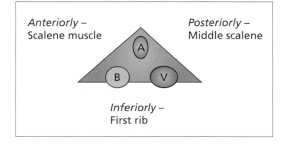

Aetiology
- **Venous:** thrombosis of the subclavian vein
- **Arterial:** subclavian artery stenosis or aneurysm
- **Neurological:** repetitive strain injury, for example keyboard typing, or trauma.

Presentation
- **Venous:** pain in the shoulder, engorgement of the veins producing a unilateral swollen arm
- **Arterial:** pulseless, pain, paraesthesia, paralysis, pallor (the '5Ps')
- **Neurological:**
  - Involvement of the roots of C8 and T1 is most common, with pain and paraesthesia in the ulnar nerve distribution.
  - The second most common root involvement is of C5, C6, C7, with pain and paraesthesia in the median nerve distribution.
- **Special tests:** elevated arm stress test (EAST):
  - The shoulder is abducted to 90 degrees and the hand alternately makes a grip and then an extended gesture for 3 minutes.
  - Positive test:
    - The patient cannot continue for a full 3 minutes due to reproduction of the symptoms.
  - Negative test
    - The patient can continue for the whole 3 minutes.
    - Patients with carpal tunnel syndrome will demonstrate paraesthesia but not shoulder pain.

Differential diagnoses
- Rotator cuff injury
- Multiple sclerosis

- Acute coronary syndrome
- Spinal cord injury

Investigations
- Imaging:
  - Chest X-ray:
    - First rib deformity
    - Clavicle deformity
    - Pancoast tumour
  - Cervical radiography: bony deformity
  - Doppler ultrasound: obstruction
  - Venography: thrombosis
  - Arteriography: emboli, aneurysm, stenosis
  - MRI: cervical spine disease
- Nerve conduction tests

Treatment
- Physiotherapy
- Anticoagulation
- Vascular surgery

Questions you could be asked

Q. How would you do a 2-minute screening test for all the major shoulder muscle groups?
Q. How would you distinguish between a rotator cuff impingement syndrome and a rotator cuff tear?
Q. What are the common nerve palsies resulting from shoulder injuries, and what are their signs?
Q. What is thoracic outlet syndrome, and how would you manage it?
A. Answers to these questions are to be found in the text above.

18 Hand

Checklist	P	MP	F
HELP			
H: 'Hello' (introduction and gains consent)			
E: Exposure (hands ideally up to elbows)			
L: Lighting			
P: Positions correctly (supine, ideally resting on a desk or table), asks if the patient is in any pain			
Washes hands			
Observation:			
• Skin: scars, colour, rashes, thinning (steroid use), bruises, wrist/elbow nodules			
• Nails: clubbing, splinter haemorrhages, pitting, onycholysis, nailfold vasculitis			
• Joints: erythema, swelling, deformity			
• Muscle: wasting, fasciculation			
• Posture: characteristic abnormalities (e.g. claw hand)			
• Observes and palpates the elbows for rheumatoid nodules			
• Looks behind the ears for psoriatic plaques			
Palpation:			
• Temperature			
• Radial pulses			
• Muscle bulk (thenar and hypothenar eminences)			
• Palmar fascia			
• Squeeze across metacarpophalangeal joints			
• Bimanual palpation of individual joints			
• Bony swellings			
• Sensation in radial, median and ulnar nerve territories			
Movement (active and passive):			
• Wrist:			
• Pronation			
• Supination			
• Flexion			
• Extension			
• Abduction			
• Adduction			

• Digits:			
• Flexion and extension at metacarpophalangeal and proximal interphalangeal joints			
• Abduction and adduction (spread fingers apart)			
• Grip (making a fist)			
• Thumb:			
• Abduction			
• Adduction			
• Extension			
• Flexion			
• Opposition with 5th digit			
Special tests:			
• Tinel's/Phalen's tests			
• Froment's sign			
Function:			
• Pincer grip			
• Squeezing student's fingers			
• Doing up buttons			
• Opening jar			
Offers to examine elbow and shoulder			
Offers to examine neurovascular function in detail			
Thanks patient			
Offers to help patient get dressed			
Washes hands			
Presents findings			
Offers appropriate differential diagnosis			
Suggests appropriate further investigations and management			
OVERALL IMPRESSION:			

Summary of common conditions seen in OSCEs

Disease	Look	Feel	Move	Special test	Function	Examiner questions
Carpal tunnel syndrome	Wasted abductor pollicis brevis Loss of sensation over median nerve territory Signs of rheumatoid arthritis (discussed below) Signs of hypothyroidism (see Chapter 9)	NAD	NAD	Positive Tinel's and Phalen's tests	Weak pincer grip	What are the causes of carpal tunnel syndrome? How is it managed?
Radial nerve palsy	Wrist drop	Reduced sensation in skin over dorsal area of root of thumb	Wrist and digit extension against resistance is weakened	NAD		What are the causes?
Ulnar nerve palsy	Claw hand	Reduced sensation over medial one-and-a-half digits Weakness of abductor pollicis brevis and dorsal interossei	Digit abduction/ adduction is weakened	NAD	Difficulty with performing any tasks, e.g. opening jar, pincer grip	What is the ulnar nerve palsy paradox?
Rheumatoid arthritis	Symmetrical red, swollen proximal interphalangeal, metacarpophalangeal and wrist joints Ulnar deviation of digits Boutonnière and swan neck deformities of digits Z-deformity of thumb Wasting of small muscles of hand	Affected joints are painful and feel boggy	Restricted movement at affected joints	NAD	Function may be restricted or lost	What are the different ways in which rheumatoid arthritis can present? What is the treatment of rheumatoid arthritis? What factors are associated with a poor prognosis in rheumatoid arthritis?

Psoriatic arthritis	Asymmetrical swelling of distal interphalangeal joints Symmetrical polyarthritis indistinguishable from rheumatoid arthritis Psoriatic plaques on extensor aspect of elbows Pitting/onycholysis of nails	Affected joints are painful and feel boggy, telescoping of digits (in arthritis mutilans)	Restricted movement at affected joints	NAD	Function may be restricted/lost	What are the patterns of joint involvement in psoriatic arthritis?
Nodal osteoarthritis	Heberden's/Bouchard's nodes Squaring of base of thumb	Bony hard swellings at nodes Pain on palpation of affected joints (wrist, 1st carpometacarpal, distal interphalangeal)	Crepitus Restricted movement at affected joints	NAD	Function may be restricted or lost	What X-ray changes are associated with osteoarthritis? How is osteoarthritis treated? What are the indications for surgery?
Systemic sclerosis	Sausage-like digits (sclerodactyly) Heliotrope rash across knuckles Microstomia with furrowing of skin around mouth on observation of face	Loss of normal skin creases Tight skin tethered to underlying structures Flexion contractures of joints	Difficulty achieving full extension of digits	NAD	NAD/difficulty forming a fist	What antibodies are associated with the two types of systemic sclerosis? How is it managed?
Dupuytren's contracture	Fifth digit held in partial flexion	Thickened palmar fascia	Difficulty extending 5th digit	NAD	NAD	What are the causes of this condition?
Trigger finger	Fixed flexion of affected finger	Palpable nodule over tendon of affected finger	Finger in fixed flexion can be 'flicked' into extension	NAD		What is the treatment of this?
De Quervain's tenosynovitis	Affected tendons are swollen (abductor pollicis longus, extensor pollicis brevis) Trigger finger or thumb	Affected tendon is tender to palpate and crepitus is felt	If nodules develop on affected tendons, finger may have to be flicked to complete movement when tendon catches	NAD	Weakened pincer grip with thumb	What is the treatment of this condition?

Hints and tips for the exams

Doing the examination

• **Careful observation** is very important because most hand diagnoses such as scleroderma, rheumatoid arthritis (RA) and common nerve palsies can often be picked up on observation alone. State what you see but do not list all the negatives.

• **Feel the temperature** using the back of your hand over the wrist and metacarpophalangeal (MCP) joints to check for joint inflammation.

• **Bimanual palpation of joints:** Squeeze gently with the index finger and thumb in an anteroposterior direction with one hand and in a mediolateral direction with the other hand.

• Get the patient to shut their eyes and familiarise them with the test for **sensation** by touching the chest.

  • **Radial nerve:** Touch over the web space between the thumb and index finger on the posterior surface of the hand.

• **Median nerve:** Touch over the thenar eminence.

• **Ulnar nerve:** Touch over the hypothenar eminence.

• Fix the elbow by pinning it to the patient's side before testing supination and pronation. Test wrist abduction and adduction with the elbow in the same position. Test flexion and extension at the wrist by asking the patient to perform the prayer and inverse prayer positions.

• When **testing movement at a particular joint,** use your other hand to **fix the joint** above that being tested.

Performing the special tests

• **Tinel's test:** Extend the wrist and tap over the carpal tunnel to see whether symptoms of carpal tunnel syndrome can be reproduced.

• **Phalen's test:** Forced flexion of the wrists for 60 seconds can reproduce the symptoms of carpal tunnel syndrome.

• **Froment's sign:** This is a test for ulnar nerve palsy. If the thumb adductor is weak, the interphalangeal joint

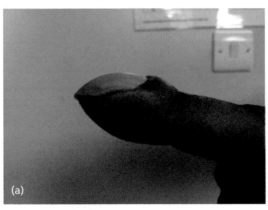
(a)

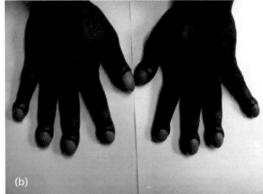
(b)

Figure 18.1 Severe clubbing

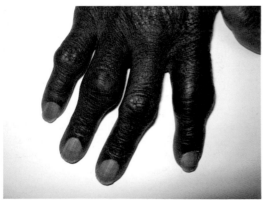

Figure 18.2 Bouchard's nodes

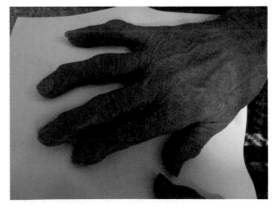

Figure 18.3 Heberden's and Bouchard's nodes in osteoarthritis

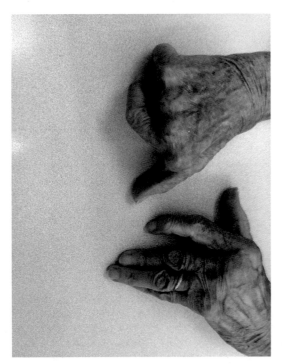

Figure 18.4 (a, b) Ulnar deviation in rheumatoid arthritis

of the thumb flexes when an attempt is made to pull out a piece of paper held between the thumb and index finger.

• **Finkelstein's test:** This is performed if De Quervain's tenosynovitis is suspected. The thumb is flexed, and the fingers are then flexed over it to form a fist (with the thumb under the fingers). The wrist is then adducted – if this causes pain, the test is positive and confirms De Quervain's tenosynovitis.

Presenting the findings

This is where most candidates slip up, especially if several hand joints are involved. As usual, it is wise to **start by stating any obvious abnormalities** that strongly point to a diagnosis. If several joints are involved, do **not** individually state each joint that is involved. This is very time-consuming, is boring for the examiner and adds little information to your presentation. A better approach is to state the groups of joints involved and the disease this pattern is consistent with, for examples 'The wrists, PIP and MCP joints are red, hot and swollen in a symmetrical distribution; this is consistent with a diagnosis of RA.'

Common variations at this station

• **Task (7–10 minutes):** *'This is a 29-year-old who complains of painful hands. Take a brief focused history and examine the patient's hands.'*
There are **some key questions** to ask in the focused history (see also Chapter 40 on history of joint pain for more detail):

  • Are your joints stiff in the morning?
  • Which joints are involved?
  • Are there any extra-articular features?
  • Is there any functional impairment?

• **Task (7–10 minutes):** *'Perform a GALS screen of this patient's musculoskeletal system and then examine the hands'.* You should aim to spend no more than 2–3 minutes performing the GALS screen at this station. Look particularly for large-joint pathology, axial involvement and psoriatic plaques.

• **Task (5–10 minutes):** *'This patient complains of pins and needles in her hand at night. Examine her hands and then give her some brief advice on management.'*

• This is probably the most difficult variation at this station. This type of scenario is frequently tested in finals OSCEs, and it is important to follow the generic structure:

  • Confirmation of diagnosis (e.g. nerve conduction studies)
  • Conservative measures: splinting, weight loss
  • Medical measures: analgesia, treatment of underlying disorders
  • Steroid injections
  • Surgery: surgical decompression of the carpal tunnel
  • Safety netting: for example, carpal tunnel syndrome can be a first presentation of RA so you must tell your patient to report development of any joint pain or extra-articular features

Questions you could be asked

Q. What are the causes of carpal tunnel syndrome?
A. Pregnancy, RA, osteoarthritis, acromegaly, diabetes mellitus, hypothyroidism, obesity and idiopathic.
Q. How is it carpal tunnel syndrome managed?
A. For management, see the main text above.
Q. What are the causes of radial nerve palsy?
A. Fracture of the humeral shaft, elbow fracture/injury, forearm injury (the posterior interosseous branch passes between the two heads of the supinator muscle) or as part of mononeuritis multiplex.
Q. What is the treatment of RA?
A. Analgesia, disease-modifying antirheumatic drugs (including methotrexate), anti-tumour necrosis factor

medications, and intramuscular or oral steroids (for exacerbations).

Q. What factors are associated with a poor prognosis in RA?

A. Rheumatoid nodules, positive rheumatoid factor, systemic symptoms and late onset of joint involvement.

Q. What are the different patterns of joint involvement in psoriatic arthritis?

A. Symmetrical polyarthritis involving the small joints of the hands, synovitis of the distal interphalangeal joints, asymmetrical oligoarthritis, axial arthritis and arthritis mutilans.

Q. What X-ray changes are associated with osteoarthritis?

A. Loss of joint space, subchondral sclerosis, subchondral cysts and osteophytes.

Q. How is osteoarthritis treated?

A. • Conservative: for example, walking aids and weight loss
 • Medical: topical or oral analgesics, steroid injections for rapid pain relief.
 • Surgical: for example, arthroscopy and partial or complete joint replacement

Q. What are the indications for surgery in osteoarthritis?

A. Persistent severe pain or stiffness not amenable to medical management, and loss of joint function.

Q. What antibodies are associated with the two types of systemic sclerosis?

A. For limited disease, anticentromere antibodies, and for diffuse disease anti-scl70 + anti-RNA polymerase in about 20–30% of patients.

Q. How is systemic sclerosis managed?

 • Conservative: for example, gloves
 • Medical: for example, immunosuppression to control disease activity, antihypertensives, angiotensin-converting enzyme inhibitors to decrease the chance of renal crisis, and drugs to reduce pulmonary hypertension

Q. What is the treatment of trigger finger?

A. Steroid injections and surgery.

Q. What is the treatment of De Quervain's tenosynovitis?

A. Thumb splinting, steroid injections and surgery.

Q. What are the predisposing factors for Dupuytren's contracture?

A. White ethnicity, family history, chronic liver disease (particularly secondary to alcohol), diabetes mellitus, chronic obstructive pulmonary disease, epilepsy and antiepileptic medication.

19 Hip

Checklist	P	MP	F
HELP			
H: 'Hello' (introduction and gains consent)			
E: Exposure (nipples to knees/down to groins)			
L: Lighting			
P: Positions correctly (supine), asks if the patient is in any pain			
Washes hands			
Inspects from the end of the bed for relevant paraphernalia: • Walking stick • Zimmer frame			
Assesses gait: • Symmetry (symmetrical – normal, parkinsonian, marche à petits pas, wide-based; asymmetrical – hemiplegic gait, antalgic, orthopaedic) • Size of paces (normal – waddling, small – parkinsonian, marche à petits pas) • Distance between feet (normal, scissoring, cerebellar, broad-based) • Knees (normal, high-stepping) • Painful gait (arthritis, trauma) • Phases of walking (heel strike, stance, push-off, swing) • Arm swing (present or absent)			
Inspection (patient standing, inspect all around patient, 360 degrees): • Skin – trophic, sinuses, scars (e.g. total hip replacement) • Muscle (gluteal muscle bulk) • Leg length (disparity) • Bony deformity (scoliosis) • Posture (lumbar lordosis for fixed flexion deformity) • Erythema/swelling (rheumatoid arthritis, osteoarthritis, trauma, tumour, septic arthritis) • Position (degree of rotation of leg, fixed flexion deformity)			

Trendelenburg test (see below)			
Measure (patient lying): • Leg length			
Palpate (patient lying): • Skin – temperature (infection, inflammation) • Bone – tenderness (fracture, trochanteric bursitis, labral tears)			
Move (patient lying): • Flexion (normal: flexion arc 0–120 degrees) • Extension (patient prone, normal: 0–10 degrees) • Abduction (normal: 0–40 degrees) • Adduction (normal: 0–25 degrees) • Rotation (normal: internal 0–45, external 0–60) • Assess pain and any reduction in range of movement (ROM)			

Special tests (patient lying):
To assess the joint:
  • FABER test
  • FAIR test
To assess the muscles and tendons:
  • Thomas test			

Thanks patient Offers to help patient get dressed Washes hands Offers to examine sacroiliac (joint above) and knee (joint below) Offers to examine neurovascular function of lower limbs Presents findings Offers appropriate differential diagnosis Offers appropriate investigations and management plan			
OVERALL IMPRESSION:			

Summary of common conditions seen in OSCEs

Painful hip

Condition	History	Symptoms and signs
Osteoarthritis	Primary Secondary – infection, trauma, developmental dysplasia of the hip	Local Pain on weight-bearing Restricted ROM Referred pain – knee, buttocks Flexion contracture
Rheumatoid arthritis	Morning stiffness Age younger than for osteoarthritis	Muscle wasting Bilateral pain Trophic skin changes
Avascular necrosis of the hip	Trauma Alcohol intake Gout Diabetes	Groin pain upon walking Stiffness
Bursitis	Repetitive movement – ballet, rowing, dancing	Trochanteric – pain on adduction Ischiogluteal – pain upon sitting for long periods
Spondyloarthropathies	Ankylosing spondylitis Inflammatory bowel disease Psoriatic arthritis	Painful sacroiliac joint referred to the lower buttock and thigh Pain elicited by extension and compression of the hip
Piriformis syndrome	Compression of the sciatic nerve	Pain upon sitting
Septic arthritis	Immunocompromised	Fever Acute pain Erythema Swelling Hot Decreased motion

Gait abnormalities you may encounter in a hip station

Type of gait	Pathology	Condition
Waddling (Trendelenburg)	Weak proximal muscles	Muscular dystrophy Congenital hip dysplasia
Parkinsonian	Basal ganglion dysfunction	Parkinson's disease Drugs – phenothiazines, haloperidol, thiothixene, metoclopramide Carbon monoxide poisoning
Scissoring	Spastic paraparesis	Multiple sclerosis Cord compression Cerebral palsy Syringomyelia Pernicious anaemia Liver failure
Cerebellar ataxia	Ipsilateral cerebellar lesion	Multiple sclerosis Alcohol Stroke/transient ischaemic attack
Foot drop	Common peroneal nerve palsy (unilateral)	Trauma to knee Fracture of fibula
Marche à petits pas	Diffuse cerebrovascular disease – lacunar state	
Sensory ataxia	Peripheral neuropathy	Diabetes Alcohol intake Multiple sclerosis
Antalgic gait	Trauma	See table above

Hints and tips for the exam

Know your anatomy

The hip is a ball and socket joint in which the acetabulum is the 'socket' and the head of the femur is the 'ball'. This musculoskeletal structure is used for weight-bearing and supporting bipedal movements. The following table exhibits the complexity of the muscular origins of the hip movements and will help in diagnosing a labral tear if one is apparent in the hip examination.

Movement	Muscles
Flexion of hip	Iliacus
	Psoas major
Extension of hip	Hamstring muscles
	Gluteus maximus
Adduction of hip	Adductor brevis
	Adductor longus
	Adductor magnus
Abduction of hip	Gluteus medius
	Gluteus minimus
Lateral rotation of hip	Tensor fasciae latae
	Gluteus medius and minimus

Special tests

Apparent limb length and true limb length

• Apparent limb length = distance from the xiphisternum to the medial malleolus bilaterally.
• True limb length = distance between the anterior superior iliac spine and the medial malleolus bilaterally.

The clinical significance of this is that a fixed adduction deformity of the hip can be diagnosed if the apparent limb lengths are different but true limb lengths are equal. In hip dislocations, Perthes disease or slipped femoral epiphysis, there is a difference in true limb length.

Trendelenburg test

Aim – To assess the abductor muscles of the hip (gluteus medius, gluteus minimus).

Technique – If you are assessing the **left hip**, the patient should stand upright, and then lift the right foot off the ground while flexing the right knee. The right hip should then move upwards as the **left hip muscles contract to pull it up**.

• If this happens, the test is *negative* as the left hip muscles are functioning normally.
• If the right hip sags down, the test is *positive* as the left hip muscles are unable to contract and pull the right hip upwards.

As easy way to remember this is that the **'sound side sags'** – is if there is sagging of the hip (i.e. it does not move upwards when the foot is raised off the floor), the defect is in the contralateral hip abductors.

FABER test

Aim – To assess hip joint pathology.

Technique –The patient lies supine with one leg flexed at the knee and externally rotated. The ankle rests upon the opposite knee joint. The patient extends the flexed knee while pressure is applied over the hip and knee joint by the examiner. This is repeated for the opposite hip joint (FABER = Flexion, Abduction, External Rotation).

Clinician's position – The clinician stands by the flexed knee and applies pressure to the medial aspect of the knee and opposite hip joint.

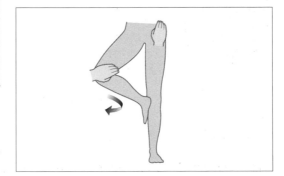

Clinical significance –
• **Negative test:** No pain upon movement, equal range of movement bilaterally, both knees are level at the end of the examination.
• **Positive test:** Hip pain upon movement and decreased ROM.

The pelvis articulates with the sacroiliac joint and the lumbar spine. The iliopsoas muscle functions as a hip flexor and external rotator of the femur. Thus, pressure exerted upon the hip joint exerts tension on these structures, causing pain if pathology is present. Articular hip pathology, for example synovitis or loose bodies, also presents with pain upon movement.

FAIR test

Aim – To assess articular pathology.

Patient's position – The patient lies in the lateral recumbent position, the upper hip and knee both flexed to 90 degrees.

Clinician's position – The clinician stands placing a stabilising pressure on the hip while depressing the flexed knee, which internally rotates and adducts the hip (FAIR = Flexion, Adduction, Internal Rotation).

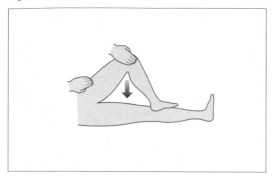

Clinical significance –
• **Negative test:** No pain upon movement or compression of the hip.
• **Positive test:** Sciatic symptoms are recreated. There is hip pain upon movement.

The piriform muscle is attached to the superior medial aspect of the greater trochanter and inserts into the obturator internus. The piriform muscle has multiple functions, including acting as a flexor, abductor and internal rotator of the hip. The sciatic nerve pierces the piriformis muscle, so trauma or strenuous activity, for example long-distance running, leading to inflammation of the muscle, may compress the nerve, producing an intense shooting pain following the distribution of the sciatic nerve. Reproduction of the symptoms is achieved by the FAIR manoeuvre.

The psoas bursa is a fluid-filled sac that lies between the psoas tendon and the lesser trochanter of the femur. Strenuous repetitive exercise, such as ballet, rowing or gymnastics, can cause psoas bursitis. The FAIR manoeuvre can indicate towards a psoas bursitis or articular pathology if pain or an audible snap from the inguinal region is elicited.

Thomas test
Aim – To assess for fixed flexion deformity.

Patient's position – The patient lies supine, holding one knee flexed.

Clinician's position – The clinician slides their hand under the spine and assesses the curvature of the lumbar spine. A normal patient will exhibit a flat plane.

Clinical significance –
• **Negative test:** No flexion of the pelvis.
• **Positive test:** Increased lumbar lordosis. The hip cannot remain extended and straight, and starts to flex.

The test is positive if a **fixed flexion deformity** is present. A variety of pathologies can cause this, osteoarthritis being a common one.

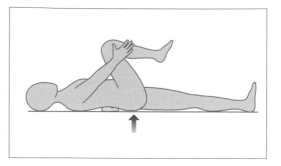

Management of hip fractures
There are some specific anatomical considerations to bear in mind when deciding how a hip fracture should be managed. The most important distinction is between intracapsular and extracapsular fractures (the numbers corresponding to the diagram below):
• **Intracapsular fractures** proximal to the capsular insertion:
  • (1) Subcapital
  • (2) Transcervical
• **Extracapsular fractures** (trochanteric and subtrochanteric – which can be further subdivided into undisplaced and displaced)
  • (3) Basicervical
  • (4) Intertrochanteric
  • (5) Subtrochanteric

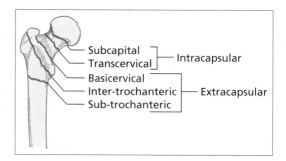

To understand the reasoning behind this, it is important to appreciate the blood supply of the hip. The femoral artery divides to form the medial and lateral circumflex arteries, which act as an arterial ring around the femoral neck. The posterior–superior retinacular arteries ascend from the arterial ring and ultimately form the lateral epiphyseal arteries. Thus, extracapsular fractures have a **decreased** risk of avascular necrosis due to the relatively extensive blood supply. In contrast, the more distal the fracture is, as with intracapsular fractures, the higher the risk of avascular necrosis – as the blood supply there is relatively limited.

Extracapsular fractures

A dynamic hip screw is implanted into the femoral head, and a plate is fixed to the shaft of the femur with further screws. The dynamic hip screw allows controlled sliding of the femoral head component along the construct.

Undisplaced intracapsular fracture

The approach is internal fixation with the insertion of parallel screws that course through the neck and into the head of the femur to hold it in position.

Displaced intracapsular fracture

• <65 years and active patients undergo an open reduction and internal fixation.
• >65 years and those with pre-existing joint pathology have a hemiarthroplasty (replacing the femoral head): Austin Moore prosthesis, which has three components:
  • Acetabular cup: cemented to the acetabulum.
  • A femoral component: stem and femoral head cemented/non-cemented to the shaft of the femur.
  • Articular interface: between the acetabular cup and the femoral component.

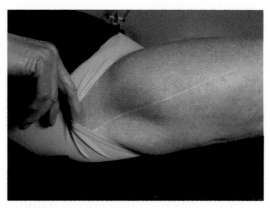

Figure 19.1 Total hip replacement

Questions you could be asked

Q. Describe the blood supply to the hip, and explain the implications for the management of a hip fracture.

Q. Explain the surgical management of a fracture of the neck of the femur.

A. The answers can be found in the text above.

20 Knee

Checklist	P	MP	F
HELP			
H: 'Hello' (introduction and gains consent)			
E: Exposure (patient should undress down to underwear, making sure the whole leg is exposed)			
L: Lighting			
P: Position correctly (supine), asks if patient is in any pain			
Washes hands			
Observation: • Paraphernalia: walking stick, joint support, wheelchair • Skin: colour, rash, bruising, scars • Joint: erythema, swelling • Muscle: wasting (measures quadriceps circumference) • Popliteal fossa: swelling, nodules • Posture: genu varus, genu valgus, flexion deformity, patellar alignment			
Palpation: • Temperature • Swellings • Muscle bulk around joint • Palpates medial joint line with knee flexed • Palpates lateral joint line with knee flexed • Palpates around borders of patella • Palpates patellotibial ligament and tibial tuberosity • Palpates in popliteal fossa for Baker's cyst • Palpates for joint effusion using patellar tap test or bulge test			
Movement: • Assesses degree of passive and active flexion possible • Assesses degree of passive and active extension possible • Assesses hyperextension • Assesses for pain and crepitus			

Special tests:
• Collateral ligaments:
  • Flexes knee approximately 30 degrees
  • Applies valgus strain to test for integrity of medial collateral ligament:
    • Technique: stabilises thigh just proximal to knee, holds lower leg with other hand just distal to knee, and moves medial aspect of lower leg laterally
    • Pain + movement indicates medial collateral ligament damage
  • Applies varus strain to test for integrity of lateral collateral ligament:
    • Technique: stabilises thigh just proximal to knee, holds lower leg with other hand just distal to knee, and moves lateral aspect of lower leg medially:
    • Pain + movement indicates lateral collateral ligament damage			

• Cruciate ligaments:
  • Inspects for posterior sag with knee flexed to 90 degrees
  • Performs anterior and posterior draw test to test anterior and posterior cruciate ligaments (respectively)
  • Technique:
    • Sits on patient's ipsilateral foot
    • Holds lower leg just distal to knee
    • Pulls lower leg forward: pain + movement indicates anterior cruciate ligament damage
    • Pushes lower leg backwards: pain + movement indicates posterior cruciate ligament damage			

- Menisci:
  - Performs McMurray's test *or* Apley's grinding test
  - Technique for Apley's grinding test:
    - Asks patient to lie on prone on their front
    - Flexes knee to 90 degrees
    - Stabilises upper leg with left hand
    - Holds lower foot with right hand
    - Pushes lower foot (and thereby tibia/fibula) down and rotates it in a 'grinding' manner
    - Pain indicates a positive test and possible meniscal injury

- Patellofemoral joint:
  - Tests for patellar apprehension
  - Technique:
    - Extends knee and pushes patella laterally
    - If patient is in pain or tries to flex the knee due to apprehensiveness, the test is positive, indicating an unstable patella and possible previous dislocations

Function:
- Comments on gait (ease of walking, speed of turn, antalgia)

Thanks patient
Offers to help patient get dressed
Washes hands
Offers to examine ankle (joint below) and hip (joint above)
Offers to examine neurovascular function of the lower limbs
Presents findings
Offers appropriate differential diagnosis
Offers appropriate investigations and management

OVERALL IMPRESSION:

Summary of common conditions seen in OSCEs

Disease	Look	Feel	Move	Special test	Function/gait	Examiner questions
Total knee replacement	Vertical scar over anterior aspect of knee	NAD	Active and passive flexion may or may not be limited	NAD	NAD	What are the indications for a total knee replacement?
Paget's disease	Varus deformity of knees. Beware of other bony lumps, particularly on femur, that may be an osteosarcoma	Warm overlying skin bilaterally	May be restricted flexion and extension and crepitus due to secondary osteoarthritis	NAD	NAD	What are the complications of Paget's disease? How is it diagnosed?
Baker's cyst	Swelling on medial side of popliteal fossa	Round, smooth, transilluminable mass	Foucher's sign is positive: knee extension tenses the swelling, flexion to 45 degrees causes disappearance or softening of the swelling	NAD	NAD, antalgic gait if severe	What are the important differential diagnoses of a Baker's cyst? How can a Baker's cyst present?
Osteoarthritis	Varus deformity. Fixed flexion. Swelling (without effusion). Wasted quadriceps	Crepitus. Joint line tenderness	Restricted flexion and extension. Locking	NAD	Antalgic gait	What are the indications for surgery in osteoarthritis of the knee?
Effusion in rheumatoid arthritis	Red, swollen, nodules on posterior aspect. Varus (most common), but can get valgus or fixed flexion deformities	Warm. Joint line tenderness. Wasted quadriceps	Limited flexion and extension	May experience pain but tests should be negative	Circumduction on affected side/ NAD	How should rheumatoid arthritis in the knee be managed?
Seronegative arthritis	Psoriatic plaques (anterior aspect of knee). Erythema nodosum (on shins). Question mark posture (associated with ankylosing spondylitis). Thin body habitus (if associated with inflammatory bowel disease)	Warm. Joint line tenderness	Painful/reduced ROM	May experience pain but tests should be negative	NAD/circumduction on affected side	What are the features of seronegative arthritides? What is the differential diagnosis in this case?
Meniscal lesions	Swollen knee	Effusion. Tender ipsilateral joint line	Decreased extension due to locking of knee	McMurray's or Apley's test	Knee gives way on turning	How can meniscal tears be treated?

Collateral ligament lesion	Swollen knee	Effusion Tender ipsilateral joint line	Pain on movement/NAD	Opening up of joint line (>5–10 degrees) on application of contralateral (varus/valgus) strain		What are the causes of collateral ligament injuries?
Torn cruciate ligament	Swollen knee	Effusion	NAD	Positive anterior draw test (if anterior ligament is torn); positive posterior draw test + posterior sag (if posterior ligament is torn)		How can torn cruciate ligaments be treated?
Osgood–Schlatter syndrome	Swollen tibial tubercle Adolescent/young adult patient	Pain/grimacing/ withdrawal on palpation of tibial tubercle	NAD	NAD	NAD	What advice do you want to give to this patient?
Recurrent dislocation of the patella	NAD	NAD	NAD	Patient grimaces/tenses muscles when patella is pushed laterally and knee is slowly flexed from full extension	NAD	What are the causes of recurrent dislocation of the patella? What is the management of recurrent dislocation of the patella?
Bursitis	Prepatellar: swelling over patella Infrapatellar: superficial swelling inferior to patella	Tenderness on palpation of swelling	NAD	NAD	NAD	What are the causes of bursitis? How can it be managed?
Fractured neck of femur (NB. This is a very easy scenario to simulate)	Affected leg appears shortened and is held in flexion (at hip and knee) and external rotation (at hip)	Poorly localised pain on palpation of knee	Poorly localised pain on movements of knee	Poorly localised pain on performing special tests	Unable to weight-bear on the affected side	What would you do next if you saw this patient in A&E?
Septic arthritis (NB. This is a very easy scenario to simulate)	The examiner may tell you to assume the joint is red and swollen	Tenderness on palpation of all areas of knee	Flexion and extension vastly restricted	Pain on performing special tests	Unable to weight-bear on affected side	What is your next step in management? What are the differential diagnoses? What investigation would you like to perform?

Hints and tips for the exam

Most students practise the knee examination thoroughly, especially the 'special tests', while preparing for finals. As important as these are, remember to stick to the 'look – feel – move – special-test – function' routine in order to look slick and avoid missing important signs of disease. Here are some tips to prevent you from committing some common errors.

One knee or both knees?

There is a lot to do in this station in the 5 or 10 minutes available. Candidates are often confused over whether they should examine one or both knees. If the instructions are not explicit, examine the knee that looks abnormal, or is said to be painful by the patient, and compare it with the other knee to interpret the findings from special tests. In the unlikely scenario that both knees appear normal, you must examine both knees fully and hence pace your work appropriately.

Don't inspect for too long

Do not spend too long looking at the knees. If they appear normal, say so and move on to avoid wasting time. Mention significant positive findings, but if time is short do not list all the negatives as there are unlikely to be many marks for doing this – and the examiner will probably ask you anything he or she deems important. If there is an obvious abnormality, state this at the start when presenting your findings. If this is not the case, follow the same routine that you used to examine when you are presenting your findings.

Joint line tenderness

Make sure you palpate the **medial and lateral joint lines one at a time** so that you can tell which side is causing pain. **Look at the patient's face** for grimacing.

Examining effusions

If there is a large effusion visible to the naked eye, perform the **patellar tap test**, and if there is no visible effusion perform the **bulge test**.

Assessing the menisci

Ask the examiner before performing McMurray's or Apley's test because many examiners will not want you to actually perform them on the patient and may instead ask you to talk through how you would perform them. **Apley's test is generally easier and quicker to do.**

Gait

If the patient is able to walk, make sure you **examine the gait**. Not only does this add valuable signs to your

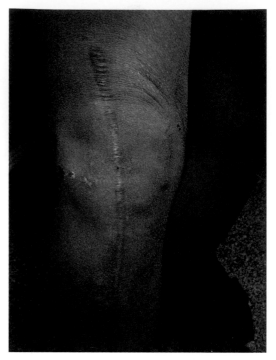

Figure 20.1 Total knee replacement

examination, but it also shows that you are thinking about the impact of the condition on the patient's **general functional ability**. Remember, an examination is *not* complete without eliciting the effect of the disease on the patient's functional ability.

Remember the joint above and the joint below

Do not forget to state that you would **finish by examining the hip and ankle joints** and the neurovascular function. Remember that hip fractures can sometimes present with knee pain.

Variations at this station

- **Task (7–10 minutes):** *'Perform a GALS screen of this patient's musculoskeletal system and then examine the knees.'* You should aim to spend no more than 2–3 minutes performing the GALS screen at this station.
- **Task (5–10 minutes):** *'This patient suffered an injury while playing football. Examine his knee and then give him some brief advice on management.'* This is the most difficult variation at this station. This type of scenario is frequently tested in finals OSCEs, and it is important to follow the generic structure:

• Confirmation of diagnosis (e.g. imaging)
• Conservative measures: **R**est, **I**ce, **C**ompression, **E**levation
• Medical measures: analgesia
• Physiotherapy
• Safety netting for complications
• Future prevention
• **Task (7–10 minutes):** *'This is a 19-year-old who recently sustained an injury playing football. Take a brief focused history and examine his knee.'* At this station, you must find out about the injury itself and how function has been limited after sustaining it. There are **three key questions** to ask in addition to this:
  • Did the knee swell up after the injury?
  • Does the knee give way when you try to turn?
  • Does the knee lock?

Questions you could be asked

Arthritis

Q. What are the indications for surgery in osteoarthritis of the knee?
A. Arthroscopy if there is knee locking, and knee replacement for refractory pain/stiffness.
Q. How should rheumatoid arthritis in the knee be managed?
A. Medical: analgesia, disease-modifying antirheumatic drugs, anti-tumour necrosis factor alpha inhibitors. Surgery is used with refractory pain/stiffness, or secondary septic arthritis.

Acutely swollen painful knee

Q. What would your next step be in the management of such a patient in A&E?
A. Admit and resuscitate the patient with respect to airway, breathing and circulation. Give empirical intravenous antibiotics (e.g. flucloxacillin or Augmentin), aspirate the joint and send the specimen for microscopy, culture and sensitivity and polarised light microscopy for crystals. Take a full history and examination to identify predisposing factors (e.g. intravenous drug use, diabetes, sickle cell disease).
Q. What are the differential diagnoses of an acutely swollen painful knee?
A. Septic arthritis, crystal arthropathy (gout or pseudogout), inflammatory disease (e.g. rheumatoid arthritis, systemic lupus erythematosus) and haemochromatosis.
Q. What investigations would you like to perform?
A. C-reactive protein level, blood culture, aspiration of the joint for microscopy, culture and sensitivity and microscopy under polarised light, and imaging (joint X-ray, MRI).

Knee fracture

Q. What would your initial management be if you saw a patient with a knee fracture in A&E?
A. • Resuscitate with respect to airway, breathing, circulation, and the examine the neurovascular status of the limb distal to the fracture.
  • Reduce the fracture under anaesthesia
  • Immobilise/restrict the fracture
  • Take a focused history to elucidate the impact of the injury, the possible underlying causes of the fall, co-morbidities and other injuries (especially head injury)
  • Request a specialist orthopaedic review
Q. What are the indications for a total knee replacement?
A. Osteoarthritis causing pain or stiffness that is refractory to medical treatment, rheumatoid arthritis with refractory joint pain, stiffness or deformity, and some cases of septic arthritis.

Patellar dislocation

Q. What are the causes of recurrent dislocation of the patella?
A. A 'high-riding' patella, joint hypermobility, family history, connective tissue disease.
Q. What is the management of recurrent dislocation of the patella?
A. Exclusion of a secondary cause (e.g. connective tissue disease) and vastus medialis strengthening exercises

Knee ligaments and menisci

Q. What are the causes of collateral ligament injuries?
A. Typically sport-related injuries, such as being tackled from the side, and also car accidents in which impact has been from the side – it is quite common to see torn lateral collateral ligaments together with a common peroneal nerve palsy.
Q. How are torn cruciate ligaments managed?
A. Arthroscopic reconstructive surgery with a prosthetic ligament. If the patient not fit for general anaesthesia, conservative management includes knee support and physiotherapy to strengthen the surrounding musculature.
Q. How can meniscal tears be treated?
A. Arthroscopic joint washout, meniscal repair, meniscectomy.

Osgood–Schlatter disease

Q. What advice do you give to a patient with Osgood–Schlatter disease?

A. Avoid painful activities such as running, squatting and jumping for up to 6 months. Analgesic medication can be used for symptom relief. Refer to physiotherapy for advice on quadriceps strengthening exercises.

Baker's cyst

Q. What are the important differential diagnoses of a ruptured Baker's cyst?

A. Deep venous thrombosis, cellulitis.

Q. How can a Baker's cyst present?

A. Popliteal fossa swelling, walking difficulty, swollen painful calf secondary to rupture.

Bursitis of the knee

Q. What are the causes of bursitis?

A. Trauma (e.g. housemaid's knee), infection, inflammatory disease (e.g. rheumatoid arthritis), idiopathic.

Q. How can it be managed?

A. Drainage of bursal fluid, treatment of the underlying cause (e.g. antibiotics, immunosuppressants), steroid injection

Paget's disease

Q. What are the complications of Paget's disease?

A. Deafness, high-output cardiac failure, osteosarcoma, pathological fractures, secondary osteoarthritis.

Q. How is it diagnosed?

A. Isolated raised alkaline phosphatase level (usually very high), characteristic radiological features.

21 Confirming death

Task (5 minutes): You are an FY1 attached to the care of the elderly firm. Sister Jones has just bleeped you regarding a terminally ill 85-year-old man who has become unresponsive and has stopped breathing. She thinks he has passed away and has asked you to come to the ward as soon as possible to confirm this and document it in the notes. Please demonstrate how you would confirm death on the manikin provided and complete the patient notes provided.

Checklist	P	MP	F
Introduces self to nurse			
Asks patient's details and whether death was expected			
Asks to see patient's notes			
Confirms patient is not for resuscitation			
Washes hands before entering room			
States intention to draw curtains/ensure privacy			
Confirms patient's identity from wristband			
Checks for a pacemaker			
Exposes patient adequately			
Attempts to elicit a response from the patient to voice and then deep stimulation			
States intention to observe for signs of life for 5 minutes from end of bed			
Palpates both carotid and femoral pulses for 1 minute to confirm absence of circulation			
States intention to auscultate for heart sounds at apex for 1 minute to confirm absence of cardiac output			
States intention to auscultate both lungs for 3 minutes to confirm absence of breath sounds			
Confirms both pupils are fixed in dilation when a light is shone into the eyes			
Confirms absence of corneal reflexes in both eyes			
States intention to visualise fundi using an ophthalmoscope to check for segmentation of retinal columns			
Covers patient up to neck and states intention to close patient's eyes			
Washes hands			
States intention to inform nurse that death can be confirmed			
States intention to make arrangements to inform next of kin			
Documents confirmation of death in the notes:			
• Date, time, name of nurse, patient's resuscitation status			
• Comments on responsiveness to voice and deep stimulation			
• Comments on signs of life after 5 minutes of observation			
• Comments on central pulses and heart sounds			
• Comments on breath sounds			
• Comments on pupils, corneal reflexes and fundi			
• States date and time that death was confirmed			
• Prints name and signs notes			
Documentation is organised and clearly legible			

Hints and tips for the exam

Confirming death is a very commonly tested OSCE station in finals. You are very unlikely to get any opportunities to practise this during clinical attachments, so it is important to practise it several times within your study groups before the OSCE.

There are several 'easy' marks to be picked up in this station so do *not* forget to pick up these up by performing simple steps such as washing your hands at the start and the end, checking the patient's identity, exposing and covering the manikin fully when appropriate and documenting your findings in the notes appropriately.

Although it may feel slightly odd, remember to treat the manikin with respect as if it were a real patient. Do *not* make the mistake of asking the 'dead' manikin for consent to perform the examination as many candidates do in the heat of the moment!

Potential variations at this station

• Confirming death on a manikin and filling out a death certificate using the information provided. This may be a 5-minute station or a 10-minute station. (NB. This station is covered separately in Chapter 70.)

• Confirming death on a manikin and answering questions on criteria for referral to the coroner.

Part 2: Histories

Top tips

Do:

• **Use SOCRATES to explore any symptom (SOCRATES = site, onset, character, radiation, associated symptoms, timing, exacerbating factors, severity):** Although this is generally used for pain, it can be used as a basis for any symptom. For example, if you are taking a history of shortness of breath, site and radiation are clearly irrelevant – but onset, alleviating/exacerbating factors, severity and character are decisively important.

• **Know your 'red flags':** In 5 or 10 minutes, it may be difficult to cover every single aspect that could possibly have even a vague relevance. This is why it is important to be as focused as possible, and to rule out serious and life-threatening problems as soon as possible – especially if you are running out of time. The key to this is to rule out 'red flag' symptoms that signify diagnoses such as cancer and other serious pathologies. Different parts of the body have different 'red flags', but in general the following symptoms are generic for all systems:

  • Weight loss
  • Loss of appetite
  • Bleeding (this applies to bleeding from virtually any part of the body, depending on the history – rectal bleeding or melaena, haematuria, vaginal bleeding, haematemesis, haemoptysis and even unexplained skin bruising)
  • Night sweats

• **Take a thorough social history:** This is important and there are lots of easy marks for it. Remember that social histories are not only about smoking and alcohol – make sure you explore the points listed below. Also find out about how the patients symptoms **affect** the patient's life.

  • Activities of daily living (ADLs): An easy way to remember the ADLs is to work through the normal activities that most people do when they wake up:

    • Get out of bed (transfer)
    • Walk to the bathroom (mobility → walking aids)
    • Use the toilet (continence → urinary and faecal)
    • Brush the teeth, wash the face (personal hygiene)
    • Use the stairs
    • Cook meals
    • Eat meals (does the patient need help with feeding?)
    • Shop
  • Work/occupation
    • Job
    • What the job involves
    • Whether the patient travels to work
  • Social activities: hobbies, meeting other people
  • Driving: the DVLA ordains driving restrictions for various conditions, such as strokes, heart attacks and epilepsy
  • Travel: this could be prove to be a 'clincher', for example for pulmonary embolism, tuberculosis, malaria or viral hepatitis

• **ICE – ideas, concerns, expectations:** Although these are not as important as they are for the communication skills stations, they usually carry significant marks even for the basic history stations.

• **Listen carefully:** Demonstrate this actively using **non-verbal skills** – nod, say 'yuh', or whatever feels comfortable and appropriate. It is vital that the patient feels you are listening and feels encouraged to give you the information you need – and it will also get you valuable marks.

• **Summarise:** There is often a specific mark for this, and it is also an excellent way for you to organise your own thoughts and identify anything you may have missed.

• **Be specific and think before you speak:** This may sound too obvious to mention, but it is always disappointing to hear candidates take excellent histories and ruin it by making silly mistakes with their words. For example, we have often heard candidates use IBS and

OSCEs for Medical Finals, First Edition. Hamed Khan, Iqbal Khan, Akhil Gupta, Nazmul Hussain, and Sathiji Nageshwaran.
© 2013 John Wiley & Sons, Ltd. Published 2013 by John Wiley & Sons, Ltd.

IBD interchangeably, despite these being fundamentally different conditions.

- **Practise reading the instructions:** Nervousness, anxiety and a rush to get cracking within the limited time may cause even the best candidate to miss the instructions and jump straight into the scenario. So when you are practising histories, make sure that whoever is assessing you gives you instructions so that you can practise the process of reading and absorbing them.
- **Practice with different colleagues:** Try to practise with different people as different actor-patients will have different ways of presenting their histories, which may make eliciting the history easier or more difficult in different ways.
- **Women's health is different from men's health:** Remember to ask about **periods** in all women with any systemic conditions. Various endocrinological, haematological and inflammatory problems can cause a change in the menstrual cycle.
- **Start with open questions, and then move on to closed specific questions:** Demonstrating your ability to utilise both types of question is important. There are usually marks for this, and they are easy to gain, so don't miss them.
- **Remember the obvious – introduce yourself properly and get consent:** Yes, it is obvious, but as examiners we have seen finalists say 'Hello' in the most pleasant manner and tell the patient that they will be taking a history. There will always be a significant number of marks for a proper introduction. This includes the following:
  - Tell the patient your name
  - Confirm the patient's name
  - Tell the patient who you are (medical student, FY2, consultant, professor!)
  - Explain what you **would like** to do (i.e. take a history)
  - Ask the patient if they are happy for you to do this
  - Ask the patient an open question (e.g. what brings you here today?)
- **Define smoking in pack–years:** This will impress the examiner. Twenty cigarettes per day for 1 year is a pack year. You can use this to calculate how many pack–years the patient's smoking history represents:
  - 20 cigarettes per day for 1 year = 1 pack–year
  - 40 cigarettes per day for 10 years = 20 pack–years
  - 10 cigarettes per day for 3 years = 1.5 pack–years
- **Know your alcohol units:** 1 unit = 8 g of pure alcohol, which is equivalent to:

- Half a pint of standard beer or lager
- Half a glass of wine
- One standard measure of spirit or sherry

Don't:
- **Don't ask leading questions:** It is important not to direct the patient towards a certain line of history or a certain diagnosis. It could push you towards the wrong diagnosis, and separately to that there will often be marks for using a line of enquiry that does not involve leading questions.
- **Don't use medical jargon:** As a student, it is terribly embarrassing when a patient asks you what you mean by 'myocardial infarction'. More importantly, you will almost definitely lose marks for doing this.
- **Don't ignore the patient's concerns:** As important as it is, it is not enough merely to elicit patients' ideas, concerns and expectations. It is absolutely imperative that you also act on them, or at least acknowledge and react to them. Ignoring them and carrying on as if the patient never said anything will lose you marks.
- **Don't ignore cues:** see the Top Tips for the communication skills station.

Generic points for all history stations

Appropriate introduction
Confirms patient's name
Explains reason for consultation
Obtains consent
Establishes rapport
Open question to elicit presenting complaint
History of presenting complaint
Past medical history
Family history
Drug history
Allergies
Social history
'Red flags'
Review of systems
Systematic approach
Explores and responds to ICE
Shows empathy
Non-verbal skills
Avoids technical jargon
Devises holistic management plan and addresses psychosocial issues as well as medical problems
Summarises
Offers to answer any questions
Thanks patient

22 General lethargy and tiredness

Checklist	P	MP	F
Appropriate introduction			
Confirms patient's name and age			
Explains reason for consultation			
Obtains consent			
Open question to elicit presenting complaint			
Allows patient to open up, listens carefully, remains silent and does not interrupt the patient			
Signposts: e.g. 'Mr Gregory, thank you for telling me about this problem. I would like to ask a few more detailed questions. Is that all right?'			
History of presenting complaint:			
• Onset (how it started) • Character (what the patient means by tiredness) • Time (duration) • Alleviating factors • Exacerbating factors • Severity (in comparison with other episodes of tiredness) • Asks if there is a pattern with activities/daily routine • Asks about menstrual disturbances (if patient female) • Establishes sleep pattern • Asks if patient is suffering from any other symptoms • Asks about any recent illnesses • Previous episodes of lethargy/tiredness			
Depression screening: asks about mood, previous history of depression and sleeping patterns			
Asks closed focused questions to rule out specific common causes of lethargy:			
• Thyroid dysfunction (sweating, tremor, dry hair, neck discomfort, eye symptoms, bowel changes, menstrual irregularities) • Anaemia (shortness of breath, chest pain, palpitations, menorrhagia) • Diabetes mellitus (polydipsia, polyuria, recurrent infection) • Cancer (weight loss, night sweats, family history of cancers, cough, diarrhoea, melaena) • Hypopituitarism (loss of appetite, nipple discharge, loss of libido) • Chronic kidney disease/nephrotic syndrome (ankle swelling, orthopnoea) • Chronic infection (fevers) • Chronic fatigue syndrome symptoms (sore throat, headaches, muscle pains, exacerbated by exertion) • Obstructive sleep apnoea (unrefreshing sleep, feeling sleepy in the day, loud snoring, waking up suddenly in the night, loss of libido, irritability) • Depression (mood, anhedonia, sleep, appetite, concentration)			
Review of systems			
'Red flags': • Night sweats • Fevers • Weight loss • Loss of appetite • Palpable lymph nodes			
Past medical history			
Family history: • Cancers • Endocrine disorders, especially thyroid disorders and diabetes • Depression			
Drug history: • Over-the-counter medication			

Allergies			
Social history: • Smoking • Alcohol • Illicit drug use • Stressors in social life (relationship, financial, etc.) • Change in work/occupation • Symptoms of depression or anxiety • Recent foreign travel			
Use of non-verbal cues, e.g. good eye contact, nodding head and good body posture			
Systematic approach			

Explores and responds to ICE: • Ideas • Concerns • Expectations			
Shows empathy			
Non-verbal skills			
Avoids technical jargon			
Devises holistic management plan and addresses psychosocial issues as well as medical problems			
Summarises			
Offers to answer any questions			
Thanks patient			

Summary of common conditions seen in OSCEs

System	Conditions
Cardiovascular	Heart failure
	Infective endocarditis
Respiratory	Lung cancer
	Tuberculosis
	Obstructive sleep apnoea
Gastrointestinal	Bowel cancer
	Coeliac disease
Liver	Viral hepatitis
	Chronic liver disease
Neurological	Myasthenia gravis
	Motor neurone disease
Endocrine	Hypothyroidism Hypopituitarism
	Addison's disease
	Pituitary adenoma
	Diabetes
Renal	Chronic kidney disease
Rheumatological	Rheumatoid arthritis
	SLE
Haematological	Anaemia from any cause
	Leukaemia/lymphoma
Genitourinary	HIV
	Sexually transmitted disease
Urological	Prostate cancer
	Bladder cancer
Gynaecological	Menorrhagia
Psychiatric	Depression
Others	Chronic fatigue syndrome
	Poor sleep hygiene
	Illicit drug use
	Benzodiazepine overuse
	Crash dieting

Hints and tips for the exam

Like weight loss, tiredness is a common non-specific symptom. GPs see several patients every day who complain of feeling tired without any other specific symptoms. There is a vast array of potential underlying causes ranging from the most serious, such as underlying malignancies, to absolutely nothing.

Like the weight loss station, this station is in many ways a vast 'review of systems' where you have to work through most of the systems and narrow down the potential causes to one of them. The most important thing is to confirm or rule out potentially serious causes, such as diabetes and cancer. **Weight loss** is a symptom that should start ringing alarm bells.

Don't forget depression and psychiatric causes

Many students forget that generalised lethargy is a common symptom of depression. The NICE guidelines (2009) suggest using the following two questions to screen for depression:

During the last month, have you often been bothered by:
• Feeling down, depressed or hopeless?
• Having little interest or pleasure in doing things?

If the patient answers yes to either of these, carry out a full assessment for depression.

Basic initial investigations for fatigue

If you have absolutely no idea about the cause of the underlying fatigue, tell the examiner that you would like to do a full systemic examination and the following investigations. They are relatively quick and non-invasive, and you could decide how to proceed after you get the results.

Blood tests

• Full blood count: anaemia, raised white cell count, abnormal white cell differential
• ESR:
  • A raised ESR could indicate an inflammatory/rheumatological aetiology
  • >100 mm/hour indicates serious causes such as malignancies, sepsis, tuberculosis, polymyalgia rheumatica/giant cell arteritis or myeloma
• Us+Es:
  • Hyponatraemia (Addison's disease)
  • Chronic kidney disease/any renal impairment
• Liver function tests: Liver or bone problems (alkaline phosphatase for bone)
• Bone profile:
  • Hypercalcaemia: This causes lethargy in itself, but more importantly it may result from ectopic parathyroid secretion from a malignancy, or a myeloma
  • Hypocalcaemia may result from malabsorption, for example due to coeliac disease
• Fasting blood glucose: for diabetes mellitus
• Thyroid function tests: hypothyroidism
• Ferritin, vitamin B12 and folate levels:
  • Dietary deficiencies, which are not uncommon in the elderly
  • Pernicious anaemia
  • A low ferritin level with a microcytic anaemia, which needs further investigation to rule out a gastrointestinal malignancy
  • Malabsorption
• Brain natriuretic hormone: for heart failure

Imaging

• Chest X-ray:
  • Lung cancer, especially if the patient is a smoker
  • Cardiomegaly in heart failure
  • Tuberculosis

Urine

• Urine dipstick:
  • Blood: bladder cancer, glomerulonephritis, infective endocarditis
  • Protein: renal impairment, nephrotic syndrome, glomerulonephritis
  • Nitrites: urinary tract infection – chronic urinary tract infections can cause general chronic lethargy in the elderly
  • Glucose: diabetes

Other

• Epstein–Barr virus/Monospot: for glandular fever

Questions you may be asked

Q. What is the key diagnostic investigation for chronic fatigue syndrome?
A. None – it's a clinical diagnosis. The most important thing is to rule out any other diagnosis.

Reference

National Institute for Health and Clinical Excellence (2009) Depression: treatment and management of depression in adults, including adults with a chronic physical health problem. Available from: www.nice.org.uk/nicemedia/live/12329/45890/45890.pdf (accessed June 2010).

23 Weight loss

Checklist	P	MP	F
Appropriate introduction			
Confirms patient's name and age			
Explains reason for consultation			
Obtains consent			
Open question to elicit presenting complaint			
Allows patient to open up, listens carefully, remains silent and does not interrupt the patient			
Signposts: e.g. 'Mr Smith, thank you for telling me about this problem. I would like to ask a few more detailed questions. Is that all right?'			
History of presenting complaint:			
• Onset (how it started) • Time (duration – over what length of period did the patient lose weight, or if it was a brief transient phase) • Severity – quantifies weight loss, either in kilograms/pounds or waist circumference • Asks if anybody else around the patient (family, work colleagues, friends) has noticed the loss of weight • Asks if patient intended to lose weight (e.g. exercise regime) • Establishes patient's appetite and eating habits • Establishes whether there has been any change in the patient's activity levels (e.g. has he or she started walking to work or taken up a new exercise regime?) • Asks about menstrual disturbances (if the patient is female) • Asks if patient is suffering from any other symptoms • Asks about any recent illnesses • Previous episodes of weight loss			

Psychiatric disorder screening:
 • Depression screening: asks about mood, previous history of depression and sleeping patterns
 • Eating disorder screening:
   • **S**ick (has the patient been vomiting?)
   • **C** = lost **c**ontrol = does the patient feel as if they have lost control over their eating habits?
   • **O**ne stone weight loss in last 3 months?
   • **F** = does the patient feel **f**at?
   • **F**= does the patient spend a lot of time thinking about **f**ood?
 • Needs further investigation if two or more of the five criteria are positive			

Asks closed focused questions to rule out specific common causes of weight loss:			
• Hyperthyroidism (sweating, tremor, neck discomfort, eye symptoms, bowel changes, menstrual irregularities) • Diabetes mellitus (polydipsia, polyuria, recurrent infection) • Addison's disease (tiredness, pigmentation, faintness) • Cancer (weight loss, night sweats, family history of cancers, cough/haemoptysis if smoker, diarrhoea/melaena if suspecting bowel cancer) • Chronic infection (fevers) • Laxative abuse/overuse			
'Red flags': • Night sweats • Fevers • Palpable lymph nodes • Symptoms of cancer (as above)			
Past medical history			

Family history: • Cancers • Endocrine disorders, especially thyroid disorders and diabetes • Bowel disorders			
Drug history : • Over-the-counter medication			
Allergies			
Social history: • Smoking • Alcohol • Illicit drug use • Stressors in social life (relationship, financial, etc.) • Change in work/occupation • Symptoms of depression • Recent foreign travel			
Review of systems			
Use of non-verbal cues, e.g. good eye contact, nodding head and good body posture			

Systematic approach			
Explores and responds to ICE: • Ideas • Concerns • Expectations			
Shows empathy			
Non-verbal skills			
Avoids technical jargon			
Devises holistic management plan and addresses psychosocial issues as well as medical problems			
Summarises			
Offers to answer any questions			
Thanks patient			

Summary of common conditions seen in OSCEs

System	Conditions
Respiratory	Lung cancer
	Tuberculosis
Gastrointestinal	Bowel cancer
	Coeliac disease
	Irritable bowel disease
Liver	Viral hepatitis
	Chronic liver disease
Neurological	Motor neurone disease
Endocrine	Hyperthyroidism
	Addison's disease
	Diabetes
Renal	Chronic kidney disease
Haematological	Leukaemia/lymphoma
	Multiple myeloma
Genitourinary	HIV
Urological	Prostate cancer
	Bladder cancer
Gynaecological	Ovarian cancer
Psychiatric	Eating disorder/anorexia
	Depression
Others	Exercise!
	Secondary metastatic cancer

Hints and tips for the exam

Weight loss should always ring alarm bells, so its vital – both for OSCEs and in clinical practice – to find the cause and deal with it swiftly.

Go through the systems

The weight loss station is fundamentally an extensive, thorough review of systems, with a specific focus on certain areas. So it is vital that you go through each of the systems and associated symptoms.

Energy in: dietary history

Although most candidates will take a thorough history to rule out important organic causes, most do not appreciate delving into the details of the patient's daily food intake. A change of job, house or other circumstances may result in a marked change in the patient's eating habits. For example, if the patient used to have a regular high-calorie meal that they now miss out, it is likely that there would be a significant weight loss resulting from this. However, such a weight loss should not persist.

Energy out: exercise

Find out whether the patient has started a new exercise regime, or if their work or leisure pursuits now require much more physical activity than before.

Don't forget possible psychiatric causes of weight loss

Many students will have had their psychiatry modules in the fourth year of their course, and finals will be largely based around medicine and surgery. However, the odd station might still have a psychiatric slant to it, and 'weight loss' is perfect for this. It is one of the key 'biological symptoms' of depression, and is naturally a result of eating disorders such as anorexia nervosa and bulimia. So make sure you ask about mood and anhedonia, and that you go through the 'SCOFF' questions listed in the checklist. The SCOFF questionnaire was published in the *BMJ* in 1999 after being devised by Dr John Morgan, a research fellow in psychiatry in the UK at the time it was published.

Questions you may be asked

Q. What questions would you ask to assess the possibility of eating disorders in a patient?

Q. What psychiatric disorders could lead to weight loss?

A. Answers to both these questions are given in the text above.

24 Chest pain

Checklist	P	MP	F
Appropriate introduction			
Confirms patient's name and age			
Explains reason for consultation			
Obtains consent			
Open question to elicit presenting complaint			
Allows patient to open up, listens carefully, remains silent and does not interrupt the patient			
Signposts: e.g. 'Mr Gregory, thank you for telling me about this problem. I would like to ask a few more detailed questions. Is that all right?'			
History of presenting complaint			
Elicits further details of chest pain: • Site • Onset: retrosternal • Character: burning, crushing, stabbing • Radiation: jaw, left arm and back (myocardial infarction), back (dissection) • Associated symptoms: asks specifically about nausea, sweating, light-headedness/loss of consciousness, shortness of breath, palpitations, fever, cough, heartburn, abdominal pain • Exacerbating factors: inspiration, lying down, coughing, physical activity • Alleviating factors: stopping physical activity, sitting up, drugs (e.g. GTN) • Time course: changes in the pain between onset and now • Severity • Asks if patient is suffering from any other symptoms • Asks about any recent illnesses • Previous episodes of chest pain			
Elicits cardiac risk factors: • Family history of myocardial infarction in first-degree relative <55 years of age • Smoking • Hypertension • Diabetes mellitus • Hyperlipidaemia			

Checklist	P	MP	F
Elicits risk factors for pulmonary embolism/deep venous thrombosis: • Calf pain/swelling • Recent travel • Recent surgery • Family history of clotting disorders • Malignancy • Oral contraceptive pill (if female patient) • Pregnancy (if female patient)			
Review of systems			
Past medical history • Myocardial infarction, angina, other heart disease • Stroke, peripheral vascular disease • Asthma, COPD • Diabetes mellitus • Lung cancer			
Family history: • Cardiac disease • Pulmonary embolism • Asthma • Lung cancer • Sudden death			
Drug history			
Allergies			
Social history • Alcohol • Smoking • Occupation • Diet and lifestyle			
Use of non-verbal cues, e.g. good eye contact, nodding head and good body posture			
Systematic approach			
Explores and responds to ICE: • Ideas • Concerns • Expectations			
Shows empathy			

Non-verbal skills				Summarises			
Avoids technical jargon				Offers to answer any questions			
Devises holistic management plan and addresses psychosocial issues as well as medical problems				Thanks patient			

Summary of common conditions seen in OSCEs

	'Red flags'	Common errors
Acute coronary syndrome (ACS)	Past medical history of ACS Central crushing pain Radiation to left arm and/or jaw Not relieved by GTN spray in a known angina sufferer	Mistaking pain from an aortic dissection for an ACS. The management of aortic dissection and ACS are completely different so it is imperative to be sure what you are dealing with before implementing a management plan. Thrombolysing a dissecting aneurysm will result in death, so if unsure mention that you would do a CT scan to rule out dissection
Aortic dissection	Tearing central pain of sudden onset radiating to the back Past medical history of hypertension Past medical history and/or family history of connective tissue disease, e.g. Marfan syndrome	
Pneumothorax	Young male typically in teens or twenties Sudden onset Associated with shortness of breath	
Pulmonary embolism	Positive risk factors Past medical history of pulmonary embolism Family history of thrombophilia Pain increased by inspiration Associated with red, swollen, painful leg	Assuming that pulmonary embolism has been ruled out if there are no symptoms of a deep vein thrombosis (DVT). Remember that a significant proportion of DVTs are initially asymptomatic or cause only mild discomfort, and most pulmonary embolisms occur without clinical evidence of a DVT
Pneumonia	Cough productive of green/blood-stained phlegm Recent upper respiratory tract infection	Chest pain alone is an uncommon presenting symptom of pneumonia so ensure you have ruled out all the other causes listed in this table before diagnosing this
Pericarditis	Pain improved by sitting forward Fever or recent viral illness Recent myocardial infarction (associated with Dressler's syndrome) Past medical history of rheumatoid arthritis, SLE, sarcoid or radiotherapy	Any of the 'red flags' may be 'red herrings' so it is important to take a thorough history to rule out ACS and other diagnoses even if pericarditis is strongly suspected from the history
Peptic ulcer disease or gastritis	Associated symptoms include dysphagia, acid reflux, weight loss and melaena Drug history includes NSAIDs, steroids or any other drugs that predispose to peptic ulcer disease Location of pain is epigastric with retrosternal radiation	About 1 in 10 patients diagnosed with 'gastritis' in A&E actually have inferior myocardial infarction, so even if gastritis is strongly suspected from the history, you must do an ECG to rule out inferior myocardial infarction
Ruptured oesophagus	Upper gastrointestinal endoscopy in the last 48 hours Violent vomiting, e.g. after an alcohol binge	Recent endoscopy could be a 'red herring' so rule out other causes before settling on this rare condition
Costochondritis	Point tenderness when asked about site of pain	Settling with these diagnoses without ruling out life-threatening differential diagnoses through appropriate questioning
Shingles	Associated with rash Pain radiating out across chest in a dermatomal distribution Pain made worse by contact with clothing	

Hints and tips for the exam

History of chest pain is an examiner's favourite because it is a common presenting complaint, there are a wide range of differential diagnoses and it should have been practised by students on numerous occasions on clinical attachments. But beware – this is not an easy station because forgetting to ask the key questions (as candidates often do) will be deemed unsafe and can prevent you passing. The essentials to pass this station and common pitfalls to avoid are as follows.

Key points to demonstrate safety

• You MUST ask questions to **rule out ALL the potentially life-threatening causes** of chest pain even if you have a good idea of what the diagnosis is after your first question.
• Establish **risk factors** for ischaemic heart disease. These are listed on the mark sheet but don't forget that the name and age of the patient can provide valuable information. Age >55 years and being of South-Asian origin substantially increases the risk of ischaemic heart disease.
• **Beware of red herrings.** A flu-like illness 3 weeks previously does not necessarily mean that a patient is suffering from pericarditis. You must rule out other causes.
• If asked about management, remember the importance of resuscitating the patient with respect to **airway, breathing and circulation** before implementing more complex management plans aimed at correcting the underlying cause of the chest pain.
• When eliciting the past medical history, beware of conditions that may **contraindicate the use of certain drugs.** For example, a patient with myocardial infarction and a past medical history of cerebral neoplasm

cannot be treated with thrombolytic drugs. Such knowledge will be expected from candidates to be considered for merits.

Key points to demonstrate good communication skills

• Start with an **open question** such as 'How can I help you?' even if an acute situation is being simulated. Allowing the actor-patient to express themselves initially will usually give you a good indication of the diagnosis. Closed questions can subsequently be used to rule out each of the other potentially life-threatening conditions and their risk factors.
• Do not forget to ask the actor-patients about their **main concerns**. You will typically be asked what you think is causing the chest pain, or what will happen next. It is important to use phrases that demonstrate empathy, but you must NOT provide false reassurance that everything is fine if you are suspecting a serious diagnosis – this could result in a fail.
• Do NOT miss out on opportunities to **demonstrate empathy**. Actor-patients often give cues such as mentioning bereavement during the family history. It is a good idea to briefly express commiseration by saying 'I'm sorry to hear that' before moving on.

Questions you may be asked

Q. If you were an FY1 doctor in A+E, how would you hand this patient with central crushing chest pain over to the cardiology team?
A. See Chapter 56 on the handover.
Q. Take a history of this patient presenting with chest pain and interpret the ECG shown to you by the examiner.
A. The answer to this obviously depends on the specific case.

25 Palpitations

Checklist	P	MP	F
Appropriate introduction			
Confirms patient's name and age			
Explains reason for consultation			
Obtains consent			
Open question to elicit presenting complaint			
Allows patient to open up, listens carefully, remains silent and does not interrupt the patient			
Signposts: e.g. 'Mr Gregory, thank you for telling me about this problem. I would like to ask a few more detailed questions. Is that all right?'			
History of presenting complaint:			

• Duration of episode(s)
• Frequency (if more than one episode)
• Precipitants and relieving factors
  • Asks about activities before onset
  • Asks about intake of caffeine and alcohol
  • Asks about learned methods of termination
• Rhythm of palpitations (regular, irregular)			

Associated symptoms: • Chest pain, shortness of breath • Loss of consciousness • Symptoms of hypoglycaemia: jitteriness, hunger, sweating, on insulin • Symptoms of anxiety: anxiety, tingling, headaches, nausea • Symptoms of hyperthyroidism: weight loss, diarrhoea, eye symptoms, agitation, sweating • Symptoms of the menopause: last menstrual period, vaginal dryness, mood changes			
Establishes cardiovascular risk factors: • Smoking • Diabetes mellitus • Hyperlipidaemia • Hypertension • Family history of premature cardiac disease			
Review of symptoms			

Checklist	P	MP	F
Past medical history: • Cardiac disease, multiple sclerosis • Thyroid disease/surgery • Anxiety disorders • Diabetes mellitus			
Establishes family history: • Cardiac disease • Thyroid disease • Sudden death • Arrhythmias			
Drug history: • Salbutamol • Over-the-counter medication			
Social history: • Smoking • Alcohol intake • Illicit drug use • Occupation • Stress levels • Exercise • Impact of symptoms on patient's lifestyle			
Use of non-verbal cues, e.g. good eye contact, nodding head and good body posture			
Systematic approach			
Explores and responds to ICE: • Ideas • Concerns • Expectations			
Shows empathy			
Non-verbal skills			
Avoids technical jargon			
Devises holistic management plan and addresses psychosocial issues as well as medical problems			
Summarises			
Offers to answer any questions			
Thanks patient			

Summary of common conditions seen in OSCEs

Condition	Key points in history	Key points in management
Atrial fibrillation	Elderly patient Past medical history of ischaemic heart disease, hypertension, congestive heart failure, mitral valve disease Recent onset coinciding with symptoms suggestive of lower respiratory tract infection	See Chapter 65 on ECGs
Supraventricular tachycardia	Past medical history of COPD (predisposes to multifocal atrial tachycardia) Associated with symptoms of compromise, e.g. chest pain, shortness of breath, pre-syncope Previous episodes terminated by vagal manoeuvres, e.g. blowing the nose	See Chapter 65 on ECGs
Ventricular tachycardia	Symptoms of compromise, e.g. chest pain, shortness of breath, pre-syncope, cold peripheries, sweating History of recent myocardial infarction Past medical history of ischaemic heart disease Family history of sudden death, known long QT syndrome	See Chapter 65 on ECGs
Thyrotoxicosis (causing sinus tachycardia or atrial fibrillation)	Weight loss, increased appetite, heat intolerance, diarrhoea, tremor, mood disturbance Past medical history of thyroid disease Past medical history of other autoimmune disease (insulin-dependent diabetes mellitus, vitiligo, Addison's disease, pernicious anaemia, etc.)	Follow protocol for atrial fibrillation Medical/surgical correction of thyrotoxicosis
Hypertrophic obstructive cardiomyopathy (HOCM)	Family history of sudden death Collapse while playing sport family history of HOCM	Amiodarone Anticoagulate if paroxysmal atrial fibrillation Implantable defibrillator Septal myomectomy
Excess caffeine intake	History of excessive caffeine intake (definition of 'excessive' varies from patient to patient) No symptoms suggesting compromise Palpitations self-limiting Past medical history of cardiac or thyroid disease	Decrease caffeine intake Rule out cardiac and thyroid-related causes
Phaeochromocytoma	Triad of episodic headache, sweating, fast palpitations Weight loss Symptoms of anxiety NB. This **must** be ruled out before ascribing symptoms to generalised anxiety disorder	Urgent referral to endocrine surgeons Investigate for multiple endocrine neoplasia type 2, neurofibromatosis, von Hippel–Lindau syndrome

(Continued)

Condition	Key points in history	Key points in management
Simple anxiety	Associated with important/stressful event No symptoms of compromise No history of cardiac or thyroid disease	Reassurance Behavioural therapy/cognitive-behavioural therapy Beta-blockers if severe symptoms
Fever	Localising symptoms of infection (e.g. cough, earache) First episode or episodes only coincide with febrile illness	Antipyrexial medication (e.g. paracetamol)
Generalised anxiety disorder	Associated with important/stressful event No symptoms of compromise No history of cardiac or thyroid disease Past medical history of depression Avoidance of predisposing situations	Referral to psychiatry Beta-blockers for symptom control
Ventricular ectopics	Recent myocardial infarction Past medical history of ischaemic heart disease Description of missed beat followed by heavier beat	Usually no treatment required if asymptomatic and infrequent Amiodarone if >10/min or symptomatic
Pacemaker failure	Past medical history of pacemaker insertion	Replacement/repair of pacemaker
Hypoglycaemia	Associated with sweating, anxiety, hunger, tremor, dizziness Past medical history of diabetes mellitus Drug history of hypoglycaemic medication (**not** metformin) History of liver disease, Addison's disease	Oral sugar followed by slow-release carbohydrate Intravenous dextrose (if unable to swallow)

Relevant investigations you may need to discuss at this station

Investigation	Justification
ECG	Instant detection of underlying rhythm
	Detection of long QT syndrome
Full blood count	Anaemia precipitates palpitations
	High white cell count suggests infection
Thyroid function tests	Diagnosis of thyrotoxicosis
Blood glucose	Diagnosis of hypoglycaemia
	Risk assessment for cardiovascular disease
Us+Es	Hypokalaemia/hyperkalaemia can cause fatal arrhythmias
Mg and Ca	Low levels of Ca and Mg predispose to long QT syndrome and therefore polymorphic ventricular tachycardia
24-hour ECG monitoring	Identification of paroxysmal arrhythmias
Echo	Identification of structural heart disease, e.g. HOCM or mitral stenosis, that may predispose to arrhythmias
Exercise ECG	Detection of arrhythmias precipitated by ischaemic heart disease

Hints and tips for the exam

Palpitations are an extremely common complaint in general practice and A&E settings so this is a popular station in the OSCE exam. The underlying causes range from being benign (e.g. anxiety prior to an OSCE) to being potentially catastrophic (e.g. paroxysmal ventricular tachycardia after a myocardial infarction). This can make the task of taking a history in 5 minutes challenging. However, your task will be made easier if you remember the following six tips:

• The importance of **starting with an open question** to get the patient talking cannot be stressed enough. The information from this alone will often go a long way towards formulating a differential diagnosis to guide further history-taking BUT . . .
• **You MUST enquire about the following 'red flag' symptoms in order to pass:**
  • Past medical history of cardiac disease
  • Family history of sudden death, cardiac disease or arrhythmias
  • Loss of consciousness, shortness of breath
  • Weight loss

Even if you are reasonably sure that the cause is benign, it is imperative to ask questions that may implicate serious pathology.
• Be careful about diagnosing 'panic attacks' when questioned by the examiner at the end. Remember that **organic causes must be ruled out before any psychiatric/psychological cause is ascribed**. Panic attacks can be caused by phaeochromocytoma and hyperthyroidism, so mention that you would like to test for this before instigating management for the panic attacks.
• **Beware of 'red herrings'** – just because a patient drinks 'a lot' of coffee, it does not necessarily mean it is the cause of the palpitations.
• **A detailed social history is key**. Remember that the actor is unlikely to offer information about stress levels, alcohol/illicit substance use and the impact on their lifestyle unless you ask in a sensitive manner. **Do NOT hurry the actor** if he or she appears to be going into 'unnecessary' detail – it is probably important.
• **Address the patient's concerns appropriately**. For example, if the patient is worried that they may be suffering from ischaemic heart disease (because a close family member suffered from a myocardial infarction), offer simple options to investigate this further or rule it out, such as an ECG and formal calculation of cardiovascular risk. This is perhaps the most difficult aspect of this station because it requires the candidate to apply basic knowledge in a clinical setting to formulate a simple plan that is in line with a patient's expectations.

You are almost guaranteed to be asked about baseline investigations and your reasons for using them – the 'investigations' table summarises this.

Potential variations at this station

• Take a history from this patient presenting to your GP surgery with palpitations and explain your steps in management to the patient. (5–10 minutes)
• Take a history from this patient presenting to your GP surgery with palpitations. Hand the patient over to the medical registrar who is on call at the local hospital. (5–10 minutes)

Questions you could be asked

Q. What is the investigation of choice for paroxysmal atrial fibrillation?
A. 24-hour ECG.
Q. What is the treatment of choice for asymptomatic ventricular ectopics?
A. Nothing – see the text above.

26 Cough

Checklist	P	MP	F
Appropriate introduction			
Confirms patient's name and age			
Explains reason for consultation			
Obtains consent			
Open question to elicit presenting complaint			
Allows patient to open up, listen carefully, remains silent and does not interrupt the patient			
Signposts: e.g. 'Mr Gregory, thank you for telling me about this problem. I would like to ask a few more detailed questions. Is that all right?'			
History of presenting complaint:			

• Onset (how it started)
• Character (dry or productive)
• Time (duration)
  • Alleviating factors: work/home
• Exacerbating factors:
  • Exertion/exercise
  • Season (worse in winter, e.g. COPD; worse in summer, e.g. allergic)
  • Pollen/chemicals (asthma)
  • Posture (worse when lying flat)
• Severity
• Variability:
  • Diurnal (worse at night/in early morning)
  • Continuous/intermittent
  • Environment (home, work, indoors, outdoors)
  • Season
• Asks if patient is suffering from any other symptoms
• Asks about any recent illnesses
• Previous episodes of coughing			

Asks about other respiratory/other relevant symptoms:
• Shortness of breath: orthopnoea
• Sputum:
  • Fresh/bright red
  • Dark clots
  • Colour (white, yellow, green, pink)
  • Offensive smell
• Wheeze
• Chest pain → pleuritic, sharp, worse with inspiration?
• Ankle oedema
• Throat symptoms/irritation
• Fevers
• Sleep disturbance			

'Red flags': • Haemoptysis • Weight loss • Night sweats • Hoarseness			

Review of systems:
• Musculoskeletal/rheumatological symptoms → related to pulmonary fibrosis
  • Arthralgia
  • Morning stiffness
• ENT symptoms:
  • Rhinitis
  • Nasal drip
  • Throat pain/symptoms
• Symptoms of gastro-oesophageal reflux disease: burning epigastric pain/heartburn			

Past medical history			

Family history:
• Atopy:
  • Asthma
  • Eczema
  • Hayfever
• Lung cancer
• Tuberculosis
• Pulmonary fibrosis			

Drug history: • Angiotensin-converting enzyme inhibitors • Beta-blockers • NSAIDs • Methotrexate • Amiodarone • Over-the-counter medication			
Allergies			
Social history: • Smoking • Alcohol • Illicit drug use • Occupation (dusty environment) • Exposure to asbestos • Pets (especially birds and cats) • Activities of daily living			

Use of non-verbal cues, e.g. good eye contact, nodding head and good body posture			
Systematic approach			
Explores and responds to ICE: • Ideas • Concerns • Expectations			
Shows empathy			
Non-verbal skills			
Avoids technical jargon			
Devises holistic management plan and addresses psychosocial issues as well as medical problems			
Summarises			
Offers to answer any questions			
Thanks patient			

Summary of common conditions seen in OSCEs

Throat/ENT	Trachea/bronchus	Lung	Others
Foreign body in ear canal	Upper respiratory tract infection	Lower respiratory tract infection, pneumonia	Angiotensin-converting enzyme inhibitor
Rhinitis	Tracheitis, bronchitis	Tuberculosis	Gastro-oesophageal reflux disease
Post-nasal drip	Obstructive airway diseases (asthma, COPD)	Malignancy	Left ventricular failure
Laryngeal cancer	Inhaled foreign body	Interstitial lung disease, pulmonary fibrosis	Diaphragmatic irritation (e.g. abscess)
Throat cancer	Bronchiectasis	Cystic fibrosis	Smoking
	Malignancy	Pulmonary oedema	Yellow nail syndrome
		Vasculitic, inflammatory causes (Goodpasture's syndrome, Wegener's granulomatosis)	Psychogenic
		Pneumonitis	

Key investigations

• Chest X-ray: to look for abnormal shadowing, areas of consolidation, bronchiectasis, cardiac failure, etc.
• Lung function tests, spirometry: to differentiate restrictive from obstructive lung disease and to assess flow–volume loops
• Peak expiratory flow rate: to look for diurnal variation in asthma
• Sputum microscopy, culture and sensitivity: to find the cause of a chest infection
• Sputum acid-fast bacillus: for tuberculosis
• Sputum cytology: for suspected lung cancer
• Full blood count: haemoglobin could be low in malignancy, raised white cell count in infection
• Us+Es:
  • Hyponatraemia in small-cell carcinomas, Legionnaire's disease
  • Hypercalcaemia in squamous cell carcinomas
• ESR raised in connective tissue diseases, any inflammatory conditions and malignancy
• High-resolution CT scan: for lung cancer and pulmonary fibrosis
• Bronchoscopy: for tracheal/bronchial carcinomas and for washings for sputum acid-fast bacillus and microscopy, culture and sensitivity
• Cardiac investigations, e.g. ECG, echocardiogram (if heart failure is a cause of cough)
• Nasoendoscopy: for ENT-related causes
• 24-hour pH manometry: for gastro-oesophageal reflux disease

Hints and tips for the exam

Everyone gets a cough at some point in their lives, and the underlying cause is not usually serious or significant. The key here is to be thorough and work through all the associated symptoms in a systematic way. Below we have summarised some key points that students often tend to forget:
• A persistent cough can often be a sign of poor asthma control so it is important to check compliance with medication and inhaler technique.
• A travel history is important to elicit, for example, atypical pneumonia and tuberculosis.
• Occupational history is equally important as irritant exposure at work could be the reason for the cough. In such cases, peak expiratory flow rate measurements at home and work would be a useful investigation.
• Nocturnal cough can occur as a result of gastro-oesophageal reflux, and a course of a proton pump inhibitor will often alleviate the symptoms.
• Remember to consider issues related to isolation and contact tracing if you suspect tuberculosis.

Questions you could be asked

Q. In which part of the lungs are you most likely to see changes associated with tuberculosis on a chest X-ray?
A. The apices.
Q. Which bronchus is a foreign body more likely to lodge in?
A. The right, as it is shorter and wider in diameter than the left.
Q. What is yellow nail syndrome?
A. A rare disorder in which patients have yellow discoloured nails, pleural effusions and lymphoedema.

27 Shortness of breath

Checklist	P	MP	F
Appropriate introduction			
Confirms patient's name and age			
Explains reason for consultation			
Obtains consent			
Open question to elicit presenting complaint			
Allows patient to open up, listens carefully, remains silent and does not interrupt the patient			
Signposts: e.g. 'Mr Gregory, thank you for telling me about this problem. I would like to ask a few more detailed questions. Is that all right?'			
History of presenting complaint:			

• Onset (how it started, gradual/sudden)
• Time (duration)
• Alleviating factors
• Exacerbating factors:
  • Exertion/exercise
  • Pollen/chemicals (asthma)
  • Orthopnoea (worse when lies flat)
• Severity:
  • Exercise tolerance on a flat surface
  • Exercise tolerance when walking upstairs/up an incline
  • Shortness of breath (SOB) at rest
• Variability: Is the SOB continuous throughout the day, intermittent or progressively worse? If intermittent, when is it worse/better?
• Asks if patient is suffering from any other symptoms
• Asks about any recent illnesses
• Previous episodes of SOB			

Asks about other respiratory symptoms: • Cough • Sputum • Wheeze • Orthopnoea • Paroxysmal nocturnal dyspnoea • Chest pain → is it pleuritic, sharp, worse with inspiration? • Ankle oedema • Fevers			
'Red flags': • Haemoptysis • Weight loss • Night sweats • Hoarseness			

Past medical history			

Family history:
• Lung cancer
• Atopy:
  • Asthma
  • Eczema
  • Hayfever
• Ischaemic heart disease/myocardial infarction
• Pulmonary fibrosis			

Drug history: • Methotrexate • Amiodarone • NSAIDs • Over-the-counter medication			
Allergies			
Social history: • Smoking • Alcohol • Illicit drug use • Occupation • Exposure to asbestos • Activities of daily living/functional assessment and impairment due to SOB			
Review of systems			
Use of non-verbal cues, e.g. good eye contact, nodding head and good body posture			
Systematic approach			
Explores and responds to ICE: • Ideas • Concerns • Expectations			
Shows empathy			
Non-verbal skills			
Avoids technical jargon			
Devises holistic management plan and addresses psychosocial issues as well as medical problems			
Summarises			
Offers to answer any questions			
Thanks patient			

Summary of common conditions seen in OSCEs

Cardiovascular	Trachea/bronchus	Lung	Neuromuscular conditions	Others
Heart failure	Obstructive airway diseases (asthma/COPD)	Lower respiratory tract infection, pneumonia	Guillain–Barré syndrome	Anaemia
Infective endocarditis	Bronchiectasis	Tuberculosis	Motor neurone disease	Anxiety, psychogenic
Primary pulmonary hypertension	Malignancy	Malignancy	Myasthenia gravis	
Aortic stenosis/other valvular heart disease	Obstructive sleep apnoea	Interstitial lung disease, pulmonary fibrosis	Obesity hypoventilation syndrome	
Arrhythmias – especially paroxysmal atrial fibrillation and superventricular tachycardia		Pulmonary embolism	Kyphosis, scoliosis	
		Pulmonary oedema		
		Pleural effusions		
		Vasculitic/inflammatory causes (Goodpasture's syndrome, Wegener's granulomatosis)		
		Pneumonitis		
		Pneumothorax		
		Primary pulmonary hypertension/pulmonary hypertension from any cause		

Key investigations
Blood tests
• Full blood count: anaemia is a common cause of SOB
• Us+Es and liver function tests: SOB can be a presenting feature of renal failure/hepatic failure if this has resulted in fluid overload and pleural effusions
• Brain natriuretic peptide: for heart failure

Cardiac investigations
• ECG: for arrhythmias and left ventricular failure
• Echocardiogram: for valvular heart diseases and heart failure
• Cardiac catheter studies: for pulmonary hypertension

Respiratory investigations
• Chest X-ray: for pneumonias, lung cancer, cardiomegaly and pleural effusions

• Lung function tests/spirometry: to distinguish between and diagnose obstructive and restrictive lung conditions
• Bronchoscopy: for bronchial/tracheal malignancies
• CT pulmonary angiogram and ventilation/perfusion scan: for pulmonary embolism
• High-resolution CT scan: for some lung cancers and pulmonary fibrosis

Others
• Nerve conduction studies: for Guillain–Barré syndrome and myasthenia gravis
• Spine/back X-rays: for kyphosis, scoliosis, etc.

Hints and tips for the exams

There may be more than one aetiology
Patients who are suffering from SOB often have more the one coexisting condition to account for their symp-

toms; for example, heart failure may be exacerbated by anaemia.

Know your emergencies

Acute SOB is a common presenting symptom in A&E, so don't be surprised if it appears as an OSCE station. You should know how to manage common medical emergencies causing SOB such as acute severe asthma, pulmonary embolism and pneumothorax.

Questions you could be asked

Q. What is yellow nail syndrome?

A. A rare disorder in which patients have yellow discoloured nails, pleural effusions and lymphoedema.

Q. If you suspect an inpatient has a deep vein thrombosis or a pulmonary embolism and you are awaiting a definitive diagnosis, what treatment should you get the patient started on?

A. Low molecular weight heparin. See the *BNF* for dosing details.

28 Haemoptysis

Checklist	P	MP	F
Appropriate introduction			
Confirms patient's name and age			
Explains reason for consultation			
Obtains consent			
Open question to elicit presenting complaint			
Allows patient to open up, listens carefully, remains silent and does not interrupt the patient			
Signposts: e.g. 'Mr Gregory, thank you for telling me about this problem. I would like to ask a few more detailed questions. Is that all right?'			
History of presenting complaint			

Elicits further details of haemoptysis:
• Onset (how did it start)
• Duration of symptoms
• Approximate quantity of blood
• Appearance of blood (and sputum)
  • Streaks
  • Fresh red
  • Dark clots
• Exacerbating factors: smoke, dust, exertion
• Alleviating factors
• Asks whether patient is suffering from any other symptoms
• Asks about any recent illnesses
• Previous episodes of chest pain			

Associated symptoms: • Weight loss • Night sweats (TB) • Fevers (TB, pneumonia, vasculitis) • Hoarseness (cancer) • Chest pain (cancer) • Shortness of breath (pulmonary embolism) • Ankle swelling • Wheeze (cancer) • Bony pains (cancer) • Throat pain (throat malignancy) • Nosebleeds • Bleeding elsewhere (haematological disorders): haematuria, haematemesis, epistaxis, bruising, blood in stool			

Elicits risk factors for pulmonary embolism/deep vein thrombosis: • Calf pain/swelling • Recent travel • Recent surgery • Family history of clotting disorders • Malignancy • Oral contraceptive pill (if patient female) • Pregnancy (if patient female)			
Review of systems			
Past medical history: • Lung disease • Heart disease • Blood disorders • Any cancer • Kidney disease, haematuria • Autoimmune conditions			
Family history: • Lung disease • Vasculitis • Bleeding/coagulation disorders • Kidney disease			
Drug history: • Anticoagulant medication • NSAIDs			
Allergies			

Social history:
• Smoking:
  • Type of cigarettes/pipes, roll-ups, 'sheesha'
  • Number
  • Duration
• Exposure to asbestos
• Alcohol
• Travel history and BCG
• Contact with possible TB patients
• Current and previous occupation(s)
• Pets			

Use of non-verbal cues, e.g. good eye contact, nodding head and good body posture			
Systematic approach			

Explores and responds to ICE: • Ideas • Concerns • Expectations			
Shows empathy			
Non-verbal skills			
Avoids technical jargon			

Devises holistic management plan and addresses psychosocial issues as well as medical problems			
Summarises			
Offers to answer any questions			
Thanks patient			

Summary of common conditions seen in OSCEs

Condition	'Red flags'	Common errors
Lung cancer	Current, ex- or passive smoker Weight loss Change in voice Bone pain Working with asbestos	Settling for a diagnosis of chest infection if there is a small amount of haemoptysis in a heavy smoker Remember that lung cancer **must be ruled out** in a smoker with any amount of haemoptysis, even if the other features from the history suggest it is not the likeliest diagnosis
TB	Weight loss Night sweats Travel to areas with high prevalence	Failing to take a travel history Failing to ask about BCG vaccination if suspecting TB (**but** remember that the BCG is only around 40% protective against TB)
Pulmonary embolism	Risk factors (see above) Red, swollen, painful leg	Insufficient questioning on risk factors Assuming pulmonary embolism is impossible if there are no clinical features of deep vein thrombosis
Pneumonia	Cough productive of rusty or green sputum with small amounts of blood mixed in Fever Recent upper respiratory tract infection	
Bronchiectasis	Recurrent chest infections Croup during childhood Presence of wheezing	
Pulmonary oedema	Ankle swelling Known mitral valve disease Pink frothy sputum Inhalation of toxic fumes Pregnancy	Failing to ask about symptoms of congestive cardiac failure, e.g. orthopnoea, paroxysmal nocturnal dyspnoea, ankle oedema, shortness of breath on exertion Insufficient questioning about coughed-up blood
Goodpasture's syndrome	Haematuria Family history	Failing to ask about haematuria
Wegener's granulomatosis	Nasal discharge and/or epistaxis Oral ulcers Purpuric skin rash Arthralgia Haematuria	Not able to recollect common clinical features Lack of time to complete a thorough systems review

Hints and tips for the exam

Haemoptysis is a very worrying symptom for patients. It is important to elicit concerns and respond to them empathically. You will get marks for doing this.

It is a potentially life-threatening symptom if blood loss is profuse. Therefore a sound knowledge of the common and serious underlying causes is essential to direct good history-taking. These can be divided into general and local causes. The most common and serious of these are tinted in red in the algorithm.

Using open questions to initiate the interview is particularly useful because these allow the actor-patient to describe the characteristics of the coughed-up blood and volunteer any other associated symptoms. This is usually enough to narrow down your differential diagnosis from the outset. You can then dedicate your efforts to focusing your questioning on this. Questions relating to other less likely causes can subsequently be asked to demonstrate that you are also thinking about them. The sample mark sheet outlines the key questions that need to be asked to rule out serious and life-threatening causes of haemoptysis.

You are likely to be asked to provide a differential diagnosis based on your history. It is worth remembering a few 'rules of thumb' that are applicable in most cases:

• Haemoptysis in a patient with a long-standing **smoking history** (usually considered to be >20 pack–years) is **lung cancer** until proven otherwise.

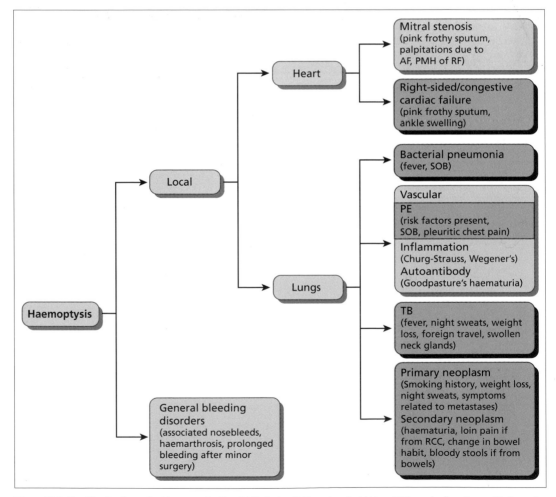

Figure 28.1 Algorithm for diagnosis of haemoptysis. AF, atrial fibrillation; PMH, past medical history; RCC, renal cell carcinoma; RF, rheumatic fever; SOB, shortness of breath

• Haemoptysis associated with **fever and weight loss** in a traveller recently returned from the tropics is likely to be caused by **TB**.

• **Acute-onset haemoptysis with pleuritic chest pain and/or shortness of breath is pulmonary embolism** until proven otherwise.

Time permitting, you may be asked to offer first-line investigations to support or rebuke your preliminary diagnosis. The list below outlines some key investigations that can be requested:

• Chest X-ray (neoplasm, consolidation secondary to infection or pulmonary oedema, TB)

• D-dimer test (pulmonary embolism)

• Ventilation/perfusion scan (pulmonary embolism)

• Sputum microbiology (bacterial pneumonia)

• Sputum auramine stain (TB)

• Echocardiogram (right heart failure)

Candidates being considered for merits or distinctions may be asked further questions, but it is difficult to predict what these may be. It is likely they will relate to more challenging aspects of the scenario, for example the limitations of the investigations. Here are a few limitations that it may be worthwhile remembering:

• A ventilation/perfusion scan can give a false-positive result when investigating for a pulmonary embolism if there is alveolar consolidation.

• The differential diagnosis for a round opacity in a lung field on a chest X-ray is vast and includes:

• Neoplasm
• Abscess
• Granuloma
• Aspergilloma
• Foreign body
• Skin tumour

• D-dimer testing has a very low sensitivity but a relatively high specificity for pulmonary embolism. In other words, it is increased above normal in several conditions, such as pulmonary embolism, pneumonia, etc., and hence is not sufficient to confirm a diagnosis of pulmonary embolism. However, a negative D-dimer result suggests that a pulmonary embolism is highly unlikely. Therefore it can be used to rule out suspected pulmonary embolism but not to confirm it.

Questions you could be asked

Q. Take a history and explain your management plan to the patient. (5–10 minutes)

Q. Take a history from this patient presenting to your GP surgery with haemoptysis and write a referral letter to the appropriate hospital team to hand the patient over. (10 minutes)

Q. Take a history from this patient presenting with haemoptysis and present the chest X-ray to the examiner. (5–10 minutes)

29 Diarrhoea

Checklist	P	MP	F
Appropriate introduction			
Confirms patient's name and age			
Explains reason for consultation			
Obtains consent			
Open question to elicit presenting complaint			
Allows patient to open up, listens carefully, remains silent and does not interrupt the patient			
Signposts: e.g. 'Mr Gregory, thank you for telling me about this problem. I would like to ask a few more detailed questions. Is that all right?'			
History of presenting complaint			

• Clarify what the patient means by diarrhoea in their own words
• Onset (how it started)
• Character:
  • Consistency:
    • Watery
    • Loose
    • Greasy and difficult to flush away
    • Well formed
    • Mucus
  • Colour:
    • Black (melaena)
    • Red (blood)
    • Green
  • Smell: offensive
  • Pellets
• Time:
  • Duration
  • Intermittent, continuous, progressive
• Frequency
• Volume (more or less than usual)
• Alleviating factors: dietary factors
• Exacerbating factors:
  • Dietary factors
  • Gluten-containing foods (coeliac disease)
• Severity
• Asks if patient is suffering from any other symptoms
• Asks about any recent illnesses
• Previous episodes of diarrhoea
• Family members/contacts with similar symptoms			

Asks about other gastrointestinal/colorectal and other relevant symptoms:
• Nausea/vomiting
• Bloating
• Abdominal pain: is it reduced with defecation?
• Abdominal swelling
• Anal pain
• Constipation
• Tenesmus
• Faecal incontinence
• Fevers
• Symptoms of IBS:
  • Constipation
  • Psychosocial stressors
  • Flatulence
• Symptoms of anaemia:
  • Lethargy
  • Shortness of breath
  • Dizziness → postural
• Symptoms of malabsorption: generalised weakness/lethargy
• Symptoms of IBD:
  • Blood
  • Arthralgia
  • Back pain (sacroiliitis)
  • Oral ulcers
  • Skin problems
    • Pyoderma gangrenosum
    • Erythema nodosum
  • Eye pain
• Risk factors for *Clostridium difficile*:
  • Recent hospital admissions
  • Recent antibiotic courses			

'Red flags':
• Rectal bleeding:
  • Mixed with stool
  • Around stool
  • Dripping from rectum, separate from stool
• Black stools (melaena)
• Weight loss
• Loss of appetite			

Review of systems: • Gynaecological symptoms: related to ovarian cancer			

Past medical history:			
• Any bowel disorders			
• Diabetes (for autonomic neuropathy)			
• Radiotherapy (for radiation colitis)			
• Previous abdominal/intestinal surgery			

Family history:			
• Colon cancer			
• IBD (Crohn's disease, ulcerative colitis)			
• Coeliac disease			

Drug history:			
• Laxatives			
• Metformin			
• Iron tablets			
• Antibiotics (e.g. erythromycin)			
• Thyroxine			
• Over-the-counter medication			

Allergies			

Social history:			
• Recent foreign travel/foreign contacts			
• Similar symptoms in other members of travelling party			
• Accommodation			
• Rural/forest exposure			
• Water consumed (mineral water, tap water, boiled water)			
• Diet:			
• Recent changes			
• Takeaways			
• Barbecues			
• Contact with anyone suffering from diarrhoea			
• Smoking			
• Alcohol			
• Occupation (dusty environment)			
• Accommodation: institution, residential home			
• Activities of daily living			

Use of non-verbal cues, e.g. good eye contact, nodding head and good body posture			
Systematic approach			
Explores and responds to ICE:			
• Ideas			
• Concerns			
• Expectations			
Shows empathy			
Non-verbal skills			
Avoids technical jargon			
Devises holistic management plan and addresses psychosocial issues as well as medical problems			
Summarises			
Offers to answer any questions			
Thanks patient			

Summary of common conditions seen in OSCEs

Condition	Key features in history	Key investigations
Infective causes		
Bacterial/viral gastroenteritis	Recent takeaway/restaurant Recent barbecue Raw/undercooked meat or seafood, unpasteurised milk Foreign contacts, travel abroad Contacts with diarrhoea	Stool microscopy, culture and sensitivity if suspecting bacterial cause Full blood count and Us+Es (for haemolytic-uraemic syndrome or *Escherichia coli*)
Clostridium difficile	Recent antibiotic use Green, foul-smelling diarrhoea	*Clostridium difficile* toxin
Malignancies		
Bowel cancer	Melaena (tarry black stool) Rectal bleeding Weight loss, loss of appetite	Colonoscopy and biopsy Full blood count + mean corpuscular volume (microcytic anaemia) Ferritin (iron deficiency)
Inflammatory		
Inflammatory bowel disease (ulcerative colitis, Crohn's disease)	Young Blood and mucus in stool Systemic symptoms of IBD: • Arthralgia • Back pain (sacroileitis) • Oral ulcers • Skin problems: • Pyoderma gangrenosum • Erythema nodosum • Eye pain	Colonoscopy and biopsy Barium studies Erythrocyte sedimentation rate
Malabsorption		
Coeliac disease	Steatorrhoea (offensive-smelling 'floaters' that are difficult to flush away) Correlation with gluten intake Failure to thrive (if child)	Anti-tissue transglutaminase antibodies Small bowel biopsy
Chronic pancreatitis	Steatorrhoea (offensive-smelling 'floaters' that are difficult to flush away)	Imaging of pancreas (ideally CT scan)
Short bowel syndrome	Steatorrhoea (offensive-smelling 'floaters' that are difficult to flush away) History of small bowel resection	Exclude other diagnoses
Drug abuse, iatrogenic		
Laxative abuse/overuse	Psychological stressors	Us+Es (hypokalaemia) Laxative screen
Excess alcohol intake	History of excess alcohol intake Symptoms of chronic liver disease	Investigations for chronic liver disease Liver function tests and gamma-glutamyl transpeptidase Ultrasound

Condition	Key features in history	Key investigations
Drugs	Recent history of drug use Common drugs that cause diarrhoea: • Antibiotics (especially erythromycin) • Metformin • Colchicine • Magnesium-based antacids • Proton pump inhibitors	None – clinical diagnosis Exclude other causes
Diet	Recent changes to diet, e.g. new vegetarians	None – clinical diagnosis Exclude other causes
Endocrine causes		
Autonomic neuropathy secondary to diabetes	Symptoms of diabetes: • Polydipsia • Polyuria • Weight loss • Lethargy Other autonomic symptoms: • Dry mouth • Constipation • Urinary retention	Fasting blood glucose HbA_{1c} if already diabetic
Hyperthyroidism	Symptoms of hyperthyroidism: • Increased appetite and weight loss • Menstrual disturbance • Tremor • Excessive sweating • Irritability • Heat intolerance	Thyroid function tests
Others/rare causes		
IBS	Both constipation and diarrhoea Abdominal pain and/or bloating Symptoms improve after opening bowels Correlation with stress	Rule out organic diseases Full blood count, erythrocyte sedimentation rate, coeliac screen
Overflow diarrhoea	Elderly History of constipation Constipation-inducing medications (e.g. codeine-based analgesia)	Rectal examination (faecal impaction)
Carcinoid	Flushing Wheezing Abdominal pain Cardiac symptoms (from right-sided valve problems)	24-hour urinary 5-HIAA CT chest/abdomen
Radiation enteritis/colitis	Enteritis: steatorrhoea Colitis: blood in stool Both: • History of radiotherapy • Abdominal pain	Barium studies Colonoscopy with histology
VIPoma	Massive volumes of diarrhoea Dehydration	Raised vasoactive peptide levels Imaging (usually CT scan) Hypokalaemia
Whipple's disease	Steatorrhoea Cognitive impairment, dementia Chest pain, cardiac symptoms (pericarditis) Lymphadenopathy Joint pains Fevers	Jejunal biopsy: macrophages with PAS stain-positive granules

Hints and tips for the exam

Diarrhoea is a very common symptom and one that absolutely everyone will suffer from at some point in their lives. The vast majority of cases are caused by viral gastroenteritis, which is self-limiting and requires only rehydration either with water or oral rehydration therapy (such as Dioralyte).

However, various other potentially serious pathologies can also cause diarrhoea, and the characteristics of the diarrhoea and its associated symptoms can vary immensely depending on the aetiology. This is why diarrhoea lends itself particularly well to OSCEs.

What does the patient mean by diarrhoea?

The patient may be referring to the character/type of stool, frequency or volume when they refer to diarrhoea. Although definitions vary, most clinicians would agree that the following features constitutes diarrhoea:

- Amount of >200–300 mL or g per day
- Stools that are liquid/loose
- Increased frequency (more than three times a day is unusual)

Acute versus chronic

Again, different clinicians have different definitions of these terms. Generally, diarrhoea that persists for more than **4 weeks** is deemed chronic.

'Red flags'

Any of the following symptoms should prompt you to request further investigations urgently:

- Rectal bleeding
- Melaena
- Weight loss
- Chronic diarrhoea

If you are in any doubt about which investigations to suggest, you can rest assured that the following will be a good answer in the vast majority of diarrhoea-related cases:

- **Colonoscopy with histological analysis/biopsy:** Visualising the lesion and getting a tissue sample will usually lead to a definitive diagnosis.
- **Full blood count and ferritin studies:** A microcytic anaemia with low ferritin levels usually indicates gastrointestinal bleeding. Severe anaemia causing symptoms and haemodynamic instability is a medical emergency that needs urgent intervention.
- **Imaging:** Barium studies, CT abdomen and CT colon may all be useful in certain cases, particularly if the patient is not fit enough for a colonoscopy.

Questions you could be asked

Q. What are the symptoms of a VIPoma, and which investigations would you do to help you diagnostically?

Q. Name some endocrinological causes of diarrhoea.

Q. What non-gastroenterological symptoms may present in a patient with IBD?

A. The answers to all of these questions can be found in the text above.

30 Abdominal pain

Checklist	P	MP	F
Appropriate introduction			
Confirms patient's name and age			
Explains reason for consultation			
Obtains consent			
Open question to elicit presenting complaint			
Allows patient to open up, listens carefully, remains silent and does not interrupt the patient			
Signposts: e.g. 'Mr Gregory, thank you for telling me about this problem. I would like to ask a few more detailed questions. Is that all right?'			
History of presenting complaint			

- Site (see also Chapter 3)
- Onset (how it started):
  - Sudden
  - Gradual
- Character:
  - Colicky (renal stones)
  - Sharp/sudden (rupture of viscus)
  - Burning (peptic ulcer disease)
  - Dull
- Radiation:
  - To back (abdominal aortic aneurysm, ruptured duodenal ulcer)
  - To testicles/groin (hernia)
  - To shoulders (gallbladder)
  - Loin to groin (renal stone)
- Time:
  - Duration
  - Intermittent, continuous, progressive
- Alleviating factors:
  - Dietary factors
  - Opening bowels
- Exacerbating factors:
  - Dietary factors
  - Swallowing (oesophagus/stomach)
  - Fatty foods (gallstones)
  - Acidic/spicy foods, hot drinks (peptic ulcer disease)
- Severity
- Asks if patient is suffering from any other symptoms
- Asks about any recent illnesses
- Previous episodes of abdominal pain
- Family members/contacts with similar symptoms

Associated symptoms:
Gastrointestinal/colorectal symptoms:
- Nausea/vomiting
- Bowel habit, diarrhoea/constipation
- Dysphagia
- Dyspepsia
- Bloating/abdominal swelling (generalised/localised)
- Flatulence
- Fevers
- IBD symptoms: arthralgia, eye symptoms, skin features, oral ulcers, bloody diarrhoea

Liver/hepatic symptoms:
- Right upper quadrant pain
- Jaundice
- Ankle swelling

Gallstone symptoms:
- Jaundice
- Right upper quadrant pain radiating to shoulders
- Dark stools
- Pale urine

Renal symptoms:
- Location and character:
  - Loin to groin + flank + colicky: renal stones
  - Flank + burning dysuria: pyelonephritis
- Generalised lethargy
- Pruritus
- Ankle swelling

Females: gynaecological symptoms:
- Correlation with menstrual periods
- Menorrhagia
- Irregular periods
- Vaginal discharge

Females: obstetric symptoms:
- **Possibility of patient being pregnant**
- Last menstrual period
- Unprotected sexual intercourse **must** signpost before taking sexual history
- Contraception
- Vaginal bleeding (with severe abdominal pain = ectopic pregnancy until proven otherwise)

'Red flags':
- Bleeding:
  - Rectal: fresh red, melaena
  - Vaginal: intermenstrual, postcoital
  - Haematemesis
  - Haematuria
- Weight loss
- Loss of appetite

Review of systems:
- Gynaecological symptoms: related to ovarian cancer

Past medical history:
- Any bowel disorders
- Diabetes (for autonomic neuropathy)
- Radiotherapy (for radiation colitis)
- Previous abdominal/intestinal surgery

Family history:
- Colon cancer
- IBD (Crohn's disease, ulcerative colitis)
- Recent abdominal surgery

Drug history:
- NSAIDs
- Over-the-counter medication

Allergies

Social history:
- Alcohol (peptic ulcer, gastritis)
- Smoking
- Illicit drug use
- Diet:
  - Spicy foods (peptic ulcer disease)
  - High-fibre foods (low intake may correlate with diverticulitis)
- Occupation
- Activities of daily living

Use of non-verbal cues, e.g. good eye contact, nodding head and good body posture

Systematic approach

Explores and responds to ICE:
- Ideas
- Concerns
- Expectations

Shows empathy

Non-verbal skills

Avoids technical jargon

Devises holistic management plan and addresses psychosocial issues as well as medical problems

Summarises

Offers to answer any questions

Thanks patient

Summary of common conditions seen in OSCEs

Causes of abdominal pain can be broadly divided into acute and chronic.

Acute abdominal pain

Lower gastrointestinal tract/colon	Upper gastrointestinal tract	Hepatobiliary tract	Kidneys/ ureter/ bladder	Obstetric and gynaecological/ genitourinary	Metabolic	Others
IBD exacerbation	Perforated peptic ulcer	Biliary colic, cholecystitis, cholangitis	Renal/ureteric stones	Ectopic pregnancy	Diabetic ketoacidosis	Any perforated viscus leading to peritonitis
Ischaemic bowel	Small bowel obstruction	Hepatitis, hepatic pain	Urinary tract infection	Ruptured ovarian cyst	Addisonian crisis	Rupture or dissection of abdominal aortic aneurysm
Appendicitis	Severe gastroenteritis	Pancreatitis	Pyelonephritis	Ovarian torsion	Hypercalcaemia	Psychogenic
Diverticulitis	Strangulated hernia			Testicular torsion	Porphyria	Myocardial infarction
Large bowel obstruction						Sickle cell crisis
						Abscess in any part of the abdomen

Chronic abdominal pain

Lower gastrointestinal tract/colon	Upper gastrointestinal tract	Hepatobiliary tract	Kidneys/ ureter/ bladder	Obstetric and gynaecological/ genitourinary	Metabolic	Others
Diverticular disease	Gastritis	Gallstones	Recurrent urinary tract infection	Endometriosis, adenomyosis	Addison's disease	Psychogenic/ functional abdominal pain
Constipation	Peptic ulcer	Chronic pancreatitis	Renal/ureteric stones	Fibroids	Porphyria	Mesenteric artery ischaemia
Malignancy	Hiatus hernia	Malignancy (gallbladder or liver)	Adult polycystic kidney disease	Pelvic inflammatory disease	Lead poisoning	Lower lobe/basal pneumonia
	Malignancy		Malignancy (renal cell, bladder)	Dysmenorrhoea		Hip joint pain
	IBS			Ovarian cyst		Psoas abscess
	Subacute obstruction (due to adhesions, etc.)			Pregnancy		
				Sexually transmitted disease		
				Testicular cancer		
				Epididymitis, orchitis		
				Malignancy (ovarian/ endometrial)		

Investigations to consider for abdominal pain

Blood tests

• Full blood count: anaemia may be present in cases of gastrointestinal malignancy or a perforated peptic ulcer. A raised white cell count would be found in infective or inflammatory conditions.
• Us+Es: renal impairment may be found in pyelonephritis or any other renal/renal tract pathology.
• C-reactive protein: raised in IBD, infections and any other pathologies causing inflammation.
• Liver function tests: deranged in hepatitis, raised alkaline phosphatase in cholecystitis (often follows biliary colic and will be associated with constant pain and fever).
• Amylase: raised levels in pancreatitis.
• Arterial blood gasses: this is very useful in an 'acute abdomen'. A low base excess and a high lactate level may indicate severe general physiological decompensation. A metabolic acidosis will help narrow down the potential causes (e.g. pancreatitis).

Urine

• Urine dipstick on midstream urine sample: to look for haematuria in renal colic due to renal stones, nitrites if a urinary tract infection or pyelonephritis is present.
• Urine beta-human chorionic gonadotropin: for pregnancy.

Imaging

• Erect chest X-ray: to look for air under the diaphragm due to a perforated viscus.
• Abdominal X-ray: to assess for abnormal fluid air levels, loops of dilated bowel, etc.
• Ultrasound/CT: for any structural hepatobiliary or gynaecological pathologies.
• MRCP: for hepatobiliary pathology.
• Intravenous urogram: for suspected ureteric obstruction due to calculi.
• Mesenteric angiogram for suspected mesenteric ischaemia (remember that this can occur in atrial fibrillation).

Others

• Oesophago-gastro-duodenoscopy/colonoscopy: for cases of suspected gastrointestinal bleeding or any pathology in the lumen of the oesophagus or colon.
• ERCP: for diagnosing cholangiocarcinoma and for close visualisation of the hepatobiliary tract.
• *Helicobacter pylori*: can be detected either by a stool antigen test or a CLO test (via oesophago-gastro-duodenoscopy); serology is of limited clinical value.
• Vaginal/endocervical swabs: if suspecting pelvic inflammatory disease/genitourinary infection.

Hints and tips for the exam

Work through the systems

Abdominal pain is potentially more difficult to manage due to the wide variety of systems from which it may originate. To help narrow down your list of differential diagnoses, it may be helpful to work your way through the different organs or systems in your mind. The following list summarises these:
• Oesophagus/stomach
• Small intestine
• Large intestine
• Liver/hepatobiliary tract
• Abdominal aorta
• Kidneys, renal tract, bladder
• Gynaecological/pelvic organs (ovaries, fallopian tubes, uterus)
• Scrotal/testicular
• Metabolic

Don't forget non-abdominal causes of abdominal pain

These could be as serious and potentially life-threatening as the classical causes that originate from the abdomen – the tables above list them in the 'Others' column.

Managing an acute abdomen

This is a common surgical emergency that every junior doctor should know inside out. Although there is an absolute plethora of possible causes, the initial management is generic for most of them:
• Make the patient nil by mouth.
• Start intravenous fluids.
• Administer adequate analgesia: remember to prescribe an antiemetic with any opioid-based analgesia.
• Take bloods for the following:
  • Full blood count, Us+Es, liver function tests, C-reactive protein level, amylase
  • Blood cultures

• Group and save
• Vaginal swabs in women.
• Do a pregnancy test.
• Do a urine dipstick.
• Do an erect chest X-ray to look for air under the diaphragm.
• Request a specialist assessment by the general surgical and/or gynaecology on-call team.

Women's health

In women, remember to consider pathologies related to obstetric and gynaecological causes – it is unusual to encounter obstetrics and gynaecology-related pathologies in a finals OSCE, but it is still possible.

Pregnancy test

This should be one of the first tests you do in a woman of child-bearing age presenting with lower abdominal pain. A urinary beta-human chorionic gonadotropin test is quick and easy to do.

Ectopic pregnancy

A pregnant woman with acute lower abdominal pain is a case of ectopic pregnancy until proven otherwise. Ectopic pregnancies can rupture, bleed, cause peritonitis and ultimately be fatal. Most women will have had their first pregnancy-related scan by around 12 weeks, which will reveal whether or not the baby is in the uterus.

Deciding where the pain originates from

The key to this lies in appreciating some basic anatomy and embryology (as distant in your training as it may sound):
• **Visceral pain:** This is the pain that the patient feels **first**. It occurs as a result of stretching of the viscera (such as the intestines, the wall of the stomach, and anything that forms the gastrointestinal or hepatobiliary tract). This pain is usually quite vague and often difficult to localise to a very specific area.

To appreciate the origin of visceral pain, one has to appreciate how the gastrointestinal tract was formed. To cut a long story short, the zygote develops in three layers – the endoderm (the innermost layer), the mesoderm (the middle layer) and the ectoderm (the outermost layer). The only one that is relevant here is the endoderm. This develops into **foregut, midgut and hindgut**, which later develop into various parts of the gastrointestinal system. This is relevant is because the area of the abdomen where the pain is first felt correlates with these three divisions – abdominal pain in the

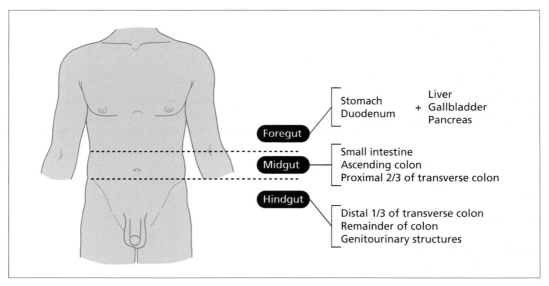

Figure 30.1 Foregut, midgut and hindgut

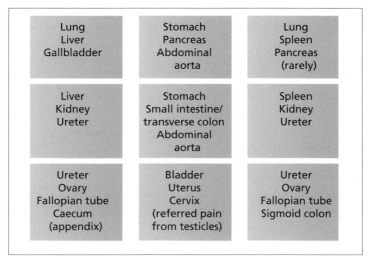

Figure 30.2 Location of organs in the abdomen

epigastric area usually originates from structures derived from the foregut, pain in the umbilical area originates from structures derived from the midgut, and pain in the suprapubic area originates from structures derived from the hindgut. Figure 30.1 illustrates this more simply.

• **Peritoneal pain:** This is the pain that the patient feels **later**. In contrast to visceral pain, peritoneal pain is more clearly defined and easier to localise. It occurs after the painful organ either touches, stretches or inflames the peritoneal peritoneum, which is why it happens after visceral pain (which is due to stretching of an organ or other structures). To localise where peritoneal pain is coming from, you need to know the structures that underlie the peritoneum, as illustrated in Figure 30.2.

Questions you could be asked

Q. If a Turkish patient presented with unexplained acute abdominal pain and had a family history of such presentations, what diagnosis might you consider?

A. Familial Mediterranean fever.

Q. What is the difference between a normal abdominal aorta and an abdominal aortic aneurysm on clinical examination?

A. A normal aorta is only pulsatile, whereas an abdominal aortic aneurysm is both pulsatile and expansile.

Q. What comprises 'triple therapy' for *Helicobacter pylori* eradication?

A. This can vary depending on local guidelines but usually includes a combination of a proton pump inhibitor, clarithromycin and amoxicillin (or metronidazole if the patient is allergic to penicillin) for 1 week (see the *BNF* for other combinations and dosages).

31 Abdominal distension

Checklist	P	MP	F
Appropriate introduction			
Confirms patient's name and age			
Explain reason for consultation			
Obtains consent			
Open question to elicit presenting complaint			
Allows patient to open up, listens carefully, remains silent and does not interrupt the patient			
Signposts: e.g. 'Mr Gregory, thank you for telling me about this problem. I would like to ask a few more detailed questions. Is that all right?'			
History of presenting complaint:			
• Site:			
• Generalised			
• Localised			
• Onset (how it started):			
• How did the patient first notice it?			
• Sudden			
• Gradual			
• Character:			
• Soft fluctuant/fluid swelling			
• Hard, mass-like swelling			
• Radiation:			
• To testicles/groin (hernia)			
• Time:			
• Duration			
• Intermittent/continuous/progressive			
• Correlation with menstrual periods			
• Alleviating factors:			
• Dietary factors			
• Opening bowels			
• Exacerbating factors:			
• Dietary factors/meals			
• Position (e.g. worse on lying down/standing – hernia), coughing (hernia)			
• Worse at the end of the day (oedema)			
• Pain/tenderness			
• Bloating/discomfort			
• Local compression-related symptoms (e.g. urge incontinence)			
• Asks if patient is suffering from any other symptoms			
• Asks about any recent illnesses			
• Previous episodes of abdominal distension			
• Family members/contacts with similar symptoms			

Associated symptoms:			
• Gastrointestinal/colorectal symptoms:			
• Abdominal pain			
• Flatulence			
• Nausea/vomiting			
• Bowel habit/diarrhoea/constipation: any correlation of distension with opening bowels?			
• Dysphagia/dyspepsia			
Ascites:			
• Facial swelling			
• Ankle swelling			
• Shortness of breath/orthopnoea			
Liver/hepatobiliary symptoms: right upper quadrant pain, jaundice, dark stools, pale urine			
Renal symptoms: urinary symptoms, frothy urine (nephrotic syndrome), lethargy, pruritus			
Heart failure symptoms: chest pain			
Hypothyroidism			
Females: gynaecological symptoms:			
• Correlation with menstrual periods			
• Irregular/painful periods			
• Intermenstrual/postcoital bleeding			
• Pelvic pain			
Females: obstetric symptoms:			
• **Possibility of patient being pregnant**			
• Last menstrual period			
• Unprotected sexual intercourse: **must** signpost before taking sexual history			
• Contraception			
'Red flags':			
• Bleeding (rectal, melaena, vaginal)			
• Weight loss, loss of appetite, night sweats (malignancy)			
Review of systems			
Past medical history:			
• Constipation			
• Abdominal surgery –especially laparoscopic surgery			
• Gynaecological history: fibroids, ovarian cysts			
• Heart failure			
Family history:			
• Colorectal cancer			
• Ovarian cancer			
• Polycystic kidney disease			
• Hernia			
• Fibroids			

Drug history:			
• Laxative history: any recent changes, stopped taking			
• Oral contraceptive pill (OCP, if patient female)			
• Over-the-counter medication			
Allergies			
Social history:			
• Alcohol (peptic ulcer disease, gastritis)			
• Smoking			
• Illicit drug use (especially intravenous drug abuse for hepatitis B/C)			
• Diet:			
• Intake of fibre			
• Recent change in diet			
• Occupation			
• Activities of daily living			
Use of non-verbal cues, e.g. good eye contact, nodding head and good body posture			

Systematic approach			
Explores and responds to ICE:			
• Ideas			
• Concerns			
• Expectations			
Shows empathy			
Non-verbal skills			
Avoids technical jargon			
Devises holistic management plan and addresses psychosocial issues as well as medical problems			
Summarises			
Offers to answer any questions			
Thanks patient			

Summary of common conditions seen in OSCEs

Condition	Key points	'Red flags'	Management
Small bowel obstruction	Adhesions (70%) Acute hernia (20%) Malignancy Stricture Foreign body – gallstone Intussusception Volvulus	Vomiting (early) Colicky abdominal pain (high in abdomen) Constipation	Investigations: full blood count, Us + Es, amylase, abdominal X-ray, erect chest X-ray, Gastrograffin follow-through, CT Strangulation (blood supply compromised) – surgery Nil by mouth Nasogastric tube insertion and intravenous fluids – drip and suck Analgesia Monitor fluid status
Large bowel obstruction	Malignancy (60%) Stricture – diverticular, Crohn's disease (20%) Volvulus – sigmoid, caecal Impacted faeces	Vomiting (late) Constant abdominal pain Constipation	Call surgeon Surgery
Hernia	See Chapter 12 on hernia examination		
Malignancy	Abdominal distension may be due to cancer mass, bowel obstruction, ascites or organomegaly	Generalised symptoms Smoker Older patient Family history	Bloods: full blood count, Us + Es, liver function tests, carcinoembryonic antigen, faecal occult blood Imaging: sigmoidoscopy, colonoscopy, CT/MRI, liver ultrasound scan Special test: genetic testing (hereditary non-polyposis rectal cancer) Management: surgery (some scope for radiotherapy and chemotherapy)

Condition	Key points	'Red flags'	Management
Irritable bowel syndrome	Abdominal pain Mucous per rectum Related to mood/stress May be postinfectious Chronic course Check the ROME III criteria	Alternating diarrhoea and constipation	Reassurance: in 50%, symptoms improve by 1 year Explore food allergies Constipation: ispaghula, methylcellulose Diarrhoea: fibre, loperamide Bloating: mebeverine Proton pump inhibitor Amytriptyline
Pregnancy	Missed period(s) History of unprotected intercourse Poor compliance with OCP Drug interaction with OCP (e.g. antibiotics and OCP)		Folic acid Follow-up in antenatal clinic
Splenomegaly	See Chapter 3 on abdominal examination		
Hepatomegaly	See Chapter 3 on abdominal examination		
Ascites	See Chapter 3 on abdominal examination		
Abdominal aortic aneurysm	Abdominal/back pain Pulsatile Expansile	Trauma Peripheral vascular disease Risk factors for atheroma	See Chapter 14 on arterial examination
Pelvic mass	Fibroids Bladder Fetus Ovarian cyst/malignancy	Cannot get below it on palpation	Pelvic ultrasound Refer to gynaecologist
Renal cell carcinoma	Haematuria Flank pain Abdominal mass	Generalised symptoms Left varicocele	Bloods: full blood count, Us + Es, alkaline phosphatase, erythrocyte sedimentation rate Urine microscopy and cytology Imaging: renal ultrasound, CT/MRI, chest X-ray, IVU Surgery Robson Staging

Hints and tips for the exam

Remember the '5 Fs and 1 T' of abdominal distension (Figure 31.1)

- Fat (hypothyroidism, Cushing's disease)
- Fluid (is this ascites?)
- Faeces (constipation, obstruction – is it complete?)
- Flatus (complete obstruction, food intolerance, irritable bowel syndrome)
- Fetus (pregnancy test)
- Tumour

Women's health

The sex of the patient will help rule out a number of pathologies that only affect women. If your patient is

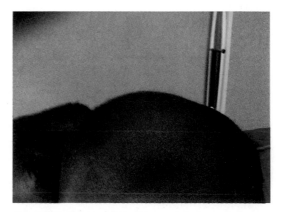

Figure 31.1 Abdominal distension

female, remember to ask about her last menstrual period and the likelihood that she is pregnant. When discussing management with the examiner, remember in your list of investigations to mention offering a pregnancy test. All women of child-bearing age with abdominal symptoms should be offered a pregnancy test. This should also be done before any radiological investigations such as an abdominal X-ray.

Elderly + bloating = high possibility of malignancy

An elderly patient should make you consider malignant processes first and aim to rule these in or out. Both colorectal and ovarian pathology can cause bloating – although constipation is quite often the underlying cause.

Acute causes

One of the aims in your history will be to assess the urgency of the situation. Is the patient in urinary retention? Does the patient have a toxic dilatation of the colon (megacolon) or are they just constipated? Know the 'red flag' signs for acute abdominal conditions.

The chronology of the symptoms is important, so make sure you are comfortable in terms of which came first (e.g. vomiting shortly after eating – high gastrointestinal obstruction; vomiting some time after eating – small bowel obstruction; constipation followed by vomiting (bilious and later faeculant) – lower gastrointestinal obstruction).

An important question commonly forgotten is to ask when the patient last opened their bowels and also if there has been a change. Be sure also to differentiate simple constipation from absolute constipation by asking whether, in addition to not passing stool, they have passed any wind. If not, this may suggest complete obstruction.

Differentiating between small bowel and large bowel obstruction on abdominal X-ray

- Small bowel:
  - Prominent loops of bowel in the centre of the abdomen
  - Valvulae conniventes that cross the entire width of the small bowel
  - No gas in the large bowel
- Large bowel:
  - Prominent bowel in the periphery of abdomen
  - Haustra do not cross the entire width of the bowel
  - There is no air distal to the obstruction

- Remember to look for loops of bowel in the hernial orifices.

Ascites – transudates versus exudates

Abdominal distension caused by fluid has a broad differential diagnosis. Fluid may collect in the peritoneal cavity or in the bowel (e.g. third-space losses as a result of obstruction or ileus). Hence the patient may have symptoms of dehydration such as a dry mouth, thirst and light-headedness. Distension may be a sign of fluid overload so be sure to ask about swelling of the ankles, orthopnoea and paroxysmal nocturnal dyspnoea.

Ascites is the term used to describe fluid in the abdominal peritoneal cavity. The most common cause is cirrhosis of the liver. When discussing the causes in your OSCE, subdivide them into transudative and exudative causes (see the table). The key investigation here is an **ascitic tap/drain.** This is both *diagnostic* (as it should be sent for microscopy, culture, sensitivity and cytology) and *therapeutic* (by offloading fluid to reduce discomfort).

In conjunction with ascites, a fever may signify spontaneous bacterial peritonitis (diagnosed by finding $>250/mm^3$ neutrophils). This is an emergency and requires antibiotic therapy.

Transudate	Exudate
<25 g/L protein	>35 g/L protein
Due to low oncotic pressure (resulting from low protein levels) or high hydrostatic pressure (e.g. right heart failure)	Local infection or inflammation
Causes	**Causes**
Cirrhosis (alcoholic liver disease)	Cancer
Heart failure	Infection – tuberculosis, spontaneous bacterial peritonitis
Constrictive pericarditis	Pancreatitis
Fluid overload	Serositis (inflammation)
Nephrotic syndrome	Budd–Chiari syndrome (hepatic vein obstruction due to thrombosis or tumour)
Malabsorption	
Hypothyroidism	
Meigs syndrome (pleural effusion secondary to ovarian fibroma)	

Splenomegaly and hepatomegaly

See Chapter 3 (abdominal examination).

Questions you could be asked

Q. What signs might you see on an examination of bowel obstruction?

A. • Distressed patient
  • Protuberant abdomen
  • Surgical scars
  • Hyperresonant percussion note
  • Tinkling bowel sounds on auscultation (absent bowel sounds may indicate ischaemia)
  • Signs of peritonism (rigid abdomen, guarding, rebound tenderness)
  • Signs of hypovolaemia and/or shock

Q. How would you differentiate between small bowel and large bowel obstruction on an abdominal X-ray?

A. The answer can be found in the text above.

Q. What are the key investigations in liver failure (cirrhosis)?

A. • Blood:
    • Liver function tests:
      • Aspartate aminotransferase, alanine aminotransferase, alkaline phosphatase, gamma glutamyl transferase (all raised early)
      • Albumin (lowered), International Normalised Ratio (raised due to reduction in liver-derived clotting factors: II, VII, IX, X) – these indicate the synthetic function of the liver and are deranged later in the course of disease
  • Liver ultrasound and duplex scan
  • Ascitic tap: microscopy, culture and sensitivity, cytology
  • Liver biopsy

Q. Describe what is involved in post-splenectomy prophylaxis?

A. • After splenectomy, patients are susceptible to infection, especially by encapsulated organisms.
  • Vaccination 2 weeks prior to elective splenectomy or at the next opportunity after an emergency splenectomy (e.g. rupture).
  • Vaccines should be given: *Haemophilus influenzae* type B, pneumococcus, meningitis C
  • Lifelong penicillin V

  • Advice on symptoms of serious infection.
  • MedicAlert bracelet.

Q. Outline the Duke's staging criteria for colorectal carcinoma.

A. • Remember the layers of the bowel wall:
    • Mucosa (innermost)
    • Submucosa
    • Muscularis propria
    • Serosa
  • Mention that staging is now usually by the TNM classification.

Dukes staging

Stage	Criteria	5-year survival after treatment
A	Beneath muscularis mucosae	90%
B	Through muscularis mucosae (no nodes)	65%
C	Positive lymph nodes	30%
D	Metastases	<10%

Q. Describe the NHS bowel cancer screening programme.

A. • All men and women between 60 and 69 years of age are seen.
  • Individuals are sent a home faecal occult blood kit.

Q. What is a colonoscopy, and what are the possible complications of the procedure?

A. • An endoscope is passed via the rectum to visualise the entire large colon.
  • It can be an outpatient or a day case.
  • Laxative is used the day before, both morning and night (sodium picosulfate).
  • Sedation is necessary (patients will need someone to take them home).
  • The procedure takes around 45 minutes.
  • A biopsy can be taken.
  • Complications are discomfort, bloating and bleeding after biopsy.

32 Haematemesis

Checklist	P	MP	F
Appropriate introduction			
Confirms patient's name and age			
Explains reason for consultation			
Obtains consent			
Open question to elicit presenting complaint			
Allows patient to open up, listens carefully, remains silent and does not interrupt the patient			
Signposts: e.g. 'Mr Gregory, thank you for telling me about this problem. I would like to ask a few more detailed questions. Is that all right?'			
History of presenting complaint:			
• Volume: **If large volume, patient needs to be assessed and resuscitated immediately** • Number of episodes • Character/colour: • Coffee grounds • Dark clots • Fresh, bright red • Mixed with vomitus • Onset (what brought it on): • Medications, alcohol • Vomiting/retching (Mallory–Weiss tear) • Precipitating factors: • Alcohol → Mallory-Weiss tear • NSAIDs • Melaena • Abdominal/chest pain • Symptoms of shock (faintness, shortness of breath) • Trauma to abdomen • Asks if patient is suffering from any other symptoms • Asks about any recent illnesses • Previous episodes of haematemesis			
Associated symptoms: • Bleeding, bruising elsewhere, epistaxis • Anaemia (lethargy, shortness of breath) • Dysphagia, odynophagia • Vomiting • Liver/hepatic symptoms: • Right upper quadrant pain • Jaundice • Ankle swelling			

	P	MP	F
'Red flags': • Weight loss, loss of appetite • Dysphagia			
Review of systems			
Past medical history: • Gastro-oesophageal reflux disease • Peptic ulcer • Liver problems, viral hepatitis, varices • Bleeding/clotting disorders			
Family history: • Oesophageal/stomach cancer • Osler–Weber–Rendu disease (telangiectasia)			
Drug history: • NSAIDs • Warfarin • Bisphosphonates • Steroids • Over-the-counter medication			
Allergies			
Social history: • Smoking • Alcohol • Illicit drug use • Ethnicity (haemophilia) • Diet (spicy foods) • Activities of daily living			
Use of non-verbal cues, e.g. good eye contact, nodding head and good body posture			
Systematic approach			
Explores and responds to ICE: • Ideas • Concerns • Expectations			
Shows empathy			
Non-verbal skills			
Avoids technical jargon			
Devises holistic management plan and addresses psychosocial issues as well as medical problems			
Summarises			
Offers to answer any questions			
Thanks patient			

Summary of common conditions seen in OSCEs

Condition	Key points	Management*
Oesophageal varices	Due to portosystemic shunting of blood Other shunts: • Caput medusae (veins around umbilicus) • Rectal varices Causes: • Cirrhosis • Schistosomiasis	Banding Sclerotherapy Balloon tamponade Transjugular intrahepatic portosystemic shunt Portocaval shunt (rare)
Peptic ulcer	Pain related to eating: • Before meals and relieved by eating: duodenal ulcer (four times more common) • Worse after eating: gastric ulcer Peritonism if perforated (**pain**, rigid abdomen) Weight loss Risk factors: • *Helicobacter pylori* • Smoking • Drugs (NSAIDs, aspirin, steroids)	Lifestyle interventions Stop NSAIDs and other offending medications if possible Eradicate *H. pylori*[†] Reduce acid production (proton pump inhibitor – omeprazole; H2 agonists – ranitidine)
Inflammation (oesophagitis, gastritis)	Alcohol Drugs (NSAIDs, corrosive ingestion) Smoking Infection (immunocompromised – HIV)	Address causative issue
Mallory–Weiss tear	Longitudinal tear in oesophageal mucosa due to forceful vomiting Alcohol binge Eating disorder	Conservative: most will have stopped bleeding and heal themselves Medical: reduce acid production (proton pump inhibitor), antiemetic (prochloperazine), endoscopy Surgical: few require oversewing of the tear
Oesophageal cancer	Risk factors: diet, alcohol, smoking, Barrett's oesophagus, achalasia, Plummer–Vinson syndrome (iron-deficiency anaemia + postcricoid web + glossitis) Dysphagia Weight loss	Multidisciplinary team Preoperative chemotherapy Surgery Palliation
Gastric cancer	Risk factors: pernicious anaemia, smoking, high-nitrate diets – Japan, blood group A Dyspepsia Weight loss Anaemia Vomiting	Multidisciplinary team Partial or total gastrectomy Chemotherapy Palliation
Bleeding diathesis	Any bleeding disorder. May be the result of anticoagulation	Treat cause
Trauma		
Dieulafoy lesion	Large arteriole in the stomach wall that erodes and bleeds	Endoscopic injection and sclerotherapy
Boerhaave's syndrome	Oesophageal rupture due to vomiting	Surgery
Peutz–Jegher syndrome	Dark freckles on the lips, and gastrointestinal polyps that can bleed	Conservative Surgery
Osler–Weber–Rendu disease	Autosomal dominant Also known as hereditary haemorrhagic telangiectasia Telangiectasias on skin and mucous membranes	
Aorto-enteric fistula	Aortic graft repair + upper/lower gastrointestinal bleed	CT abdomen Endoscopy

40% of patients referred for upper gastrointestinal endoscopy for haematemesis have no identifiable cause of bleeding.
*Remember that the management of all these conditions begins with resuscitation (**a**irway, **b**reathing and **c**irculation).
[†]*Helicobacter pylori* eradication: 7-day regime comprising a proton pump inhibitor (e.g. omeprazole 20 mg twice daily) and two antibiotics (e.g. metronidazole, amoxicillins, clarithromycin). See the *BNF* for further details.

Hints and tips for the exam

Before attempting to practise this station, make sure you have a sound knowledge of the causes of haematemesis, how to differentiate between them and the early management of the condition. The station is likely to be set in an emergency department so remember to address resuscitation first; you can state this on entering the station before beginning the history. One way to give your differential diagnosis for haematemesis is to group by region of bleeding (e.g. oesophageal, gastric, duodenal).

Make sure it is definitely haematemesis

As always begin with an open question. An important point of call in the history is to delineate whether the patient has experienced haematemesis or haemoptysis. They are similar in presentation but have different differential diagnoses. Be clear and ask whether the patient coughed up (haemoptysis) or vomited the blood.

Aim early on to comfort the patient as vomiting blood is undoubtedly a very worrying symptom. Gaining the patient's trust early on will make the station smoother and also earn their preference marks. Ask early on whether they have any questions as cancer is a common worry; marks will be awarded for addressing patients' anxieties. Not addressing the patient's agenda is a common error in such a station when faced with a possible emergency.

Don't forget the blood in your blood tests!

Students often forget to 'group and save' and/or cross-match.

Group and save (also known as 'group and hold' and 'type and screen')

• The patient's blood is tested to determine the ABO type and the rhesus D status. It can also be tested for antibodies to red cells in the serum (e.g. anti-A, anti-B, anti-D or anti-Duffy).
• This test is indicated if a blood transfusion will be necessary in the near future, for example postoperatively.
• The sample is kept in the laboratory for a few days.
• On collection, the bottles should be completely filled and hand-labelled.

Cross-match

• This is used if there is an imminent need for transfusion.
• The patient's blood is tested for ABO and antibodies (as in group and save).
• The patient's blood is tested against the donor sample to assess whether they are compatible.

Risk-scoring systems

Know about the risk scoring scales for upper gastrointestinal bleeding and aim to elicit the relevant aspects from the history (see below). If you are able to give a Rockall score in your summary and hence an indication for rebleeding, endoscopy or surgery, this will separate you from other candidates and guide the examiner to question you on this, which you should be prepared for.

The Rockall scoring system was devised to predict the **risk of rebleeding** in patients presenting with upper gastrointestinal bleeds, and to help estimate mortality. Remember that the greatest risk of rebleeding exists is in the **first 48 hours**, so bear this in mind when considering whether or not to admit the patient.

A common presentation in this station is of bleeding oesophageal varices due to chronic liver disease. Hence, it is fundamental that you assess possible causes of chronic liver disease (e.g. alcohol, medications, viral hepatitis) in your history. It is important that you are also aware of the **Child–Pugh grading system** and how to calculate it. This is a score used to grade the severity of liver cirrhosis and the likelihood of variceal bleeding – a score >8 indicates a high risk of bleeding.

You should bear the criteria in mind when you are asked which blood tests you would like to run. The scoring is outlined in the table. Binge drinking is often associated with Mallory–Weiss tears so remember to ask about the patient's drinking habits (e.g. do they drink 'binge drink' on the weekend and not drink on weekdays?, etc.) in addition to how much they drink (with respect to quantity). Do **not** waste time assessing dependency (i.e. applying a CAGE questionnaire) – this is not the aim of this station.

Rockall score for upper gastrointestinal bleed

A score >6 may indicate a need for surgery.

	Points			
	0	1	2	3
Before endoscopy				
Age (years)	<60	60–79	>80	
Systolic blood pressure and heart rate	>100 mmHg <100/min	>100 mmHg >100/min	<100 mmHg	
Co-morbidity		Heat failure Ischaemic heart disease	Kidney failure Liver failure	Metastases
After endoscopy				
Diagnosis	1. Mallory–Weiss tears, idiopathic 2. Potentially any cause 3. Malignancy	Everything else	Malignancy	
Signs of recent bleeding	None		Blood, clot, vessel	

Child–Pugh grading for cirrhosis and variceal bleeding

	Points		
	1	2	3
Bilirubin (μmol/L)	<34	34–51	>51
Albumin (g/L)	>35	28–35	<28
Prothrombin time (number of seconds longer than normal)	1–3	4–6	>6
Ascites	None	Slight	Moderate
Encephalopathy grade	None	1–2	3–4

Kings College Hospital criteria for liver transplantation

Paracetamol-related	Not paracetamol-related
• Arterial pH < 7.3 24 hours after ingestion	• Prothrombin time >100 s
OR all of the below:	OR **three** of the criteria listed below:
• Prothrombin time >100 s	• Drug-induced liver failure
• Creatinine >300 μmol/L	• Age <10 or >40 years
• Grade 3–4 encephalopathy	• >1 week from jaundice to encephalopathy
	• Prothrombin time >50 s
	• Bilirubin >300 μmol/L

Questions you could be asked

Q. How would you investigate and manage this patient?

Q. What is their Rockall Score? What does it mean?

Q. When would you refer the patient for an endoscopy? How urgently? (Start with the golden phrase: 'I would consult the local hospital guidelines.')

Q. Describe the endoscopy procedure.

A. Answers to these questions can be found in the text above.

Other possible topics include:
• Questions related to managing shock (e.g. parameters and appropriate fluids)
• Transfusion reactions
• Liver disease
• Liver transplant (the King's College Transplant Criteria are included in the text)

33 Rectal bleeding

Checklist	P	MP	F
Appropriate introduction			
Confirms patient's name and age			
Explains reason for consultation			
Obtains consent			
Open question to elicit presenting complaint			
Allows patient to open up, listens carefully, remains silent and does not interrupt the patient			
Signposts: e.g. 'Mr Gregory, thank you for telling me about this problem. I would like to ask a few more detailed questions. Is that all right?'			
History of presenting complaint:			
• Site:			
• Mixed with stool			
• Around stool			
• Dripping from anus			
• Spotting on tissue paper			
• Onset (what brought it on)			
• Character:			
• Fresh, bright red			
• Dark, melaena			
• Clots			
• Liquid			
• Mucus			
• Smell – offensive			
• Time:			
• Duration			
• Intermittent, continuous, progressive			
• Alleviating factors			
• Exacerbating factors:			
• Dietary factors			
• Constipation (fissure)			
• Anal intercourse			
• Foreign bodies, sexual devices			
• Amount, volume			
• Frequency			
• Trauma			
• Straining when opens bowels			
• Asks if patient is suffering from any other symptoms			
• Asks about any recent illnesses			
• Previous episodes of rectal bleeding			
• Family members/contacts with similar symptoms			

Asks about other colorectal/anal symptoms:			
• Pain/soreness			
• Itching			
• Tenesmus			
• Lumps, swellings, piles			
• Rectal prolapse			
• Change of bowel habit:			
• Constipation			
• Diarrhoea			
• Frequency of opening bowels			
• Faecal incontinence			
• Abdominal pain			
• Symptoms of inflammatory bowel disease:			
• Blood			
• Arthralgia			
• Back pain (sacroiliitis)			
• Oral ulcers			
• Skin problems:			
• Pyoderma gangrenosum			
• Erythema nodosum			
• Eye pain			
• Symptoms of anaemia			
• Lethargy			
• Shortness of breath			
• Dizziness – postural			
'Red flags':			
• Weight loss			
• Loss of appetite			
Review of systems:			
• Bleeding elsewhere (vomiting, ears, bruising, epistaxis)			
Past medical history:			
• Any bowel disorders			
• Any rectal disorders			
• Polyps			
• Recent anorectal surgery			
• Radiotherapy (for radiation colitis)			
• Constipation			
Family history:			
• Colorectal cancer			
• Colorectal polyps			
• Haemorrhoids			
• Inflammatory bowel disease			
• Angiodysplasia			

Drug history:			
• NSAIDs			
• Warfarin			
• Over-the-counter medication			
Allergies			
Social history:			
• Recent foreign travel/foreign contacts			
• Diet:			
• Recent changes			
• Lack of high-fibre foods			
• Takeaways			
• Barbecues			
• Smoking			
• Alcohol			
• Activities of daily living			
Use of non-verbal cues, e.g. good eye contact, nodding head and good body posture			

Systematic approach			
Explores and responds to ICE:			
• Ideas			
• Concerns			
• Expectations			
Shows empathy			
Non-verbal skills			
Avoids technical jargon			
Devises a holistic management plan and addresses psychosocial issues as well as medical problems			
Summarises			
Offers to answer any questions			
Thanks patient			

Summary of common conditions seen in OSCEs

Condition	Key symptoms	Investigations	Treatment
Upper gastrointestinal tract cancer	Melaena – black tarry stool Characteristic foul smell	Oesophago-gastro-duodenoscopy Full blood count CT chest, abdomen and pelvis for staging	Blood transfusion if anaemic Surgical resection or chemotherapy
Colorectal cancer	If source of bleeding is after terminal ileum, bleeding is more likely to be fresh/red rather than melaena	Colonoscopy Full blood count CT chest, abdomen and pelvis for staging	Blood transfusion if anaemic Surgical resection or chemotherapy
Distal rectal tumour	Fresh red bleeding/red blood mixed with stool	Full blood count Sigmoidoscopy Colonoscopy CT, MRI, liver ultrasound scan for staging	Abdominoperineal resection if less than 8–10 cm from the anus
Haemorrhoids	Protruding tissue from the anus Fresh red blood drips, often separate from the stool	Proctoscopy	Conservative: increase dietary fibre and fluid intake Medical: topical anaesthetic, band ligation Surgery NB. Treatment of acutely thrombosed external piles is conservative if the patient presents after 72 hours of symptoms. If they present within 72 hours of the start of symptoms, best treatment is surgical repair/excision

(Continued)

Condition	Key symptoms	Investigations	Treatment
Anal fissure	Severe pain on defecation Streaks of blood often around stool	Rectal examination Proctoscopy Examination under anaesthesia if required	Classified as acute if present for <4–6 weeks: • Conservative: dietary advice • Medical: bulk-forming laxatives, lubricants prior to defecation, topical anaesthetic Classified as chronic if present for >4–6 weeks: In addition to treatment for acute fissure: • Topical GTN • Refer for surgery if GTN ineffective at 8–10 weeks
Inflammatory bowel disease (ulcerative colitis and Crohn's disease)	Young Blood and mucus in stool Systemic symptoms of inflammatory bowel disease: • Arthralgia • Back pain (sacroileitis) • Oral ulcers • Skin problems: • Pyoderma gangrenosum • Erythema nodosum • Eye pain	Colonoscopy and biopsy Barium studies Erythrocyte sedimentation rate	See Chapter 3 on abdominal examination
Bleeding/clotting disorders	Bleeding elsewhere: • Haematuria • Bleeding gums • Bruising	Full blood count International Normalised Ratio Blood film	Transfuse if anaemic Replace platelets if necessary Vitamin K if International Normalised Ratio is high

Hints and tips for the exam

Be sensitive

Patients are often reluctant to discuss rectal bleeding as they see it as a topic that is both intimate to them as well as somewhat unpleasant to discuss. This is why it is important to spend some time putting the patient at ease, expressing empathy, exploring their ideas and concerns, and reassuring them that it is a common complaint and that you are used to seeing patients with it.

Type of bleeding

This is fundamental to locating the site of the bleeding (see the table).

Characteristics of rectal bleeding	Location of source of bleeding
Melaena	Colon proximal to terminal ileum
Red blood mixed with stool or coating stool	Colon distal to terminal ileum
Fresh red blood dripping separately from stool	Anus (e.g. fissure) or haemorrhoid

Remember to take a general gastroenterological history

It can be easy to take a history that focuses on the anorectal area. Remember, however, that many serious causes of rectal bleeding (such as inflammatory bowel disease and colon cancer) could result in pathology elsewhere in the gastrointestinal tract, so it is important that you enquire about the entire gastroenterological system and any 'red flags' that may be unrelated to the presenting complaint (such as weight loss).

Questions you could be asked

Q. Above which point in the gastrointestinal tract does bleeding cause melaena (as opposed to fresh red bleeding)?

A. Although there is no specific point immediately after which fresh red blood suddenly becomes melaena, generally speaking bleeding from an area **proximal to the terminal ileum is more likely to be melaena**, as there is scope for significant 'digestion' in that part of the gastrointestinal tract.

Q. How would you manage a bleeding haemorrhoid?

A. See the chapter text.

34 Jaundice

Checklist	P	MP	F
Appropriate introduction			
Confirms patient's name and age			
Explain reason for consultation			
Obtains consent			
Open question to elicit presenting complaint			
Allows patient to open up, listens carefully, remains silent and does not interrupt the patient			
Signposts: e.g. 'Mr Gregory, thank you for telling me about this problem. I would like to ask a few more detailed questions. Is that all right?'			
History of presenting complaint:			

• How was the jaundice discovered – did the patient notice it, or was it someone else?
 • Onset (what brought it on, how it started)
 • Time:
  • Duration
  • Intermittent (e.g. Gilbert's syndrome), continuous, progressive
 • Fevers
 • Asks if patient is suffering from any other symptoms
 • Asks about any recent illnesses
 • Previous episodes of jaundice
 • Family members/contacts with similar symptoms			

Asks about other relevant symptoms:
 • Gallstones, biliary duct obstruction:
  • Abdominal pain
  • Pale stools
  • Itching
  • Steatorrhoea
  • Dark urine
 • Liver symptoms:
  • Abdominal swelling
  • Ankle swelling
  • Bleeding, bruising (liver failure and impaired synthetic function)
 • Autoimmune conditions:
  • Arthralgia
  • Vitiligo
  • Skin rashes (systemic lupus erythematosus)			

	P	MP	F

• Risk factors for viral hepatitis
  • Hepatitis B and C
  • Contaminated needles:
   • Intravenous drug abuse
   • Blood transfusions (and any transfusions outside the UK)
   • Tattoos
   • Ear/body-piercing
   • Needlestick injuries (if healthcare professional)
  • Foreign travel/contacts
  • Sexual history:
   • **Must signpost and gain explicit consent for this**
   • Number of sexual partners
   • New sexual partners
   • Type of intercourse (anal, oral, vaginal)
   • Use of barrier contraception
  • Hepatitis A
  • Swimming, diving
 • Pregnancy (HELLP, intrahepatic cholestasis of pregnancy)
 • Heart failure			

'Red flags': • **No** abdominal pain • Weight loss			
Review of systems			
Past medical history: • Previous jaundice • Autoimmune conditions (for primary biliary cirrhosis and autoimmune hepatitis) • Haemolytic anaemia • Heart failure (for congestive liver failure) • Inflammatory bowel disease (for primary sclerosing cholangitis)			
Family history: • Viral hepatitis • Autoimmune hepatitis • Hepatobiliary cancer			

Drug history:
- Hepatitis B and C immunisations
- Antibiotics
- Statins
- Antiepileptics
- Paracetamol
- Tuberculosis medications
- Cytotoxic agents
- Herbal medication
- Over-the-counter medication

Allergies

Social history:
- Alcohol intake
- Recent foreign travel/foreign contacts:
  - Jaundice in other members of the travelling party
  - Water consumed (mineral water, tap water, boiled water)
- Diet:
  - Recent changes
  - Takeaways
  - Barbecues
- Smoking
- Intravenous drug abuse (as above)

Use of non-verbal cues, e.g. good eye contact, nodding head and good body posture

Systematic approach

Explores and responds to ICE:
- Ideas
- Concerns
- Expectations

Shows empathy

Non-verbal skills

Avoids technical jargon

Devises holistic management plan and addresses psychosocial issues as well as medical problems

Summarises

Offers to answer any questions

Thanks patient

Summary of common conditions seen in OSCEs

Underlying mechanism	Condition	Bilirubin in blood		Bilirubin in urine	Liver function tests	Haemoglobin
		Unconjugated	Conjugated			
Prehepatic	Haemolysis Thalassaemia Haematological malignancies Gilbert's syndrome	↑	↔	Nil	↔	↓
Hepatic	Any liver causes (see Chapter 3 on abdominal examination)	↑	↔	Nil	↑ (AST > ALP)	↔
Obstructive	Gallstones Cholangitis Primary sclerosing cholangitis Biliary atresia Lymphadenopathy around inferior aspect of liver Benign cyst Cholangiocarcinoma Pancreatic cancer Duodenal cancer	↔	↑	↑	↑ (ALP > AST)	↔

Hints and tips for the exam

Many of the causes of jaundice have been covered in the 'abdominal examination' station (Chapter 3), so we have not discussed them at any great length here.

Jaundice is yellow pigmentation of the skin and occurs when the serum bilirubin level exceeds 35 μmol/L. There are many causes of jaundice, so familiarise yourself with the common ones and know what questions to ask as well as the relevant investigations. The causes of jaundice can be divided into prehepatic, hepatic and obstructive.

Taking a thorough social history, including the use of recreational drugs and needle-sharing, as well as a sexual history, is fundamental to this station. Remember to signpost before you ask these questions, for example 'I would now like to ask you some personal questions/questions of an intimate nature/questions about your personal life to find the cause of this problem. Is that all right?'

Questions you could be asked

Q. Which type of jaundice would cause a raised urinary urobilinogen level?
A. Prehepatic jaundice.
Q. What is one of the most common non-fatal causes of jaundice and splenomegaly?
A. Hereditary spherocytosis.
Q. What are the most common hepatic causes of jaundice, and what investigations would you utilise to find a cause?
A. See Chapter 3 on abdominal examination.

35 Dysphagia

Checklist	P	MP	F
Appropriate introduction			
Confirms patient's name and age			
Explain reason for consultation			
Obtains consent			
Open question to elicit presenting complaint			
Allows patient to open up, listens carefully, remains silent and does not interrupt the patient			
Signposts: e.g. 'Mr Gregory, thank you for telling me about this problem. I would like to ask a few more detailed questions. Is that all right?'			
History of presenting complaint			

• Onset (how it started):
   • Sudden
   • Gradual
 • Character:
   • Fluids
   • Solids
 • Time:
   • Duration
   • Intermittent, continuous, progressive
 • Level: where does food/liquid feel like it is getting 'stuck' – throat/gullet/stomach
 • Alleviating factors
 • Exacerbating factors
 • Define at which stage the dysphagia occurs:
   • When initiating swallowing
   • After swallowing has been initiated
 • Pain (oesophageal/abdominal), odynophagia
 • Trauma, foreign body
 • Feeling of a lump in the throat
 • Asks if patient is suffering from any other symptoms
 • Asks about any recent illnesses
 • Previous episodes of dysphagia
 • Family members/contacts with similar symptoms			

Associated symptoms:
 • Gastrointestinal:
   • Nausea, vomiting
   • Dyspepsia
 • ENT:
   • Hoarseness
   • Speech problems
 • Neuromuscular:
   • Motor weakness, muscle wasting
   • Sensory symptoms
   • Diplopia
 • Pharyngeal pouch:
   • Regurgitation
   • Halitosis
 • Mitral stenosis, left atrial hypertrophy:
   • Palpitations, symptoms of congestive cardiac failure
   • Haemoptysis
 • Thyroid gland symptoms:
   • Neck discomfort
   • Symptoms of hyperthyroidism
 • Lung cancer symptoms:
   • Cough, weight loss, haemoptysis
 • Xerostomia:
   • Dry mouth			

'Red flags': • Weight loss • Loss of appetite • Haematemesis, melaena • Progressive and persistent			
Review of systems			
Past medical history: • Stroke • Thyroid problems • Mitral stenosis • ENT surgery			
Family history: • Upper gastrointestinal tract cancer			
Drug history: • NSAIDs • Bisphosphonates			
Allergies			

Social history: • Alcohol (peptic ulcer disease, gastritis) • Smoking • Illicit drug use • Diet: spicy foods (peptic ulcer disease) • Occupation • Activities of daily living			
Use of non-verbal cues, e.g. good eye contact, nodding head and good body posture			
Systematic approach			
Explores and responds to ICE: • Ideas • Concerns • Expectations			

Shows empathy			
Non-verbal skills			
Avoids technical jargon			
Devises holistic management plan and addresses psychosocial issues as well as medical problems			
Summarises			
Offers to answer any questions			
Thanks patient			

Summary of common conditions seen in OSCEs

System	Conditions	Key investigations
Neurological	Stroke Bulbar palsy Myasthenia gravis Motor neurone disease Parkinson's disease	CT/MRI brain Electromyogram Acetyl choline receptor antibodies, CT thymus
ENT	Throat cancer Pharyngeal pouch	Nasal endoscopy
Xerostomia/Sjögren's syndrome	Dry mouth Symptoms of rheumatological disorders	Schirmer's test Anti-Ro and anti-La antibodies
Oesophageal: motility	Achalasia CREST Chagas disease	Barium swallow Oesophageal manometry Serology for Chagas disease Scl-70, anticentromere and antinuclear antibodies for CREST
Oesophageal: structural	Malignancy Benign stricture Hiatus hernia	Barium swallow Oesophago-gastro-duodenoscopy + biopsy Full blood count
Gastrointestinal	Stomach cancer Gastritis Gastro-oesophageal reflux disease Peptic ulcer	Oesophago-gastro-duodenoscopy
External compression: thyroid	Goitre Thyroid cancer	Fine-needle aspiration + biopsy Ultrasound neck/thyroid Thyroid function tests Radioiodine studies
External compression: heart	Mitral stenosis Left atrial hypertrophy Aortic aneurysm	Echocardiogram Chest X-ray CT chest
External compression: lungs	Lung cancer	Chest X-ray CT chest
External compression: mediastinum	Mediastinal lymphadenopathy	Chest X-ray CT chest
Globus hystericus	Anxiety Psychological symptoms	Rule out organic causes

Hints and tips for the exam

Malnutrition

Dysphagia is a very concerning symptom, and it is understandable for any candidate to get fixated on the diagnosis and treatment. Do not, however, forget that eating is essential for a patient's health and well-being, and a patient who is unable to eat may start to suffer from the effects of malnourishment if dysphagia is severe and prolonged. This is especially so in the elderly. So, in your management plan, make sure you talk about the importance of carrying out a nutritional assessment of the patient, and about considering ways of managing it while a definitive diagnosis and management plan are established. You could consider liquid supplements such as Ensure (if the patient is able to take liquids), as well as nasogastric and PEG feeding.

Liquids or solids or both?

This is often forgotten by students despite being absolutely fundamental to the diagnosis. Patients who have dysphagia for both solids and liquids are more likely to have a problem with motility (e.g. achalasia), whereas patients with dysphagia only for solids are more likely to have a structural defect (e.g. cancer or a mass).

Questions you could be asked

Q. What changes associated with dysphagia might you see on barium swallow?
A. 'Tapering' with achalasia, or an 'apple core lesion' with oesophageal cancer.
Q. What is 'Chagas disease'?
A. An infectious disease predominantly found in South America. As it is an infectious disease, the investigation of choice is microscopy, culture and sensitivity of the blood or cerebrospinal fluid. It is treated with an antiparasitic agent.

36 Headache

Checklist	P	MP	F
Appropriate introduction			
Confirms the patient's name and age			
Explains reason for consultation			
Obtains consent			
Open question to elicit presenting complaint			
Allows patient to open up, listens carefully, remains silent and does not interrupt the patient			
Signposts: e.g. 'Mr Gregory, thank you for telling me about this problem. I would like to ask a few more detailed questions. Is that all right?'			
History of presenting complaint:			

- Site:
  - Unilateral (migraine)
  - Scalp or temporal (temporal arteritis)
  - Face/in front of ear (trigeminal neuralgia)
- Onset (how it started):
  - Sudden (subarachnoid haemorrhage)
  - Gradual
- Character:
  - Throbbing (migraine)
  - Dull
- Radiation:
  - To neck (subarachnoid haemorrhage)
- Time:
  - Duration of headaches
  - Duration of pain-free periods
  - Intermittent/continuous/progressive (raised intracranial pressure)
- Alleviating factors:
  - Darkness
- Exacerbating factors:
  - Touching scalp (temporal arteritis)
  - Worse in early morning (raised intracranial pressure)
  - Light (migraine, meningism)
- Severity
- Asks if patient is suffering from any other symptoms
- Asks about any recent illnesses
- Previous history of headaches

Associated symptoms:
- Raised intracranial pressure:
  - Nausea, vomiting (increased intracranial pressure)
  - Worse on straining/bending down/coughing
- Meningitis:
  - Fever
  - Photophobia
  - Neck stiffness
  - Haemorrhagic rash
- Subarachnoid haemorrhage:
  - Sudden onset (like being hit on the head with a cricket bat)
  - Occipital
  - 'Worst' pain the patient has ever had
- Temporal arteritis:
  - Scalp tenderness
  - Ipsilateral visual disturbance
  - Shoulder/hip muscle aches (polymyalgia rheumatica)
- Migraine:
  - Nausea, vomiting
  - Photophobia
  - Periodic (e.g. every month), correlation with menstrual periods
  - Visual disturbance (zigzag lines, flashing lights)
  - Aura
- Trigeminal neuralgia:
  - Like 'electric shock'
  - Short duration (seconds to a few minutes)
  - Face/in front of ear
  - Chewing makes it worse
- Cluster headache:
  - Pain around one eye
  - Lacrimation/eye watering
  - Excruciatingly severe
  - Attacks lasting 30–60 minutes persist for a few weeks to 1–2 months and then stop for 6–12 months
- Tension headache:
  - 'Tight' headache
  - Diffuse, not localised
  - Related to stress
- Chronic analgesic-dependent headaches:
  - Long-term extensive use of high-dose analgesics
  - Daily occurrence

'Red flags':
- Recent trauma
- Focal neurological symptoms, loss of consciousness, seizures
- Vomiting
- Worst in the morning/on waking up
- Sudden onset
- Fevers
- Scalp tenderness
- Past medical history of cancer

Review of systems

Past medical history:
- Malignancy
- Hypertension

Family history:
- Migraines
- Berry aneurysms, subarachnoid haemorrhage
- Malignancy

Drug history:
- Analgesics
- Oral contraceptive pill (contraindicated in certain types of migraine)
- Over-the-counter medication

Allergies

Social history:
- Alcohol (peptic ulcer disease, gastritis)
- Smoking
- Illicit drug use
- Caffeine intake
- Diet
- Occupation
- Effect of headaches on activities of daily living
- Stressors – financial, occupational, relationship

Use of non-verbal cues, e.g. good eye contact, nodding head and good body posture

Systematic approach

Explores and responds to ICE:
- Ideas
- Concerns
- Expectations

Shows empathy

Non-verbal skills

Avoids technical jargon

Devises holistic management plan and addresses psychosocial issues as well as medical problems

Summarises

Offers to answer any questions

Thanks patient

Summary of common conditions for OSCEs

Condition	Key points	Key investigations
Migraine	Nausea, vomiting Photophobia Periodic (e.g. every month), correlation with menstrual periods Visual disturbance (zigzag lines, flashing lights) Aura	None – clinical diagnosis
Tension headaches	'Tight' headache Diffuse, not localised Related to stress	None – clinical diagnosis
Meningitis	Fever Photophobia Neck stiffness Haemorrhagic rash	Lumbar puncture and cerebrospinal fluid analysis Microscopy, culture and sensitivity on blood sample
Trigeminal neuralgia	Like 'electric shock' Short duration (seconds to a few minutes) Face/in front of ear Chewing makes it worse	Could consider electrophysiological studies Largely a clinical diagnosis

Condition	Key points	Key investigations
Chronic analgesia overuse headaches	Long-term extensive use of high-dose analgesics Daily occurrence No 'red flags'	None – clinical diagnosis
Cluster headaches	Pain around one eye Lacrimation/eye watering Excruciatingly severe Attacks of 30–60 minutes persist for a few weeks to 1–2 months and then stop for 6–12 months	None – clinical diagnosis
Intracerebral haemorrhage	Recent trauma Features of raised ICP Subdural haemorrhage: • Acute or chronic • In chronic subdural haemorrhage, symptoms often fluctuate and could take days or weeks to develop • Common in elderly and alcoholic patients • Could result from relatively minor trauma Extradural haemorrhage: • Acute • Associated with more severe trauma and skull fractures	CT/MRI brain
Subarachnoid haemorrhage	Sudden onset (like being hit on the head with a cricket bat) Occipital 'Worst' pain the patient has ever had	Lumbar puncture and cerebrospinal fluid analysis CT brain
Increased intracranial pressure	Nausea, vomiting (increased intracranial pressure) Worse on straining/bending down/coughing Focal neurological signs History of malignancy	CT/MRI brain
Temporal arteritis	Scalp tenderness Ipsilateral visual disturbance Shoulder/hip muscle aches (polymyalgia rheumatica)	Temporal artery biopsy Erythrocyte sedimentation rate
Sinusitis	Pain and tenderness around temples/sinuses Recent upper respiratory tract infection	None – clinical diagnosis
Referred pain	Pain in teeth or temporomandibular joint	None – clinical diagnosis Rule out other causes

Hints and tips for the exam

Headaches are a very common presentation in both primary and secondary care settings. The history may be very vague, and unless you ask all the relevant questions you may miss a serious cause, especially with children and forgetful elderly patients. The importance of meticulously working through the acronyms and red flags cannot be underestimated.

Combined oral contraceptive pill and migraines

Always ask a woman with suspected migraines if she is taking the combined oral contraceptive pill as it may well be contraindicated, especially if she suffers from auras or focal neurological symptoms. If you are not sure, it is reasonable to tell the patient that you will check and get back to her, and to advise her to withhold the pill and use barrier contraception in the interim.

Don't forget trauma

Trauma is often forgotten by students, but is vitally important. A chronic subdural haemorrhage can present days after the initial trauma in alcoholics and elderly patients.

Questions you could be asked

Q. What are the cerebrospinal fluid findings after a subarachnoid haemorrhage?

A. Xanthochromia (4–5 hours after the episode), red blood cells and bilirubin.

Q. Give a non-bacterial cause of meningitis.

A. A fungal cause is *Cryptococcus*. Viral causes are Epstein–Barr virus, mumps, enterovirus and herpes virus.

37 Loss of consciousness

Checklist	P	MP	F
Appropriate introduction			
Confirms the patient's name and age			
Explains reason for consultation			
Obtains consent			
Open question to elicit presenting complaint			
Allows patient to open up, listens carefully, remains silent and does not interrupt the patient			
Signposts: e.g. 'Mr Gregory, thank you for telling me about this problem. I would like to ask a few more detailed questions. Is that all right?'			
History of presenting complaint:			
• **Expresses intent to get a collateral history from a witness** • **Defines the loss of consciousness:** • **Does the patient remember what happened when they were unconscious?** • **Could the patient see or hear anything while unconscious?** • Duration • Frequency • What was the patient doing prior to loss of consciousness? • Was the patient sitting, standing or lying flat? • Where was the patient? • Trauma to head • Fall • Symptoms before loss of consciousness • Dizziness: • Faintness • Vertigo • Lateral instability • Symptoms after loss of consciousness • Asks if patient is suffering from any other symptoms • Asks about any recent illnesses • Previous episodes of loss of consciousness			

Asks about other associated symptoms: • Seizure: • Tongue bitten • Urinary incontinence • Confusion (>30 minutes) after regaining consciousness • Aura ('feeling funny', smell of burning) • Neurological symptoms: • Headaches • Motor weakness • Sensory symptoms • Visual disturbance • Speech problems • Coordination/balance difficulties • Hypoglycaemia: • Sweating • Anxiety • Palpitations • Faintness • Vascular/hypotensive: postural • Vasovagal symptoms: • Crowded/warm environment • Nausea immediately prior to loss of consciousness • Short duration (<5 minutes) • Cardiovascular symptoms: • Chest pain • Palpitations • Carotid sinus hypersensitivity: after turning head • Micturition syncope: during or immediately after urination			
'Red flags': • Headache with features of raised intracranial pressure: • Early morning headaches • Vomiting • Worse on coughing/bending down/straining			
Review of systems			

Past medical history:
- Diabetes
- Seizures/epilepsy
- Febrile convulsions (during childhood)
- Cerebrovascular disease, strokes, transient ischaemic attacks
- Cardiovascular problems:
  - Aortic stenosis
  - Heart failure
  - Arrhythmias

Family history:
- Same as past medical history

Drug history:
- Diabetes medication or insulin
- Sedatives (e.g. benzodiazepines)
- Over-the-counter medication

Allergies

Social history:
- Alcohol
- Illicit drug use
- Smoking
- Occupation
- Driving
  - Activities of daily living – especially related to mobilisation and stairs if elderly

- Effect of symptoms on activities of daily living
- **Safety assessment if vulnerable** (e.g. lives alone, dangerous occupation, elderly)

Use of non-verbal cues, e.g. good eye contact, nodding head and good body posture

Systematic approach

Explores and responds to ICE:
- Ideas
- Concerns
- Expectations

Shows empathy

Non-verbal skills

Avoids technical jargon

Devises holistic management plan and addresses psychosocial issues as well as medical problems

Summarises

Offers to answer any questions

Thanks patient

Summary of common conditions seen in OSCEs

System	Condition	Key investigations
Cardiovascular	Aortic stenosis Arrhythmias (e.g. supraventricular tachycardia) Acute coronary syndrome	Echocardiogram 24-hour ECG
Respiratory	Pulmonary embolism	Ventilation–perfusion scan or CT pulmonary angiogram
Neurological	Brain tumour Seizure Stroke/transient ischaemic attack Trauma to head (causing contusion, intracerebral bleed)	CT/MRI of brain EEG Carotid Doppler scan (carotid stenosis)
Endocrine	Hypoglycaemia Addison's disease	Blood glucose Us + Es Serum cortisol/Synacthen test
Hypotensive	Vasovagal attack Heart failure Antihypertensive medications	Lying and standing blood pressure Tilt-table testing Echocardiogram
Haematological	Anaemia	Haemoglobin
Other	Carotid sinus hypersensitivity Micturition/cough syncope Anxiety, hyperventilation	

Hints and tips for the exam

Collateral/witness history

Both in clinical practice and for exams, an accurate history is invaluable in determining the cause of loss of consciousness and how to investigate it further. Patients may be able to give a good history of the events before and after losing consciousness, but they will not be able to tell you what happened during the episode itself. This is important as the actual period of unconsciousness may reveal clues about the underlying aetiology, such as jerking of the limbs in an epileptic seizure.

To demonstrate this to your examiner, ask the patient if anyone saw them while they were unconscious, and then ask whether they would mind you speaking to the witness later on. You could also ask the patient what any witnesses said about what the patient was doing the episode of unconsciousness.

Rare symptoms

• Beware of severe aortic stenosis as a cause of syncope or loss of consciousness – this is a poor prognostic sign as severe aortic stenosis can be associated with sudden death.
• Recurrent syncopal episodes can be a feature of myocardial infarction in elderly patients, who often do not present with typical chest pain.
• Syncope can be the first sign of a leaking abdominal aortic aneurysm.

Questions you could be asked

Q. What are the regulations for driving after an episode of loss of consciousness?
A. See the official DVLA guidelines, which can be downloaded from www.dft.gov.uk/dvla/medical/ataglance.aspx.

38 Tremor

Checklist	P	MP	F
Appropriate introduction			
Confirms patient's name and age			
Explain reason for consultation			
Obtains consent			
Open question to elicit presenting complaint			
Allows patient to open up, listens carefully, remains silent and does not interrupt the patient			
Signposts: e.g. 'Mr Gregory, thank you for telling me about this problem. I would like to ask a few more detailed questions. Is that all right?'			
History of presenting complaint:			
• Site (hands, arms, head) • Bilateral, unilateral, symmetrical			

• Onset:
  • On deliberate movement (e.g. turning on a light switch, reaching for a cup of tea)
  • At rest
  • When anxious/worried			

• Constant or intermittent: • If intermittent, duration and frequency of episodes			
• Time of day			
• Alleviating factors: alcohol			

• Exacerbating factors:
  • Stress, fatigue
  • Anxiety			

• Caffeine (how many cups of coffee?)			
• Coordination, gait			
• Previous episodes			

• General neurological symptoms:
  • Headaches
  • Motor weakness, sensory symptoms
  • Loss of consciousness			

• Asks if patient is suffering from any other symptoms • Asks about any recent illnesses • Previous episodes of tremor			
Associated symptoms:			

	P	MP	F
• Parkinson's disease (slowing, rigidity, falls, depression)			
• Hyperthyroidism (palpitations, weight loss, heat intolerance)			
• Benign essential tremor (family history, eased by alcohol, exacerbated by stress)			
• Cerebellar disease (slurred/staccato speech, incoordination, imbalance)			
• Anxiety (sweating, palpitations)			
• Salbutamol overuse (frequency of inhaler use, poorly controlled asthma)			
• Alcohol withdrawal (excess intake, sudden recent reduction)			
'Red flags': • Headache with features of raised intracranial pressure (early morning, vomiting, worse on coughing, bending down) • Loss of consciousness			
Review of systems			
Past medical history: • Hyperthyroidism • Alcohol/drug addiction			
Family history: • Benign essential tremor • Parkinson's disease			
Drug history: • Salbutamol • Thyroxine • Benzodiazepines (withdrawal) • Over-the-counter medication			
Allergies			

Social history:
• Caffeine
• Alcohol
• Illicit drug use
• Smoking
• Occupation
• Driving
• Activities of daily living, functional impairment:
  • Drinking from a cup
  • Doing buttons
  • Writing			

Use of non-verbal cues, e.g. good eye contact, nodding head and good body posture		
Systematic approach		
Explores and responds to ICE: • Ideas • Concerns • Expectations		
Shows empathy		

Non-verbal skills		
Avoids technical jargon		
Devises holistic management plan and addresses psychosocial issues as well as medical problems		
Summarises		
Offers to answer any questions		
Thanks patient		

Summary of common conditions seen in OSCEs

Bold type denotes the specific and important points that help to distinguish the cause.

Condition	Key points	'Red flags'	Common errors
Hyperthyroidism/ Graves disease	**Bilateral** Swelling in neck Hot all the time Palpitations Weight loss Medication overuse Atrial fibrillation Graves disease: • Pretibial myxoedema • Thyroid acropachy • Eye problems (exophthalmos, ophthalmoplegia) – Graves-specific	Swelling in the neck with voice change – malignancy Nodular goitre – malignancy, adenoma Drugs – amiodarone, lithium Angina, heart failure Thyroid storm	Goitre can be hyper/hypothyroid or euthyroid
Parkinson's disease	**Resting tremor (3–6 Hz)** Often described as 'pill-rolling' **Unilateral** Bradykinesia (slowing) Rigidity (unable to turn in bed, turning en bloc) – 'lead pipe' rigidity Loss of postural reflexes (retropulsion test) Gait – festinant (trouble initiating and stopping) Falls (NB. falls *backwards* = progressive supranuclear palsy) Mood – depression Handwriting – micrographia Soft speech and hypomimia	Loss of arm swing Bilateral onset = unlikely to be Parkinson's disease; look at Parkinson-plus syndromes	Cogwheel rigidity – rigidity with superimposed tremor (best elicited at the wrist: catch–release–catch–release)
Cerebellar disease	**Intention tremor** **Bilateral**	Features of stroke/ cerebrovascular accident	Treat the cause
Benign essential tremor	**Postural tremor** **Titubation (head tremor)** **Bilateral** Family history – autosomal dominant	Alcohol – reduced after a drink	
Anxiety	Nervous person Psychiatric co-morbidities	Identify precipitants and underlying concerns	Manage any psychosocial stressors. Involve a counsellor/psychotherapist
Salbutamol overuse	Poorly controlled asthma Poor inhaler technique	Palpitations (arrhythmias) Hypokalaemia (rare)	

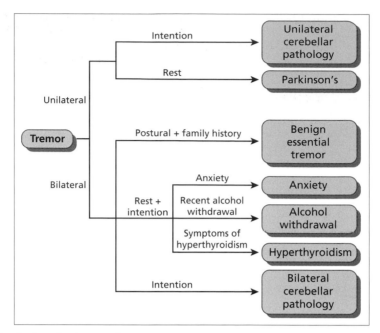

Figure 38.1 Flowchart for diagnosing the cause of a tremor

Hints and tips for the exam

Keep an open mind, and don't forget that there are several non-neurological causes of a tremor (e.g. thyroid disease, anxiety and caffeine).

If the cause turns out to be neurological (e.g. Parkinson's disease), remember to ask about the psychological features (depression) and whether the patient has support at home. These patients have an increased risk of falls so addressing this issue in the history and also in your discussion of management will be important. Mentioning a multidisciplinary review (e.g. a physiotherapist and occupational therapist) will grab those few marks for considering a holistic approach that are earmarked for better candidates.

Parkinson-plus syndromes

To grab those extra few marks for a merit or distinction, you should consider knowing the salient features of the most common Parkinson-plus syndromes as well as lithium toxicity:

• **Progressive supranuclear palsy:** a Parkinson's-plus syndrome in which patients exhibit asymmetrical Parkinsonism with early falls (often backwards) and a ver-

tical supranuclear gaze palsy. The latter is the result of a failure to initiate vertical gaze above the level of the brainstem nuclei. To confirm a pure supranuclear palsy, vertical gaze can be elicited by assessing for the presence of vestibular ocular reflexes by turning the patient's head down, with resultant upward eye deviation (the upward eye deviation is possible despite the vertical gaze palsy because the reflex does not require the supranuclear pathways).

• **Multiple system atrophy:** early autonomic dysfunction (e.g. postural hypotension), cerebellar signs (DANISH – dysdiadochokinesis, ataxia, nystagmus, intention tremor, scanning dysarthria, heel–shin test positive).

• **Corticobasal syndrome:** a very rare atypical parkinsonian syndrome. It is classically unilateral with rapid motor and cognitive decline. Patients develop apraxia and alien hand phenomenon.

• **Lewy body dementia:** early dementia is associated with visual hallucinations and fluctuating cognition.

• **Vascular Parkinsonism (multi-infarct dementia):** in this condition, there is a step-by-step decline. Cardiovascular risk factors (hypertension, diabetes, hypercholesterolaemia) are apparent.

• **Lithium toxicity:** depends on blood level:
  • >1.5 mmol/L – mild tremor
  • >2.0 mmol/L – coarse tremor, arrhythmias, fitting, renal failure (may require haemodialysis)

Questions you could be asked

Q. What level of blood lithium is needed for symptoms of lithium toxicity to develop?

Q. Name some common Parkinson-plus syndromes.

Q. What are the salient features of the most common Parkinson plus syndromes?

A. The answers to all of the questions can be found in the text above.

39 Dizziness

Checklist	P	MP	F
Appropriate introduction			
Confirms the patient's name and age			
Explains reason for consultation			
Obtains consent			
Open question to elicit presenting complaint			
Allows patient to open up, listens carefully, remains silent and does not interrupt the patient			
Signposts: e.g. 'Mr Gregory, thank you for telling me about this problem. I would like to ask a few more detailed questions. Is that all right?'			
History of presenting complaint:			
• Clarifies/defines what the patient means by dizziness: • Rotational – vertigo • Side-to-side – horizontal instability • Faintness – prior to loss of consciousness			
• Onset (gradual/sudden): what is the patient usually doing prior to the dizziness?			
• Duration of episode			
• Frequency of episodes			
• Falls or trauma to head			
• Loss of consciousness			
• Exacerbating factors/precipitating triggers: • Position (turning head – carotid sinus hypersensitivity) • Extending neck, e.g. hanging washing or painting a ceiling (vertebrobasilar insufficiency) • Standing (postural hypotension)			
• Alleviating factors: • Posture/lying down (postural hypotension) • Eating (hypoglycaemia)			
• Recent head/ear trauma			
• Asks if patient is suffering from any other symptoms • Asks about any recent illnesses • Previous episodes of dizziness			

Asks about other associated symptoms:
 • For faintness:
   • Vascular/hypotensive: postural
 • Anaemia:
   • Bleeding/bruising
   • Menorrhagia
 • Hypoglycaemia:
   • Sweating
   • Anxiety
   • Palpitations
 • Cardiovascular, arrhythmias:
   • Chest pain, palpitations
 • For vertigo:
   • Cerebellar symptoms:
     • Slurred/staccato speech
     • Coordination difficulties
     • Gait/balance problems
 • ENT symptoms:
   • Hearing loss, tinnitus
   • Nausea
   • When tilt/turn head (benign paroxysmal positional vertigo)
   • Pain, blood, discharge from ear
   • Recent viral illness (labyrinthitis)
 • For lateral instability:
   • Neurological symptoms:
     • Headaches
     • Motor weakness
     • Sensory symptoms
     • Visual disturbance
     • Speech problems
   • Carotid sinus hypersensitivity – after turning head
   • Anxiety			

'Red flags': • Headache with raised intracranial pressure features (early morning, vomiting, worse on coughing/bending down) • Loss of consciousness • Weight loss, night sweats			
Review of systems			

Past medical history:			
• Diabetes			
• Strokes (in particular cerebellar strokes)			
• Cardiovascular problems (aortic stenosis, heart failure, arrhythmias)			
• Recurrent ear infections, grommets			
Family history:			
• Same as past medical history			
Drug history:			
• Any recent changes to medication			
• Antihypertensive agents, GTN			
• Antidiabetic medication, insulin			
• Sedatives (e.g. benzodiazepines)			
• Over-the-counter medications			
Allergies			
Social history:			
• Alcohol			
• Illicit drug use			
• Smoking			
• Occupation			
• Driving			
• Activities of daily living			
• **Safety assessment if vulnerable** (e.g. lives alone, dangerous occupation, elderly)			

Use of non-verbal cues, e.g. good eye contact, nodding head and good body posture			
Systematic approach			
Explores and responds to ICE:			
• Ideas			
• Concerns			
• Expectations			
Shows empathy			
Non-verbal skills			
Avoids technical jargon			
Devises holistic management plan and addresses psychosocial issues as well as medical problems			
Summarises			
Offers to answer any questions			
Thanks patient			

Summary of common conditions seen in OSCEs

Vertigo

Condition	Key points	'Red flags'	Key examinations, investigations and treatment	Common errors
Benign paroxysmal positional vertigo	Vertigo for **seconds** after moving head Debris in semicircular canal	May have history of trauma	Diagnose with the Hallpike manoeuvre, which causes nystagmus Epley manoeuvre to treat	
Vestibular neuronitis, acute labyrinthitis	Abrupt onset Severe vertigo May last for **hours** Nausea and vomiting Hearing not affected	Recent viral illness Vertigo resolves over days Complete recovery in 3–4 weeks	Reassurance May require sedation (antihistamine – prochlorperazine)	Confused with Ménière's disease. NB. Hearing is unaffected
Ménière's disease	increased pressure in the endolymphatic system Recurrent Prolonged episodes **(20 minutes)** Nausea and vomiting Tinnitus	Fluctuating sensorineural hearing loss (may become permanent) May complain of dropping suddenly to the floor (no loss of consciousness)	Antihistamine (cinnarizine or prochlorperazine) Surgery if severe (destruction of the vestibular organ with gentamicin)	Intermittent hearing loss is the defining characteristic

(*Continued*)

Condition	Key points	'Red flags'	Key examinations, investigations and treatment	Common errors
Drug toxicity (ototoxic)	Aminoglycoside (gentamicin) Furosemide (reversible) Cisplatin	Elderly Renal failure	Us + Es (raised creatinine and low glomerular filtration rate) Stop the offending drug	Elderly people require lower doses Check Us + Es prior to starting these drugs
Ramsay Hunt syndrome	Latent varicella zoster virus reactivated in geniculate ganglion Pain Possible deafness, tinnitus and vertigo	Palsy of cranial nerve VII	Painful vesicles in the external auditory meatus	

Faintness

Condition	Key Points	'Red flags'	Key examinations, investigations and treatment	Common errors
Vasovagal syncope	Fear, pain Not sudden (seconds) May fall to ground Rapid recovery	Standing for a long time Pre-syncope: • Nausea • Pallor • Sweating • Tunnel vision Clonic jerks may occur (not epilepsy) No tongue biting	Lying and standing blood pressure (postural hypotension) Reassure: may have to explain that clonic jerks are just brains reaction to lack of blood, i.e. not epilepsy	Due to bradycardia and vasodilatation If patient remains on floor, they may jerk. This could be confused with epilepsy
Carotid sinus hypersensitivity	Excessive bradycardia and vasodilatation when baroreceptors are stimulated Elderly individuals	Faint on turning head or shaving	Management depends on frequency Education Lifestyle (increase fluid intake and salt) Pacemaker	
Epilepsy	Variable depending on type of epilepsy Tonic-clonic movements Triggers (TV, flashing lights)	History of poor sleep the previous night Incontinence Tongue biting Confusion and drowsiness after the episode Wants to sleep	Us + Es Glucose EEG MRI	May be confused with vasovagal syncope but recovery is not rapid
Hypoglycaemia	Hunger Sweating History of diabetes May be presentation of diabetes mellitus Type 1 diabetes mellitus: weight loss, polyuria and polydipsia, tiredness	Insulin Oral hypoglycaemic agents Binge drinking Liver disease	Glucose – BM sticks are not accurate at low sugar levels C-peptide – not present if exogenous insulin used	

Condition	Key Points	'Red flags'	Key examinations, investigations and treatment	Common errors
Anaemia	Low haemoglobin level Tiredness	Elderly Heavy periods Haemorrhage (any reason) Vegetarian diet	Full blood count and mean corpuscular volume Blood pressure	
(Postural) hypotension	Low blood pressure Causes: • Medications (antihypertensives, alpha-blockers, anti-parkinsonian agents) • Addison's disease/pan-hypopituitarism • Autonomic dysfunction • Parkinson's disease • Dehydration Elderly	Antihypertensives • New medication • Overuse Worse on standing	Standing and sitting blood pressure: • >20 mmHg fall in systolic blood pressure • >10 mmHg fall in diastolic blood pressure Tilt-table testing	Causes: • Addison's disease • Elderly • Medication (tricyclic antidepressants, alpha-blockers, anti-parkinsonian medication) • Hypopituitarism
Stokes–Adams attacks	Falls to ground Palpitations Pale Trauma due to fall Several attacks a day	Recovery in seconds	ECG, 24-hour ECG Pacemaker	
Anxiety	Hyperventilation Sweating Palpitations Paraesthesia	Perioral tingling Young female	Thyroid function tests, calcium ECG Reassurance Counselling	

Lateral instability

Condition	Key points	'Red flags'	Key examinations, investigations and treatment	Common errors
Acoustic neuroma	Arises from cranial nerve VIII and is actually a schwannoma May involve cranial nerves V, VI, IX and X Ipsilateral cerebellar signs (DANISH – dysdiadochokinesis, ataxia, nystagmus, intention tremor, scanning dysarthria, heel–shin test positive)	Early loss of hearing on ipsilateral side and later vertigo Neurofibromatosis type 2 (chromosome 22, autosomal dominant, café-au-lait spots, bilateral acoustic neuromas)	MRI Surgical removal Risk of damage to cranial nerve VII during surgery as both are in close proximity as they enter the internal auditory canal	Cranial nerve VII is very rarely affected by tumour
Cerebellar disease	Multiple sclerosis Stroke, transient ischaemic attack Posterior fossa tumour (gradual onset) Alcohol Phenytoin toxicity	Ipsilateral signs DANISH	See Chapter 7 on cerebellar examination MRI	

(*Continued*)

Condition	Key points	'Red flags'	Key examinations, investigations and treatment	Common errors
Peripheral nerve	Loss of peripheral sensation Pins and needles in the feet Walking on cotton wool Pain (worse at night) Long history of diabetes mellitus Chemotherapeutic medication (platinum-based)	Worse in the dark or with eyes shut	See Chapter 4 on peripheral nervous examination Absent ankle reflex Nerve conduction studies	
Dorsal column	Trauma Vitamin B12 deficiency Friedreich's ataxia	Worse in the dark or with eyes shut	Serum vitamin B12 level MRI Genetic testing	

Hints and tips for the exam

As you can see from the tables above, the differential diagnosis of 'dizzy' is extensive. Therefore your first goal should be to clarify exactly what the patient means by use of word 'dizzy.' If they cannot clearly describe the sensation, provide possible examples such as:

- Do you feel the room is spinning around you?
- Do you feel unsteady on your feet?
- Do you feel faint?

Do not assume you know what the patient means by feeling 'dizzy' – each meaning will lead you down a different diagnostic path.

Addressing the social issues in this history and your management is important. If an elderly patient or someone living alone is complaining of dizziness and/or falls, are they safe in their current environment? In a hospital setting, admitting this patient might be the best and safest next step. Mentioning a multidisciplinary team review is likely to score a mark. This will involve an occupational therapist (who will check safety and provide aids), a physiotherapist (to help improve mobility) and a carer. Mentioning this will look impressive as you will be highlighting the holistic approach to managing the case.

Offer to conduct a full neurological and cardiovascular examinations in your presentation to the examiner.

Questions you could be asked

Q. What symptoms should you consider when a patient complains of dizziness?

A.
  - Vertigo
  - Faintness
  - Instability

Q. What commonly used medications are ototoxic?

A.
  - Gentamicin
  - Furosemide (reversible)

Q. What is the definition of postural hypotension?

A. Postural hypotension is a drop in blood pressure on standing that is sufficient to cause reduced perfusion of the brain. It is usually said to occur if there is a drop greater than 20 mmHg systolic or 10 mmHg diastolic. Patients' blood pressure should be measured after lying down.

40 Joint pain

Checklist	P	MP	F
Appropriate introduction			
Confirms patient's name and age			
Explains reason for consultation			
Obtains consent			
Open question to elicit presenting complaint			
Allows patient to open up, listens carefully, remains silent and does not interrupt the patient			
Signposts: e.g. 'Mr Gregory, thank you for telling me about this problem. I would like to ask a few more detailed questions. Is that all right?'			
History of presenting complaint:			
• Site:			
• Which joints specifically			
• Small/large joints			
• Symmetrical			
• Proximal/distal			
• Onset:			
• Trauma			
• Injection			
• Chronic/gradual			
• Acute, severely painful (septic, gout, fracture)			
• Radiation			
• Time:			
• Duration of joint pain			
• Intermittent, continuous, progressive (raised intracranial pressure)			
• Alleviating factors:			
• Movement (inflammatory)			
• Exacerbating factors:			
• Movement (mechanical/degenerative)			
• Worse in morning (inflammatory)			
• Severity (excruciating pain with complete immobility: ? septic arthritis)			
• Limitation of movement/activity			
• Morning stiffness: **duration of morning stiffness – an easily forgotten point**			
• Redness, swelling (gout, septic arthritis)			
• Locking (cartilage injury), giving way (ligament injury)			
• Fevers			
• Asks if patient is suffering from any other symptoms			
• Asks about any recent illnesses			
• Previous history of joint pains			

Associated symptoms/review of symptoms:			
• Skin:			
• Erythematous patches with silver scaly patches (psoriasis)			
• Butterfly rash (SLE)			
• Nodules, calcinosis (CREST)			
• Raynaud's syndrome (CREST)			
• Skin tightness (CREST)			
• Dry mouth (Sjögren's syndrome)			
• Nails: pitting, onycholysis (psoriasis)			
• Eyes: pain (anterior uveitis in ankylosing spondylitis), dry eyes (Sjögren's syndrome)			
• Heart: pain (pericarditis)			
• Lungs: cough (sarcoid, fibrosis), shortness of breath (pulmonary fibrosis), pleuritic pain (pleurisy)			
• Gastrointestinal: diarrhoea (Reiter's syndrome), bloody diarrhoea (inflammatory bowel disease)			
• Renal: haematuria, ankle swelling (nephritis)			
• Peripheral nervous system:			
• Sensory disturbances, motor weakness (mononeuritis multiplex)			
• Pain, tingling, numbness in the first 3.5 fingers (carpal tunnel syndrome)			
• Central nervous system: nerve palsies			
• Genitourinary: urethritis, ulcers, discharge, dysuria (Reiter's syndrome)			
• Generalised: fever, weight loss, tiredness, myalgia			
'Red flags': • Weight loss, night sweats			
Past medical history:			
• Traumatic injury, fractures			
• Recent joint injection (septic arthritis)			
• Joint surgery			
• Cancer			
• Osteoporosis			
• Autoimmune conditions: inflammatory bowel disease, glomerulonephritis, psoriasis, Sjögren's syndrome			
• Osteoarthritis			
• Diabetes (pseudogout, septic arthritis)			

Family history:
- Rheumatoid arthritis, ankylosing spondylitis, inflammatory arthropathy
- Osteoporosis
- Osteoarthritis
- Cancer

Drug history:
- Long-term steroids (osteoporosis)
- Thiazide diuretics (gout)
- NSAIDs (gout)
- Over-the-counter medication

Allergies

Social history:
- Occupation
- Manual labour, lifting (osteoarthritis)
- Sports, exercise, strenuous activity (osteoarthritis)
- Effect on activities of daily living, loss of function (dressing, writing, eating, stairs)
- Alcohol (gout)
- Smoking
- Illicit drug use

Use of non-verbal cues, e.g. good eye contact, nodding head and good body posture

Systematic approach

Explores and responds to ICE:
- Ideas
- Concerns
- Expectations

Shows empathy

Non-verbal skills

Avoids technical jargon

Devises holistic management plan and addresses psychosocial issues as well as medical problems

Summarises

Offers to answer any questions

Thanks patient

Summary of common conditions seen in OSCEs

Condition	Key points	Investigations and management
Osteoarthritis	Primary or secondary to earlier joint disease (trauma, obesity) Pain on movement Worse at the end of the day Stiffness after rest Heberden's nodes (distal interphalangeal) Bouchard's nodes (proximal interphalangeal) Joints: distal interphalangeal, thumb metacarpophalangeal, knees	X-ray: • Osteophytes • Subchondral sclerosis • Bone cysts • Joint space narrowing Exercise Physiotherapy Analgesia (paracetamol/NSAIDs) Intra-articular steroid injection Joint replacement
Rheumatoid arthritis (Aletaha et al. 2010)	Symmetrical Swollen Morning stiffness Hands and feet Metacarpophalangeal, proximal interphalangeal, wrist, metatarsophalangeal Carpal tunnel syndrome Ulnar deviation Dorsal subluxation	Rheumatoid factor positive (70%) Anti-CCP (98%) Anaemia of chronic disease C-reactive protein, ESR, platelets (all raised) X-ray: • Soft tissue swelling • Osteopenia • Loss of joint space Refer to rheumatologist

Condition	Key points	Investigations and management
	Boutonnière deformity Swan neck deformity Z thumb Elbow nodules Felty syndrome: rheumatoid arthritis + neutropenia + splenomegaly Increased cardiovascular risk – ask about risk factors (e.g. smoking)	28 Joint Disease Activity Score (DAS28) DMARDs : ask about history of tuberculosis (personal and in family; reactivation on biological treatments) Steroids (oral or intra-articular) NSAIDs Exercise Joint replacement
Gout	Monoarthropathy Metatarsophalangeal joints Pain Inflammation Diuretics Alcohol Tumour lysis syndrome Renal disease	Polarised light microscopy of joint fluid: **negatively** birefringent Raised urate X-ray: • Periarticular erosions • Soft tissue swelling Acute: • NSAIDs • Colchicine Chronic: • Allopurinol Avoid alcohol and purine-rich foods (meat, seafood)
Pseudogout (CPPD)	Similar to gout Knee, hip, wrist Diabetes mellitus Hypothyroidism Hyperparathyroidism Wilson's disease	Polarised light microscopy of joint fluid: **positively** birefringent X-ray: chondrocalcinosis Analgesia NSAIDs
Ankylosing spondylitis	Spine Sacroiliac joints HLA B27 Gradual onset of low back pain Worse at **night** Morning stiffness Improves during day Question mark posture Enthesitis (inflammation at tendon insertion into bone): Achilles tendon Iritis Aortic regurgitation Apical lung fibrosis	X-ray: bamboo spine (syndesmophytes) Normocytic anaemia C-reactive protein, ESR (raised) Exercise Physiotherapy NSAIDs Anti-tumour necrosis factor alpha (etanercept, adalimumab)
Systemic sclerosis	**Limited**: CREST (**c**alcinosis, **R**aynaud's syndrome, o**e**sophageal dysmotility, **s**clerodactyly, **t**elangiectasias): • Face, hands, feet, pulmonary hypertension • Anti-centromere 70–80% **Diffuse**: skin and organs (lungs, kidneys, heart) • Anti-topoisomerase-1 (anti-Scl70) 40% • Anti-RNA polymerase 20%	Diffuse: echocardiogram, spirometry Intravenous cyclophosphamide Angiotensin-converting enzyme inhibitor Gloves, hat Prostacyclin

(*Continued*)

Condition	Key points	Investigations and management
Relapsing polychondritis (rare but somehow finds its way into OSCEs)	Floppy ears Stridor (nasal septum, larynx) Aortic valve disease Polyarthritis Vasculitis	Steroids Immunosuppression
Polymyositis, dermatomyositis (same as polymyositis + skin)	Symmetrical Proximal muscle weakness May be paraneoplastic phenomenon (lung) Fever Raynaud's disease Lung fibrosis Myocarditis Skin: • Macular rash • Heliotrope rash (eyelids) • Dilated nailbed capillary loops • Gottron's papules • Subcutaneous calcification • 'Mechanic's hands'	Creatine kinase (raised) EMG (fibrillation potentials) Muscle biopsy Anti-Mi-2 Anti-Jo-1 (acute onset) Chest X-ray (? malignancy) CT (chest, abdomen, pelvis) Prednisolone Immunosuppression
SLE	Women of child-bearing age Afro-Caribbean Relapsing and remitting Fever, malaise, myalgia Malar rash Discoid rash Photosensitivity Mouth ulcers Serositis (pleura, pericardia) Renal Central nervous system (seizures, psychiatric) Drugs: isoniazid, hydralazine, phenytoin	Anti-dsDNA (60%) C3, C4 (low) ESR (raised) C-reactive protein (**normal**) ANA (95%) ENA (20%): • Anti-Ro • Anti-La • Anti-Sm • Anti-RNP Rheumatoid factor (40%) Anti-histone antibodies (drug-induced SLE) False-positive VDRL Blood: • Haemolytic anaemia • Lymphopenia • Leukopenia • Thrombocytopenia Maintenance: • NSAIDs • Hydroxychloroquine • Steroid-sparing agents (methotrexate, mycophenalate, azathioprine)

Condition	Key points	Investigations and management
Reactive arthritis	Lower limbs After infection: sexually transmitted disease: *Chlamydia*, *Ureaplasma*; gastroenteritis: *Campylobacter*, *Salmonella*, *Shigella*, *Yersinia* Reiter's syndrome: • Urethritis • Arthritis • Conjunctivitis Iritis Keratoderma blenorrhagica (palms and soles) Circinate balanitis Mouth ulcers Enthesitis	ESR C-reactive protein Stool culture Referral to genitourinary medicine clinic X-ray
Psoriatic arthritis	Presentations: • Like rheumatoid arthritis • Distal interphalangeal joints • Asymmetrical oligoarthritis • Like ankylosing spondylitis • Arthritis mutilans	Dactylitis (sausage fingers) X-ray: pencil-in-cup deformity NSAIDs Sulfasalazine Methotrexate Ciclosporin Anti-tumour necrosis factor alpha
Septic arthritis	Fever Pain – cannot move joint Swelling Acute onset Intravenous drug user	Joint fluid aspiration and culture Intravenous antibiotics Joint washout under general anaesthetic
Behçet's disease	Mediterranean Oral ulcers Genital ulcers Uveitis Erythema nodosum Central nervous system Pathergy test: papule forms after needle prick	Immunosuppression, steroids
Charcot's joint	Peripheral neuropathy (diabetes mellitus) Deformed joint	X-ray Analgesia Surgery
Wegener's granulomatosis	Medium-vessel vasculitis Upper airways (epistaxis, saddle-nose, sinusitis) Lungs (cough, haemoptysis) Kidneys (rapidly progressive glomerulonephritis) Eyes	cANCA PR3 Urinalysis (proteinuria, haematuria) Chest X-ray Steroids Cyclophosphamide Plasma exchange Azathioprine, methotrexate
Trauma	Important to know mode of injury (high- or low-energy) Bones, ligaments torn, dislocations – knee/hip trauma is common in the history	'RICE' (rest, ice, compression, elevation) Analgesia Physiotherapy Steroid injection Surgery

'Surgical sieve'

Vitamin C D E	
Vascular	Haemophilia
Infective/inflammatory	*Staphylococcus, Streptococcus, Neisseria gonorrhoeae*, tuberculosis
Trauma	Fracture, secondary osteoarthritis
Autoimmune	Rheumatoid arthritis, SLE, rheumatic fever
Metabolic	Gout, pseudogout
Iatrogenic	High-dose steroids (avascular necrosis)
Neoplastic	Osteosarcoma
Congenital	Congenital dislocation of the hip
Degenerative	Osteoarthritis
Endocrine	Diabetes (pseudogout), postmenopausal osteoporosis

Hints and tips for the exam

Taking a history for joint pain is quite straightforward. As with any pain, you will gain marks by running through SOCRATES (**s**ite, **o**nset, **c**haracter, **r**adiation, **a**lleviating factors/associated symptoms, **t**iming, **e**xacerbating factors, **s**everity/signs/symptoms) and then following up with a standard history proforma. The marks to separate you from other candidates will come from asking about extra-articular manifestations of disease (assess this in the body systems) and the effect of the condition on the patient's life and work. If faced with an elderly patient presenting with worsening pain in the hip due to osteoarthritis, you should aim to address their social and safety issues. Are they at risk of falls? Do they need help around the house? How has their mood been affected?

Remember to ask about the joint above and the one below in all cases. For example, pain in the knee can be referred pain from the hip and vice versa.

Do not forget occupation – more often than not, the patient's job will involve use of their affected joint. Opening the station for questioning on how they are coping and what their employer feels about the situation can bring out the patient's concerns early and build a stronger rapport. Hobbies and sports activities should also be addressed.

Management will require an multidisciplinary approach with involvement of a physiotherapist (depending on the level of dysfunction), occupational therapist, surgeons (if replacement of the joint is considered), rheumatologist and GP. If there is chronic illness such as rheumatoid arthritis, mention that there are support groups and charities that the patient can contact.

Questions you could be asked

Q. What are the features of seronegative arthritides?
A. Absence of rheumatoid factor, HLA B27-positive, involvement of the axial skeleton, enthesitis, dactylitis, extra-articular features such as oral ulcers, aortic regurgitation and anterior uveitis, and asymmetrical oligoarthritis/large joint monoarthritis (e.g. in the knee).
Q. What are the differential diagnoses of seronegative arthritides?
A. Psoriatic arthritis, reactive arthritis, enteropathic arthritis, osteoarthritis, rheumatoid arthritis, haemochromatosis, SLE and septic arthritis.
Q. What are the diagnostic criteria for rheumatoid arthritis?
A. New criteria were released in 2010 from the American College of Rheumatology:
  • Presence of synovitis in at least one joint
  • Absence of an alternative diagnosis better explaining the synovitis
  • Score greater than 6/10 on:
    • Number and site of involved joints (range 0–5)
    • Serological abnormality (range 0–3)
    • Elevated acute-phase response (range 0–1)
    • Symptom duration (two levels; range 0–1)
Q. How can you monitor disease activity in rheumatoid arthritis?
A. Frequent follow-up, 28 Joint Disease Activity Score (DAS28) – repeat monthly, C-reactive protein and joint X-ray.
Q. How do you manage rheumatoid arthritis?
A. The answers can be found in the summary table above.

Reference

Aletaha D, Neogi T, Silman AJ *et al.* (2010) Rheumatoid arthritis classification criteria: an American College of Rheumatology/European League Against Rheumatism collaborative initiative. *Ann Rheum Dis* 69: 1580–8.

41 Back pain

Checklist	P	MP	F
Appropriate introduction			
Confirms patient's name and age			
Explain reason for consultation			
Obtains consent			
Open question to elicit presenting complaint			
Allows patient to open up, listens carefully, remains silent and does not interrupt the patient			
Signposts: e.g. 'Mr Gregory, thank you for telling me about this problem. I would like to ask a few more detailed questions. Is that all right?'			
History of presenting complaint:			
• Site: which part of back (cervical/thoracic/lumbar/sacral)			
• Onset (how it started):			
• Sudden			
• Gradual			
• After trauma/sudden movement			
• Character: sharp shooting			
• Radiation:			
• To legs:			
• **Which side? Bilateral?**			
• To buttocks			
• To feet			
• To groin (loin to groin pain – the classical kidney/ureteric stone pain that radiates from the back to the groin)			
• Around chest			
• Time:			
• Duration			
• Intermittent, continuous, progressive (raised intracranial pressure)			
• Alleviating factors			
• Exacerbating factors:			
• Flexion/extension			
• Walking			
• Coughing			
• Morning, with inactivity			
• Night			
• Heavy lifting			
• Severity			
• Limitation of movement, problems walking			
• Any motor weakness/sensory symptoms in the legs			
• Asks if patient is suffering from any other symptoms			
• Asks about any recent illnesses			
• Previous history of back pain			
Associated symptoms:			
• Mechanical back pain: worse on movement/flexion/extension			
Spinal cord compression (intrinsic/extrinsic – secondary):			
• Rigidity of legs			
• Motor weakness and sensory disturbance in the legs			
Myeloma: night sweats, weight loss			
Spinal stenosis:			
• Pain radiating down to thighs/buttocks, worse on extension, better with flexion			
• Motor weakness and sensory disturbance in legs			
Herniated spinal and nerve root compression:			
• Pain radiating down leg and thigh			
• Tingling down leg (rarely motor weakness)			
Spondylolisthesis: similar to nerve root compression, onset more acute			
Discitis, myelitis, abscess:			
• Immunosuppression (HIV, chemotherapy)			
• Fevers			
• Gradual onset of pain and motor weakness and sensory disturbance in the legs			
Vertebral fracture, ligament tears: trauma			
Ankylosing spondylitis:			
• Early morning stiffness, pain improves with activity as the day progresses			
• Disease of the As: **a**nterior uveitis (eye pain), **A**chilles tendinitis (Achilles pain), **a**ortic stenosis (heart symptoms), **a**pical pulmonary fibrosis (lung symptoms)			
Spinal cord infarct:			
• Sudden motor weakness + sensory disturbance (pain/temperature affected first and more severely, light touch/vibration sensation relatively spared or unaffected)			
Kyphosis/scoliosis: prolonged strain on posture (e.g. lifting a heavy rucksack for many years)			
Referred pain: renal stones (back/loin to groin), rupture of abdominal aortic aneurysm (abdomen to back)			

'Red flags':
- Cauda equina symptoms:
  - Perianal/'saddle' numbness (numb when wiping one's bottom)
  - New incontinence of faeces/urine
- Sudden motor weakness
- Weight loss
- Fevers, night sweats
- Night pain
- Recent trauma
- Past medical history of cancer
- Age <20 or >55 years

Review of systems

Past medical history:
- Cancer
- Spinal surgery
- Ankylosing spondylitis
- Osteoporosis
- Osteoarthritis

Family history:
- Cancer

Drug history:
- Over-the-counter medication

Allergies

Social history:
- Alcohol (peptic ulcer disease, gastritis)
- Smoking
- Illicit drug use
- Occupation:
  - Posture at work
  - Manual labour
  - Time off work
- Effect on activities of daily living
- Sports, exercise, strenuous activity

Use of non-verbal cues, e.g. good eye contact, nodding head and good body posture

Systematic approach

Explores and responds to ICE:
- Ideas
- Concerns
- Expectations

Shows empathy

Non-verbal skills

Avoids technical jargon

Devises holistic management plan and addresses psychosocial issues as well as medical problems

Summarises

Offers to answer any questions

Thanks patient

Summary of serious causes of back pain

Condition	History and examination	Pathology	Investigations	Management
Disc protrusion and nerve root compression	Lumbar or neck pain, limb pain, weakness, wasting, sensory disturbance Very rare at thoracic levels as less mobility there Myelopathic clinical picture. **This may not cause back pain but only lower limb neurology**	Degenerative disease causing intervertebral disc herniation and impingement on nerve roots	MRI scan Nerve conduction studies	Conservative: physiotherapy, analgesia – smaller disc protrusions without major root compression may resolve with conservative treatment Surgery: when clear compression is seen on MRI – laminectomy and removal of disc with adequate decompression of nerve roots
Cauda equina syndrome	**This may not cause back pain but only lower limb neurology** Bilateral leg pain/weakness, bladder or bowel disturbance, saddle anaesthesia Look specifically for perianal sensation, anal tone and lower limb neurology	Compression of thecal sac below conus medullaris, usually by disc herniation	Urgent MRI scan Bladder scan to assess residual volume	Emergency lumbar decompression and discectomy
Spinal stenosis	Lower back pain, neurogenic claudication (fixed distance, relieved by bending forward)	Congenital or degenerative osteoligamentous hypertrophy Can be associated with slipping of one vertebra over the next (spondylolisthesis)	Dynamic X-rays/CT to evaluate bony structures MRI to evaluate neural structures	Failing conservative management, surgical options include laminectomy to remove bony compression and occasionally spinal instrumentation to correct slipped vertebrae
Spinal infection	Progressive localised back pain, worse on movement, fever, systemically unwell	Can affect disc space and adjacent vertebrae (spondylodiscitis) Usually caused by staphylococci and streptococci, and occasionally by *Mycobacterium tuberculosis*	MRI to evaluate neural structures and any epidural/paraspinal/psoas pus collections CT to assess bony integrity Blood cultures, tests for tuberculosis Open or CT-guided biopsy to identify organism	Intravenous antibiotics for at least 6 weeks – more if tuberculosis is present Drainage (usually radiologically guided) of any psoas abscess May require surgical washout and stabilisation if extensive

(*Continued*)

Condition	History and examination	Pathology	Investigations	Management
Trauma	Mechanism of injury – flexion/compression; hyperextension/distraction; axial loading Pain at site on injury, limited range of motion, neurological compromise, associated injuries Pre-existing conditions where pathological fracture may occur if trauma is minor	Injury can affect bones, ligaments and neural structures Spinal fractures defined by how many of these are affected according to three-column theory of Denis	Cervical spine: anteroposterior/lateral and peg view X-rays or CT – **must** go to C7/T1 junction; MRI if neurological symptoms Rest of spine: CT and, if neural compromise, MRI Cardiovascular monitoring for neurogenic shock	**Immobilise** with collar, blocks, tape and spinal board until spine is cleared clinically, or radiologically if patient is unconscious Spinal board associated with high risk of pressure sores so patient should not remain on a board for more than 2 hours For stable fractures, treatment can include analgesia, mobilisation and interval X-rays to assess fusion For unstable fractures, stabilisation and reduction can be performed externally though halo stabilisation and traction or open surgery
Metastatic disease	Localised, unremitting pain, nocturnal pain, progressive, neurological symptoms May have known history of malignancy	Metastatic disease affecting spine may be sclerotic or lytic May also infiltrate extradural and intradural spaces Common cancers that metastasise to spine are prostate (Batson's valveless venous plexus) and breast	Whole-spine CT/MRI to evaluate spinal cord, multiplicity of lesions, spinal stability and integrity of bone at adjacent levels CT chest/abdomen/pelvis to stage cancer Oncology review to assess prognosis Tissue diagnosis confirmed Blood tests such as prostate-specific antigen and myeloma screen	Palliative radiotherapy or surgery (surgery cannot be performed after radiotherapy) Surgery if limited disease and reasonable prognosis Steroids

Examination of a patient with back pain

Although this is a station related to *history* of back pain, it is quite common to be asked to examine a patient with back pain, either briefly after taking a history or as part of an extended musculoskeletal station. Below is a brief checklist to guide in examination of a patient with back pain within this station.

Checklist	P	MP	F
Introduce yourself to the patient with your full name and designation			
Explain that you are going to examine their back and limbs. Obtain their consent			
Offer to provide analgesia if the patient is in obvious distress			
General inspection – pain, posture, mobility, deformity, scars, orthoses, medical aids			
Palpate spinous processes for tenderness. In the presence of trauma and spinal tenderness, the patient must remain immobilised in a hard collar and blocks until the spine has been radiologically cleared with an X-ray/CT that shows the area from the skull base to the T1 vertebra			
Movements: neck flexion, extension, lateral movements and rotation. Trunk flexion, extension and rotation. Lumbar flexion and extension (Schober's test at this stage if limited flexion is suspected)			
Full neurological examination of the upper and lower limbs			
Straight leg raise			
Femoral stretch test			
Kernig's and Brudzinski's tests if infection/ meningism suspected			
Rectal examination – a CHAPERONE is needed. Check buttock and perianal sensation to pinprick and light touch on the left and right. Check anal tone and comment on whether the rectum is full or empty. Test the abdominal, anal, cremasteric and bulbocavernosus reflexes			
Bladder: palpate for a full bladder. Check if a catheter tug is felt. Offer a hand-held bladder ultrasound scan to record residual volume.			
Gait			
Functional assessment – getting to the toilet, able to dress self			
Thank patient and help them dress			
Offer differential diagnoses			
MRI scan if there are neurological findings			

Assessing possible cauda equina syndrome: what information to have at hand when referring the patient to neurosurgery

Making referrals to other specialities and colleagues is increasingly being assessed in OSCEs, and a serious neurosurgical emergency such as cauda equina syndrome would be a perfect case to test this with. Here are the details that you should be ready with when making a referral:

· Age
· Co-morbidities
· Pre-existing back pain
· History of trauma/spinal surgery
· Detailed time course of symptoms
· Results of full lower limb neurological examination
· Can the patient walk?
· Anal tone
· Bilateral perianal sensation to light touch and pinprick
· Is the patient catheterised or passing urine?
· If catheterised, can the patient feel a strong tug of the catheter?
· Post-void/catheter residual bladder volume
· Use of antiplatelet agents/anticoagulants
· Time last ate and drank
· MRI results if available.

Clearing the cervical spine

Patients with suspected neck injury will be immobilised at the scene. Before they can be mobilised, their cervical spine has to be cleared. In unconscious patients, more

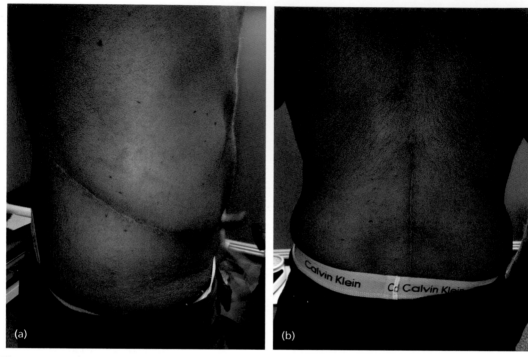

Figure 41.1 Scars from L2 vertebrectomy to treat a giant cell tumour

reliance is placed on the radiological investigations. To clinically clear a spine, the patient must have a Glasgow Coma Scale score of 15, not be intoxicated and have no distracting injuries. Patients must have no neurological deficit and no midline bony tenderness. They should be able to rotate their neck. Radiologically, the films must show the C7/T1 junction to be valid. Interpretation of cervical spine films in the trauma patient is covered in the ATLS guidelines and involves checking for correct alignment and soft tissue spaces within normal limits. In unconscious patients, in whom clinical assessment is lost, MRI may be needed to assess the ligaments.

Immobilising the spinal patient

To be correctly immobilised, the patient must be placed on a hard spinal board at the scene, with a properly fitting hard collar, blocks and tape. Without all these components, the patient cannot be said to be immobilised. To move these patients for secondary survey and imaging, they must be log-rolled. If there is an unstable spinal injury and immobilisation must continue, the patient should be placed in a Miami J or Philadelphia collar and complete bed rest ensured. Definitive immo-

bilisation is then performed with a halo vest or operative intervention.

Neurogenic shock versus spinal shock

Neurogenic shock is a cardiovascular consequence of spinal injury and can occur in spinal cord injuries above T6. It refers to disruption of the sympathetic outflow. This leads to bradycardia and hypotension as there is unopposed parasympathetic activity. It can be distinguished from hypovolaemic shock by warm vasodilated peripheries in neurogenic causes, whereas a patient who is bleeding will be peripherally shut down. Neurogenic shock should be managed in a setting where cardiovascular monitoring is available, and pressor drugs and fluids may be required. Note that ATLS guidelines require cardiovascular compromise to be treated as hypovolaemic shock until this is excluded, so never assume that a known spinal injury patient is compromised due to neurogenic shock until bleeding has been absolutely excluded.

Spinal shock is not related to the cardiovascular system. It refers to a flaccid paralysis and areflexia that occurs after spinal injury and can be reversible.

Ankylosing spondylitis

This is a seronegative multisystem disease. It usually starts as sacroiliac joint stiffness in young men that progresses to involve the whole back. It is usually worse in the morning. The pathological process includes ossification of ligaments leading to a rigid brittle spine that is vulnerable to trauma. Radiologically, an ossified 'bamboo spine' is seen, as well as characteristic Andersson lesions of the endplates on MRI where the ligaments insert. Spinal deformity such as kyphoscoliosis can occur. Systemic features of ankylosing spondylitis include aortic disease, apical lung fibrosis, uveitis, psoriasis and gastrointestinal inflammation.

Key investigations: when in doubt about the integrity of neural structures, go for an MRI

The examiner may ask you what investigations you would like to request. Unless there is a specific indication, do not request X-rays as most of the time they will come back as appearing normal or with mild osteoarthritic changes – and they also expose the patient to large volumes of radiation. The investigation of choice to investigate any structural or inflammatory pathology in the back is an MRI scan.

You could justify routine blood tests, for example full blood count, Us+Es, ESR, C-reactive protein and bone profile, as these could indicate a primary or secondary malignancy and inflammatory causes of back pain.

'Yellow flags'

'Yellow flags' are psychosocial risk factors for developing chronic back pain. These may include the following:
- Problems at work, for example the patient is bullied at work and therefore uses back pain as an excuse to be not working
- Social withdrawal or lack of social integration
- A past or current medical history of depression, stress or anxiety, or mental health problems
- Low self-motivation and failure to actively participate in activities that may help them, for example physiotherapy

Cauda equina syndrome

This a neurosurgical emergency due to compression of the nerve roots in the thecal sac below the level of the conus medullaris – untreated, it can lead to paralysis and loss of bladder and bowel control; this has been covered in detail in Chapter 11 on rectal examination. It is one of the most common causes of medicolegal action by patients.

Common causes of 'simple' musculoskeletal back pain

Back pain could underlie a very serious pathology, but the vast majority of patients suffering from back pain have 'simple/musculoskeletal' back pain. Some of the common causes of this are described in the table.

Type	Comments
Mechanical	The most common cause of lower back pain. It is commonly due to age-related disc degeneration or musculoskeletal injury after minor trauma. You may want to suggest a trial of analgesia and physiotherapy
Posture	Bending forwards to lift a heavy box or standing all day, for example with a job as a security guard, can lead to back pain. Suggest that the patient reports this problem to the occupational health department where they work
Sciatica	Caused by irritation of the sciatic nerve. Patients will describe pain that shoots down their legs and can be severe. Physiotherapy assessment will be helpful, and if the pain does not resolve, MRI can be used to assess nerve root impingement.

Questions you could be asked

Q. What would you advise a patient with mechanical lower back pain in a GP appointment?
A. It is important that patients do not take to their beds in the belief that movement will damage their back. Encourage them to go about their normal activities at work and at home. A referral for physiotherapy is also useful.

Q. Why is degenerative disc disease less common in the thoracic spine?
A. Degenerative disease and trauma occur at the most mobile segments of the spine, i.e. the cervical spine and thoracolumbar junction. The thoracic spine is relatively immobile and is well supported by the ribs, making it less vulnerable to degeneration and injury.

Q. What is an ASIA chart?
A. This is a standardised method developed by the American Spinal Injury Association to assess motor function, sensory function and anal tone. It classifies spinal cord injury as complete or incomplete, which has prognostic value. Clinically, it is useful to assess neurology serially and detect improvements or deteriorations, even when the tests are carried out by different examiners.

Q. What are some differential diagnoses for back pain?
A. Serious and common pathologies can masquerade as back pain. These include abdominal aortic aneurysm, urinary tract infections and upper tract renal disease, aortic dissection, myocardial infarction, ectopic pregnancy, pancreatitis and other retroperitoneal pathology, and duodenal ulcers.

Q. Which scan is useful in osteoporosis?
A. A DEXA scan.
Q. Which scan is useful for distinguishing between infection and malignancy?
A. Positron-emission tomography.

42 Pyrexia of unknown origin

Checklist	P	MP	F
Appropriate introduction			
Confirms the patient's name and age			
Explains reason for consultation			
Obtains consent			
Open question to elicit presenting complaint			
Allows patient to open up, listens carefully, remains silent and does not interrupt the patient			
Signposts: e.g. 'Mr Smith, thank you for telling me about this problem. I would like to ask a few more detailed questions. Is that all right?'			
History of presenting complaint:			
• How do the patient know they had pyrexia? • What was the temperature (if measured)?			
• Onset (how it started)			

• Pattern:
   • Day/night/intermittent/continuous/progressive
   • Peaks and troughs			

• Frequency			
• Exacerbating factors			
• Alleviating factors (paracetamol)			
• Rigors/shivers			
• Lethargy			
• Night sweats			
• Weight loss			
• Reduced urine output (septic shock)			
Associated symptoms that may indicate a focus:			
• Respiratory:			
• Cough, sputum (pneumonia)			
• Haemoptysis (cancer, tuberculosis)			
• Shortness of breath			
• Gastrointestinal:			
• Diarrhoea (gastroenteritis)			
• Bloody stools (inflammatory bowel disease) • What/when did the patient last eat?			

• Liver/gallbladder:
   • Right upper quadrant pain
   • Jaundice			

• Neurological:
   • Headache (abscess, meningism)
   • Neck stiffness, rash (meningism)
   • Focal neurological symptoms (abscess, encephalitis)			

• Cardiovascular: chest pain, shortness of breath, haematuria (infective endocarditis)			

• Urological:
   • Haematuria
   • Dysuria (urinary tract infection)
   • Loin pain (pyelonephritis)			

• Rheumatological, musculoskeletal:
   • Severely painful single joint (septic arthritis)
   • Pain in small joints (rheumatoid arthritis, systemic lupus erythematosus)
   • Muscle pain (myositis)			

• ENT: throat pain (upper respiratory tract infection, tonsillitis)			
• Dental: tooth pain (tooth abscess)			
• Skin: rash, inflammation, redness (cellulitis)			
• Calf pain/swelling (deep vein thrombosis)			
• Lumps (lymphadenopathy)			

• Gynaecological symptoms:
   • Vaginal bleeding/discharge (pelvic inflammatory disease)
   • Use of tampons			

• Risk factors for HIV:
   • Multiple/new sexual partners, contact with sex workers (**must signpost**)
   • Contraception
   • Intravenous drug abuse			

• Recent recurrent boils/other infections			
• Asks if the patient is suffering from any other symptoms • Asks about recent illnesses • Previous episodes of pyrexia of unknown origin (PUO)			
Past medical history:			
• HIV			
• Tuberculosis			
• Cancer			

• Valvular heart disease/replacement (infective endocarditis)			
• Organ transplants			
• Rheumatic fever			
• Blood transfusions			
• Diabetes			
• Immunisations			
• Recent hospital admissions			
• Recent surgery: any healing wounds?			
Family history:			
• Tuberculosis			
• Cancer			
• Immunosuppressive illnesses			
• Familal Mediterranean fever			
Drug history:			
• Immunosuppressants: cytotoxic agents, chemotherapy, steroids			
• Malaria prophylaxis			
• Over-the-counter medications			
• Herbal remedies			
Allergies			
Social history:			
• Recent travel history:			
• Where/when/what country?			
• Accommodation			
• Food, water, restaurants			
• Did others on holiday have same symptoms?			
• Swimming in rivers, at coasts or in possible contaminated waters			

• Fever on holiday			
• Insect/tick bites			
• Recent diet:			
• Unpasteurised dairy products			
• Barbecues			
• Drinking water abroad			
• Recent contact with farm animals			
• Foreign contacts			
• Alcohol, smoking, illicit drug use			
• Sexual history (if appropriate **and only** after signposting clearly)			
• Occupation			
• Accommodation: any recent changes			
Review of systems			
Use of non-verbal cues, e.g. good eye contact, nodding head and good body posture			
Systematic approach			
Explores and responds to ICE: • Ideas • Concerns • Expectations			
Shows empathy			
Non-verbal skills			
Avoids technical jargon			
Devises holistic management plan and addresses psychosocial issues as well as medical problems			
Summarises			
Offers to answer any questions			
Thanks patient			

Summary of common conditions seen in OSCEs

Causes of PUO can be divided into:
- Infection
- Malignancy
- Inflammatory/rheumatological diseases
- Miscellaneous
- Unknown

Infections (25%)

Condition	Key points
Tuberculosis	Cough
	Night sweats (drenched)
	Haemoptysis
	Weight loss
	Tuberculosis contact
	South Asian
Abscess	Spiking fever
	Temperature chart looks like a zig-zag line
Endocarditis	New murmur and fever
	Weight loss
	Anaemia
	Embolic phenomena (stroke)
	Janeway lesions
	Osler's nodes
	Splenomegaly
	Prosthetic valve
	Intravenous drug use
	Requires blood cultures and
	transoesophageal echocardiogram
Osteomyelitis	Pain, tenderness
	Swelling
	Heat
Pneumonia	Elderly
	Alcohol
	Previous tuberculosis
	Smoking
	Immunosuppression
Urinary tract	Frequency
infection	Dysuria
	Haematuria
Intracerebral	Delirium
– meningitis,	Cognitive ± neurological features
encephalitis,	Lumbar puncture
abscess	CT brain
HIV	Non-specific symptoms
	Opportunistic infections
	Endemic area
	Risk factors
Hepatitis	Abdominal pain
	Jaundice
	Alcohol
	Obesity
	Intravenous drug user
Tropical	Foreign travel
infections	Malaria prophylaxis (compliance)
	Immunisation history
	Consider the wider public health aspect also
	(contacting the CCDC, notifiable diseases)

Neoplasms (20%)

Condition	Key points
Lymphoma	Tiredness
	Lymphadenopathy
	Night sweats
	Pruritus
	Weight loss
Leukaemia	Bruising
	Infections
	Anaemia

Connective tissue disease (20%)

Condition	Key points
Rheumatoid	Symmetrical
arthritis	Swollen
	Painful
	Small joints of hands (metacarpophalangeal,
	proximal interphalangeal)
Systemic lupus	Non-specific symptoms (malaise, tiredness)
erythematosus	Weight loss
	Alopecia
	Malar rash
	Photosensitivity
	Mouth ulcers
	Arthralgia
	Young women
Giant cell arteritis	Elderly
	Associated with polymyalgia rheumatica
	Headache
	Temporal tenderness
	Jaw claudication
	Amaurosis fugax
Polymyalgia	Morning stiffness in the proximal limb
rheumatica	muscles
	Tiredness
	Anorexia
	Weight loss
Still's disease	Joint pain and swelling
	Salmon pink skin rash
	Fever peaks in afternoon

Miscellaneous (15%)

Condition	Key points
Drug fever (3%)	Beta-lactam antibiotics (penicillin)
	Isoniazid
	Sulphonamide (sulphasalazine)
Pulmonary embolism	Shortness of breath
	Chest pain
	Haemoptysis
	Recent surgery, immobility
Inflammatory bowel disease	Abdominal pain
	Weight loss
	Diarrhoea (ulcerative colitis – bloody)

Occupation-associated illness

Occupation	Condition
Sewage worker	Leptospirosis
Farm worker	Zoonosis
Healthcare worker	Hepatitis, HIV
Forestry worker	Lyme disease
Abattoir workers	Q fever (*Coxiella burnetii*)

Remember that 25% of patients with a PUO never receive a diagnosis for why it has occurred.

Hints and tips for the exam

Definition of PUO

The definition of PUO is a **temperature over 38.3°C for longer than 3 weeks with no obvious source despite investigation**.

Devising a list of differential diagnoses

PUO has a vast differential diagnosis so approaching this station can be tricky. Cast your net wide. Only home in on a possible diagnosis after you have asked all the key questions (i.e. even if it is clear that a connective tissue disorder is the cause, do not forget the travel and sexual histories). There is a lot to cover so be succinct, but give the patient enough time to respond so that you can gain the most marks.

In this station, one of your goals is to differentiate between whether the patient should be admitted for further investigation or can be monitored and treated in the community.

Structure your questioning according to different body systems. This will ensure you do not miss anything obvious.

Asking for the patient's personal thoughts on the cause is imperative and more often than not gives the diagnosis away in this station. This should also be used as an opportunity to allay the patient's fears if the diagnosis is clear.

In cases of PUO, the history and examination should be repeated at intervals to see if further information can be gleaned to achieve a diagnosis. This should be mentioned to the examiner when you present the case.

Examining patients with PUO

Examining a patient with a PUO involves a thorough examination focusing on possible causes that were highlighted within the history. Pay particular attention to the patient's skin, mucous membranes and lymphatic system, and the presence of abdominal masses.

Key investigations for patients with PUO

Be prepared with a number of investigations at the PUO station. Be able to justify each test based on your history, examination findings and likely differential diagnosis:
- Bedside tests: measure the temperature!
- Full blood count, white cell count and differential, Us+Es, C-reactive protein, liver function tests, ESR, blood film, amylase
- Blood cultures (×3, taken at different times from different sites using an aseptic technique.)
- Urine microscopy, culture and sensitivity
- Swabs (throat, ear, penile, high vaginal/endocervical)
- Autoantibody screen – antinuclear antibody, ANCA, rheumatoid factor
- HIV test, PPD, interferon-gamma release assay for TB
- Chest X-ray
- Abdominal ultrasound scan
- CT/MRI – the site will be dictated by what you find from your history and examination

In your management plan, first decide whether the patient needs to be admitted. A multidisciplinary approach is key in PUO (as with every OSCE).

Questions you could be asked

Q. What are the common symptoms of tuberculosis?
Q. What initial investigations would you consider in a patient presenting with a PUO?
A. The answers can be found in the chapter text.

43 Ankle swelling

Checklist	P	MP	F
Appropriate introduction			
Confirms patient's name and age			
Explains reason for consultation			
Obtains consent			
Open question to elicit presenting complaint			
Allows patient to open up, listens carefully, remains silent and does not interrupt the patient			
Signposts: e.g. 'Mr Gregory, thank you for telling me about this problem. I would like to ask a few more detailed questions. Is that all right?'			
History of presenting complaint:			
• Details about swelling:			
• Duration, extent (e.g. mid-shins, knees), changes since onset, presence of erythema/pain/itching, previous episodes of swelling			
• Change in relation to time of day			
• Associated symptoms:			
• **Related to heart failure:** shortness of breath, paroxysmal nocturnal dyspnoea, orthopnoea, past medical history of ischaemic heart disease or chronic lung disease			
• **Related to chronic liver disease:** abdominal distension, jaundice, changes to sleep–wake cycle			
• **Related to kidney disease:** swelling of face, haematuria, frothy urine, oliguria			
• **Related to venous insufficiency:** eczema, ulceration, pigmentation, risk factors, e.g. prolonged standing, high heels			
• **Related to hypothyroidism:** decreased tolerance of cold, weight gain, mood changes			
• **Related to a pelvic mass:** abdominal distension, constipation			
• **Related to a deep vein thrombosis:** severe pain			
• Asks in a sensitive manner about the possibility of being pregnant			

Checklist	P	MP	F
• Asks about risk factors for deep vein thrombosis: recent surgery, past deep vein thrombosis, immobility, thrombophilia, cancer			
Asks about constitutional symptoms: fever, weight change			
• Asks if patient is suffering from any other symptoms			
• Asks about any recent illnesses			
• Previous episodes of ankle swelling			
• Family members/contacts with similar symptoms			
'Red flags':			
• Weight loss, loss of appetite, night sweats (malignancy)			
Review of systems			
Past medical history:			
• Ischaemic heart disease and heart failure			
• Liver disease			
• Diabetes			
• Hypertension			
• Cancer			
• Pelvic surgery			
Family history:			
• Ischaemic heart disease			
Drug history:			
• Current medication			
• Recent changes to dose			
• Over-the-counter drugs			
• Intravenous drug use			
Allergies			
Social history:			
• Smoking			
• Alcohol			
• Illicit drug use (especially intravenous drug abuse – hepatitis B/C)			
• Occupation			
• Activities of daily living			
• Effect of ankle swelling on patient's mobility			
Use of non-verbal cues, e.g. good eye contact, nodding head and good body posture			
Systematic approach			

Explores and responds to ICE: • Ideas • Concerns • Expectations			
Shows empathy			
Non-verbal skills			
Avoids technical jargon			

Devises holistic management plan and addresses psychosocial issues as well as medical problems			
Summarises			
Offers to answer any questions			
Thanks patient			

Summary of common conditions seen in OSCEs

Condition	Clues from the history	Investigations
Renal failure	Risk factors, e.g. diabetes mellitus, hypertension, use of nephrotoxic drugs, Associated symptoms, e.g. tiredness, metallic taste, yellow tinge to the skin, brown discoloration of the nails	Full blood count, Us+Es, bone profile, 1,25-hydroxy vitamin D levels Renal ultrasound scan Albumin:creatinine ratio
Nephrotic syndrome	Periorbital swelling Frothy urine Diabetes, hypertension, features of connective disease (e.g. arthralgia, Raynaud's phenomenon, photosensitive rash) Haematuria	Urine dipstick Us+Es Albumin:creatinine ratio (or 24-hour urine collection) Clotting screen Lipid profile Autoantibody screen ASO titre Oral glucose tolerance test Hepatitis serology Renal biopsy
Right-sided/ congestive cardiac failure	Shortness of breath on exertion Chronic long-standing lung disease (e.g. COPD, severe asthma, fibrotic lung disease)	Plasma brain natriuretic protein Echocardiogram Chest X-ray Lung function tests High-resolution CT chest
Pulmonary hypertension	Shortness of breath Chest pain	Cardiac catheter studies ECG Echocardiogram
Chronic liver disease	Presence of associated symptoms, e.g. jaundice, ascites, confusion Past medical history of excess alcohol intake Risk factors for chronic liver disease, e.g. past medical history or family history of haemochromatosis/ Wilson's disease, intravenous drug use	Liver function tests Clotting screen Liver screen (see Chapter 3 on abdominal examination) Ultrasound abdomen
Hypothyroidism	Past history of thyroid surgery Past medical history of other autoimmune conditions Symptoms related to hypothyroidism	Thyroid function tests Thyroid ultrasound scan
Venous insufficiency	Prolonged standing Previous deep vein thromboses Presence of brown pigmentation, eczema, dilated tortuous veins	Doppler ultrasound scan Ankle–brachial pressure index Abdomen + pelvic examination + ultrasound scan to screen for venous compression from an abdominal/pelvic mass

Condition	Clues from the history	Investigations
Pelvic mass causing venous compression	Abdominal distension Constipation Vaginal bleeding Menstrual disturbance	Full blood count, Us+Es, liver function tests, ESR Ultrasound abdomen + pelvis CT abdomen + pelvis
Cellulitis	Erythema, history of penetrating injury Fever History of immunosuppression Spreading of erythema	Clinical diagnosis Raised inflammatory markers/C-reactive protein
Pregnancy	Child-bearing age Sexually active and not using contraception Vomiting	Urinary beta-hCG Pelvic ultrasound scan
Pre-eclampsia	Pregnancy >20 weeks' gestation Features due to hypertension: headache, frothy urine (proteinuria), vomiting	Urine dipstick (proteinuria) Blood pressure (>140/90 mmHg or significant rise from booking blood pressure)
Deep vein thrombosis	Presence of risk factors (outlined above)	Lower limb Doppler ultrasound studies
Hereditary lymphoedema	Family history No symptoms to suggest a secondary cause	Investigations to screen for secondary causes
Secondary lymphoedema	Radiotherapy Symptoms of intra-abdominal/pelvic malignancy	Ultrasound abdomen + pelvis Tumour markers
Iatrogenic	Amlodipine	Investigations to rule out other possible causes apart from the drug in question that may be contributing

Hints and tips for the exams

Ask about the duration of ankle swelling

Ankle swelling of rapid onset is more likely to be caused by an acute process (e.g. deep vein thrombosis), whereas swelling that has developed over the course of weeks or months is more likely to be caused by one of the failures (renal, liver, cardiac or thyroid).

Remember to take a thorough drug history

Ankle swelling is, for example, a common side effect of amlodipine.

Work through the history systematically

As you can see from the summary table, ankle swelling can be caused by pathology affecting various organ systems. Hence, it is important to 'throw the net wide' early on in your history to screen for pathology related to each of these systems.

Do NOT forget pregnancy and pre-eclampsia

Obstetrics is examined in the fourth year at most UK medical schools, so the majority of students do not revise this topic for finals. However, contrary to popular belief, obstetric emergencies **can** be examined in finals. It is thus important to remember that worsening or new-onset ankle swelling in a pregnant female beyond 20 weeks' gestation should be treated as pre-eclampsia until proven otherwise.

Potential variations at this station

• History of unilateral ankle swelling + examination of venous system of the lower limbs
• History of ankle swelling + focused examination. The 'focused examination' should include the following:
  • **Hands**: signs of chronic liver disease, clubbing (liver cirrhosis, fibrotic lung disease)
  • **Eyes**: conjunctival pallor (NB. anaemia can be related to chronic kidney disease or cardiac failure)
  • **Chest**: observation for deformities (e.g. Harrison's sulcus, barrel chest), auscultation of lung fields for crepitations associated with fibrosis or wheeze associated with COPD, auscultation of heart sounds (various murmurs can be associated with congestive heart failure)
  • **Abdomen**: hepatomegaly, palpable pelvic masses, distension (e.g. ascites, pregnancy)
  • **Legs**: other signs associated with chronic venous insufficiency (outlined above)

• **Bedside tests:** urine dipstick, peak expiratory flow rate

Questions you could be asked

Q. What else might you find on examination of the ankles in a patient with ankle swelling secondary to hypothyroidism?

A. • Pretibial myxoedema (see Chapter 9 on thyroid examination for an illustration)
   • Erythema ab igne (arising from large periods of time spent near a fire or heater as a result of cold intolerance)
   • Slow-relaxing reflexes

Q. What features would support a diagnosis of chronic rather than acute renal failure?

A. • Anaemia
   • Secondary hypoparathyroidism (low calcium, low 1,25-hydroxy-vitamin D, elevated phosphate, elevated parathyroid hormone)
   • Renal osteodystrophy (osteomalacia, osteoporosis, osteosclerosis causing a 'rugger-jersey' spine on X-ray)
   • Small kidneys on ultrasound scan
   • Lack of symptoms despite severe uraemia

44 Needlestick injury

Task (5 minutes): You are an SHO working in occupational health. You have received a phone call from an FY1 working with the infectious disease team about a needlestick injury. Advise the FY1 on what steps need to be taken.

Checklist	P	MP	F
Appropriate introduction and establishes identity of colleague			
Instructs colleague about dealing with injury appropriately:			
• Induce bleeding			
• Do not suck blood			
• Wash thoroughly under running water without use of soap or bleach			
Obtains details of injury:			
• Location and time			
• Approximate depth of needlestick penetration			
• Presence of visible blood/other fluid on needle			
• Splashes to eye or mouth			
Assesses risk and communicates this appropriately to the patient in a clear empathetic manner			
Informs colleague about risk of contracting blood-borne viral illness without post-exposure prophylaxis (PEP):			
• HIV <1%, hepatitis B up to 30%, hepatitis C 3%			
• Explains clearly that these risks are an average and depend upon risk of exposure			
Provides appropriate details about PEP:			
• PEP is offered if donor has one or more significant risk factor(s) for HIV or is known to have HIV, or if it is not possible to exclude that the donor has HIV			
• Most effective if started within the hour (but can will still have benefit if started within 72 hours of exposure)			
• Minimum course is 28 days			
• Explains side effects (myalgia, rash, pancreatitis, deranged liver function tests, neutropenia)			
• Recipient needs to avoid drinking alcohol			
Explains blood tests that need to be done:			

• Liver function tests immediately, at 3 months and at 6 months			
• HIV testing immediately and at 3 months			
• Hepatitis B testing immediately, at 3 months and at 6 months			
Enquires about previous immunisation against hepatitis B, offers immunisation/booster if appropriate, offers hepatitis B immunoglobulin if the donor is a known hepatitis B sufferer with high infectivity			
Advises colleague to refrain from obtaining consent for blood-borne virus testing from the donor themselves and explains this has to be done by a colleague			
Advises colleague to avoid unprotected intercourse and donation of blood until HIV testing has been completed or PEP has been completed			
Provides safety netting for regarding acute seroconversion illness, telling colleague to look out for:			
• Swollen glands			
• New rashes			
• Throat/mouth infections			
• Shingles			
Provides safety netting for hepatitis B, advising colleague to look out for:			
• Jaundice			
• Right upper quadrant pain			
Instructs colleague to inform supervisor and complete an incident form			
Maintains sympathetic tone throughout consultation			
Provides information clearly			
Checks colleague's understanding of information regularly and invites questions at the end			
Arranges follow-up by the occupational health department			

Hints and tips for the exam

This is a relatively difficult OSCE station because it tests candidates in three separate domains and you are unlikely to encounter many opportunities to practise it during your clinical attachments:

• **Knowledge:** You need to know *what steps need to be taken* following a sharps accident and what constitutes a *high-risk exposure* for blood-borne viral illness. Also, you should be able to construct an appropriate *safety net* with regard to signs of HIV seroconversion illness.

• **Communicating with a worried colleague:** You need to be *empathetic and calm* while trying to impart a *large volume of information* in a manner that is easily understood by your colleague.

• **Ethics and law:** You need to know that *fully informed consent* must be taken by a health professional other than the recipient of the needlestick injury before the patient's blood can be tested.

You are unlikely to get exposure to this type of scenario during clinical attachments, so the most effective way of preparing for this station is to practise it several times with colleagues before the OSCE.

There are a number of key points that will help to ensure that you cover all the necessary points at this station:

• What constitutes a high-risk exposure?:
  • Patient is known to be a carrier of a blood-borne viral infection
  • Patient has a history of sexual intercourse with a carrier of a blood-borne viral infection
  • Patient is a male with a history of sex with men
  • Patient has lived in Africa or was born there
  • Patient is/has been an intravenous drug user
  • Patient received a blood transfusion before 1991
• What are the common side effects of PEP?:
  • Gastrointestinal disturbance (nausea, vomiting, diarrhea, anorexia)
  • Pancreatitis
  • Neutropenia
  • Stevens–Johnson syndrome
  Interactions with drugs metabolised by the P450 liver enzyme system are common so the patient must be given information about which drugs are safe to use.
• What happens if the recipient is pregnant?
  • If pregnancy has not already been confirmed, carry out a pregnancy test prior to initiating PEP.
  • Pregnancy does not contraindicate the use of PEP.
  • There is limited evidence regarding any adverse effects of drugs used in PEP on the developing fetus.
  • The risk of vertical transmission of HIV should be balanced against the risk of adverse effects on the fetus by PEP.
  • Drugs used in PEP are contraindicated while breast-feeding.
• Does the recipient of the injury have to stay away from work until tests are complete at 6 months?
  • As long as seroconversion illness does not develop, healthcare workers are **not** required to stay off work or avoid exposure-prone procedures.
  • This is why it is so important at this station to construct a safety net for the signs and symptoms of seroconversion illness.

Potential variations at this station

You may encounter the following, all of which are 5-minute stations:

• A telephone conversation with an actor behind a curtain
• Face-to-face role-play with an actor
• A viva with an examiner asking questions regarding sharps incidents

45 Preoperative assessment

Checklist	P	MP	F
Appropriate introduction			
Confirms patient's name and age			
Explains reason for consultation			
Obtains consent			
Confirms operation to be performed			
Open question to find out if patient understands the purpose of the history			
Allows patient to open up, listens carefully, remains silent and does not interrupt the patient			
Enquires about cardiovascular health, asking specifically about symptoms of: • Ischaemic heart disease • Hypertension • Arrhythmias • Syncope • Peripheral vascular disease			
Enquires about respiratory health, asking specifically about: • Asthma • COPD • Sleep apnoea • Pneumonia			
Establishes exercise tolerance			
Enquires about other medical problems, in particular: • Cerebrovascular accidents • Epilepsy • Diabetes mellitus • Rheumatoid arthritis (and which joints are affected) • Renal disease (and if there is renal failure, details of dialysis) • Liver disease • Sickle cell disease			
Enquires about previous facial/head and neck surgery			
Asks about any history of hiatus hernia or gastro-oesophageal reflux			

Asks about any previous operations, general anaesthesia and associated problems			
Enquires about any family history of any problems associated with general anaesthesia			
Establishes what regular medication the patient is taking, and whether it has been taken that day			
Establishes any allergies/adverse reactions			
Asks specifically about adverse reactions to penicillin, NSAIDs, latex			
Establishes smoking history			
Establishes alcohol intake			
Establishes any history of illicit drug use			
Asks about dentition, i.e. loose teeth, caps, crowns, fillings, dentures, plates			
Asks the time when patient last had anything to eat or drink			
If the patient is young and female, establishes the possibility of the patient being pregnant			
Use of non-verbal cues, e.g. good eye contact, nodding head and good body posture			
Systematic approach			
Mentions would examine the patient, including cardiorespiratory and airway assessment			
Intention to order relevant preoperative tests as per local or national guidelines: ECG, bloods, echocardiogram, chest X-ray			
Explores and responds to ICE: • Ideas • Concerns • Expectations			
Shows empathy			
Non-verbal skills			
Avoids technical jargon			
Summarises			
Offers to answer any questions			
Thanks patient			

Summary of key points for OSCEs

Having an anaesthetic and undergoing surgery represents a major physiological challenge for the human body. The preoperative assessment is designed to anticipate any problems that might be encountered in the perioperative period and to take steps to minimise their impact as much as possible. In the emergency setting, this is not always achievable, but in designated pre-assessment clinics, patients who are scheduled for elective procedures can be 'optimised' to a large extent before the operation.

Pre-assessment clinics are increasingly nurse-led, but in many NHS trusts the surgical FY1 carries out the pre-assessment for their consultant's lists a few weeks in advance. If you get a preoperative assessment in the OSCE, it is almost certain that you will see a patient for an elective procedure.

The ASA classification

The American Society of Anaesthesiologists has developed 'grades' to classify patients in terms of their general fitness for anaesthesia (see the table).

ASA grade	Description
1	Normal, fit, healthy patient
2	Patient with mild systemic disease
3	Patient with severe systemic disease
4	Patient with severe systemic disease that is a constant threat to life
5	Moribund, not expected to survive more than 24 hours
6	Brainstem death, organ donation
E	Suffixed to any grade, E indicates an emergency operation, e.g. 1E, 2E, etc.

This grading system is the one that is most widely used; it essentially classifies a patient according to his or her functional limitation. If a patient is classified as ASA1, they are completely fit and well. The presence of mild systemic disease implies that patients are not significantly limited in their day-to-day activity; for example, patients with diabetes mellitus, mild asthma or even stable angina would all be ASA2 patients. However, those patients who are limited, for example by shortness of breath, angina, etc., such that they are unable to continue their daily activity without disturbance are classed as ASA3. This classification is thought to give some indication of how such a patient's physiology would cope with the great stress of general anaesthesia and surgery.

There are, however, several drawbacks to this system. It is unclear how to classify a patient with several co-morbidities: one individual's definition of a 'mild' disease may be 'severe' in someone else's eyes – it is largely open to interpretation. Anyone over the age of 80 cannot be classified any better than ASA2.

Preoperative investigations

Remember to tell the examiner of your intention to request relevant preoperative investigations. In most cases, those in the list below will suffice, although patients with specific co-morbidities may need other specific investigations – for example, patients with rheumatoid arthritis will usually need cervical spine X-rays to assess atlantoaxial instability.

- Blood tests:
  - Full blood count, Us+Es, liver function tests
  - Clotting screen
  - Group and save
  - Haemoglobinopathy screen (especially important with certain ethnicities, such as Afro-Caribbean, Mediterranean and Asian patients)
- ECG
- Chest X-ray
- Echocardiogram

If you encounter problems

You must be prepared to highlight any potential problems you detect in your patient assessment to the anaesthetist allocated to do the list, as well as the surgeon or their team, since this is the whole point of the preoperative assessment. If in doubt, ask! That way, a plan can be made to optimise the patient in time for the operation, whether this means referral to a specialist or a visit back to the GP. It also allows time, if required, to admit the patient a day before the planned surgery to sort out their medical conditions. You should make it clear to the examiner, if your patient presents problems, that this is what you intend to do.

Premedication

You will often be asked to prescribe the patient the medications for their drug chart in advance. This will usually consist of simple prescriptions such as preoperative drinks, enoxaparin, bowel preparation and diabetic medications. Again, there are usually local protocols for this.

Postoperative review

As a surgical FY1, it may be your responsibility to see patients postoperatively either in the recovery area or when they get back to the ward. You should assess the following.

Type of anaesthetic used

If, for example, they have had an epidural or spinal, they will not be able to move their legs and should have been catheterised. Their urine output and blood pressure need to be watched, and they may need fluid boluses to maintain these.

Type of operation

• It is important to know exactly what procedure has been carried out. For example, if the patient has had a wide local excision involving a guidewire and dye, they may have a distinctly grey appearance, which can lead to a sense of panic in the doctor if the patient is asleep!
• Familiarise yourself with the patient's medical background.
• Check the vital signs, such as heart rate, blood pressure, oxygen saturations, respiratory rate, BM values and temperature. These will all have been checked in the recovery area and any problems sorted out before the patient returns to the ward, but there may be specific instructions in terms of what is to be done if any further problems are encountered.
• Check the operative site and any drains/catheter output.
• Check the drug chart: ensure pain medications, fluids, antibiotics, diabetic medications, enoxaparin, etc. have all been adequately prescribed.
• Check whether or not the patient is in pain. Ensure there is a suitable analgesic plan.
• Check whether the patient is allowed to eat and drink, and encourage early enteral intake if allowed.

Hints and tips for the exam

• This is a station that can provide really easy marks, so you should score highly here.

• It is essentially a detailed systems review, but with far more attention to detail in terms of cardiorespiratory functional status.
• Establishing exercise tolerance is important. If somebody can walk only 10 m and then needs to stop as they are short of breath, their outcome after being subjected to major surgery is unlikely to be good, and more precautions certainly need to be in place for them.
• Asking about previous facial and neck surgery has implications for a potentially difficult airway.
• Quantify smoking and alcohol consumption.
• In certain patients, further questioning may be indicated, for example relating to pregnancy in young women of child-bearing age, or sickle cell disease in those of Afro-Caribbean descent.
• It is important to ask about previous episodes of general anaesthesia as patients may tell you that they woke up very sick last time, or that the anaesthetist could not get a tube down their throat and told them to tell all future anaesthetists. They may have also had previous problems such as malignant hyperpyrexia. Previous anaesthetic problems are valuable warnings for future anaesthetic encounters.
• It is also important to ask about a family history of problems with general anaesthesia. If anyone in the family has needed postoperative ventilation for no apparent reason, they may have conditions like 'suxamethonium apnoea' or malignant hyperpyrexia, and it is then important to check that the patient has been investigated for this.
• All preoperative assessments should include a good airway assessment, but this is probably beyond what can be achieved in 5 minutes. You should, however, mention that you would do this.

Part 3: Communication skills

Do:

• **Start with two open questions and a minute of silence:** In 10-minute OSCE stations, it can be easy to become fixated on covering all the points as soon as possible. But by giving the patient ample time and space to speak, especially at the beginning of the consultation, you will not only get plenty of marks for open questioning, but will also be able to establish the patient's tone, underlying concerns, and hopefully expectations and agenda.

• **Apply 'ICE':** this is the one of the most important mantras of communication in medicine. Apply it, and make sure it is obvious to the examiner that you are doing so:

   • **Ideas:** This refers to the patient's ideas, views and feelings about the issue being discussed. This is fundamental as these ideas may be realistic or unrealistic and you will have to pitch your information at an appropriate level:

   'What do you understand about XYZ?'
   'Have you heard of XYZ before?'
   'Did you have any ideas of why you might be having this cough?'

   • **Concerns:** Uncovering the patient's concerns will allow you to address their underlying anxieties. It is quite common for patients to present with something relatively non-serious, such as a chest infection, and actually be worried about something much more significant, such as lung cancer. They will usually have had an experience that justifies those concerns – such as a relative who recently died of lung cancer. You could use these statements to probe any underlying concerns:

   'Was there anything you were particularly worried about?'
   'Was there anything at the back of your mind that was worrying you?'
   'What concerns you most about XYZ?'

• **Expectations:** Establishing the patient's expectations is the key to identifying their agenda and establishing what they want out of the consultation. This will subsequently help to ensure that consultation remains 'patient-centred' rather than 'doctor-centred', and make the patient feel satisfied that they have got what they wanted from the consultation. Establishing the patient's expectations will also help you prepare them for any unexpected surprises – if a patient diagnosed with lung cancer was actually expecting just to get some antibiotics for a perceived chest infection, you will need to utilise all your 'breaking bad news' communication skills to recalibrate the consultation.

• **Acknowledge 'cues' and emotions:** Cues are small snippets of information underlying more major issues that patients give without elaborating much further. The onus is on the candidate to identify cues and then tease out the more important underlying issues. An excellent candidate will go on to devise a management plan to help solve the problems – or at the very least organise a follow-up appointment to explore the issues in more detail. Cues could be verbal as well as non-verbal. For example, a patient looking very anxious when you talk about cancer may have an underlying anxiety due to a recent similar diagnosis in a close relative. The following are some examples of cues you may encounter:

   • *'It's definitely not the heart/cancer is it?'* (a patient who is worried about a heart attack/cancer).
   • *'I won't have to go to hospital, will I?'* (a patient who is worried about being admitted).
   • *'Will I be able to work?'* (a patient who has financial difficulties and is worried that they will not receive sick pay when off work).
   • *'It's not serious is it?'* (a patient worried about any serious condition – a good candidate will tease out exactly what condition the patient is worried about).
   • *'So I don't have rheumatoid arthritis then, do I doctor?'* (a patient who is worried about rheumatoid

OSCEs for Medical Finals, First Edition. Hamed Khan, Iqbal Khan, Akhil Gupta, Nazmul Hussain, and Sathiji Nageshwaran.
© 2013 John Wiley & Sons, Ltd. Published 2013 by John Wiley & Sons, Ltd.

arthritis, who may have an underlying anxiety about their hands becoming deformed and subsequently impairing their ability to carry out essential tasks, such as caring for an elderly, debilitated relative).

• **Say some clear unambiguous 'empathy' sentences:** There is often one mark for 'empathy' or 'empathetic approach'. Your manner and tone are obviously decisive in this, but you can make the examiner's job easier by using some statements that clearly and obviously empathise with the patient. Sentences like 'I can see how difficult this is for you' or 'I can't even begin to understand what you must be going through right now' will help convince an ambivalent examiner of your communication skills.

• **Use non-verbal communication:** This is a vital part of any communication skills station:
  • Make facial expressions that reflect those of the patient and the mood of the station.
  • Nod when appropriate.
  • Maintain good eye contact.
  • Adopt a posture that makes you look interested, leaning slightly forwards.

• **Identify any hidden agenda:** This could be a 'concern', as discussed under 'ICE' above, or it could be something else. A patient may actually be after a sick note, or may need respite from caring for an elderly debilitated relative, or may be worried about the effect their illness might have on their work. Make sure you ask probing questions and pick up all the cues.

• **Employ signposting:** This refers to the process of telling the patient what you are going to talk about, before talking about it. In certain stations such as 'breaking bad news' (see Chapter 46), this may constitute a 'warning shot' with which you warn the patient that you will be giving them some distressing news, or it may be merely be an explanation of what you intend to cover during the consultation.

• **Remember psychosocial aspects:** This is the key to providing holistic care. Find out about your patient's life – what they do, where they work, where they live, who they live with, and what they do socially. Most importantly, explore how their condition affects all these aspects of their life – and what you can do to help them.

• **Be 'patient-centred':** Don't be too rigid when devising a management plan. Find out about your patient's needs and preferences, and orientate your plan around the patient. Remember that the communication skills station is not primarily testing your clinical skills – it is highly important to ensure that the patient is at ease and feels happy with your plan.

• **Summarise:** There is often a specific mark for this, and it is also an excellent way for you to organise your own thoughts and identify anything you may have missed.

• **Involve the multidisciplinary team:** Utilise everyone in your team – social workers, dietitians, physiotherapists, occupational therapists, pharmacists, specialists, GPs and so on.

• **Use patient information leaflets:** This is easy and consumes very little time – and it also makes your patient's life easier. There are leaflets for everything, so use them!

• **Follow the patient up:** It is unlikely that your station will mark the end of the patient's story, so always arrange a follow-up appointment.

Don't:

• **Don't miss the point:** Avoid overindulging in empathy and being nice to the extent that you miss the aim of the station. Read the scenario carefully and make sure that, by the end, you have done what the instructions asked you to do.

• **Don't be pedantic about the clinical minutiae:** As mentioned before, the primary aim of communication skills stations is not to test your clinical knowledge, so don't get too hung up on the minute details.

• **Don't get impatient:** This can be difficult when you are pushed for time, but rushing the patient may upset them and lose you marks. For example, your empathy and listening skills will be unconvincing if you keep one eye on the clock. Take your time, and don't worry if you do not quite finish – most examiners will forgive this if you have been empathetic and you have demonstrated all the other relevant communication skills.

• **Don't sound paternalistic:** As your communication skills are being tested, don't be surprised if you have patients who are difficult to communicate with – such as those who are vague, unreasonable, overdemanding or just plain rude! Patiently persist, continue to be nice, and always negotiate and compromise where you need to.

Ethics and law

There is at least one ethics and law station in the final-year OSCE at the vast majority of medical schools. The main themes that you should have a thorough knowledge of are:
• Confidentiality
• Mental capacity
• Best interests
• DNAR orders
• Euthanasia

The way to go about ethical scenarios is to always go through the four key principles of ethics:
- Beneficence: doing good
- Non-malevolence: not doing harm
- Autonomy: the right to self-determination
- Justice/law: consideration of the law, with respect to the underlying legal frameworks and legal implications

The vast majority of candidates have a sound knowledge of ethical principles and medical law, and score well on MCQs on these topics. However, a large proportion of medical students find the ethics and law station one of the most difficult to score well on in the OSCE. Frequent reasons for encountering difficulty are:
- Failure to recognise that the station is testing ethics and law
- Failure to establish a plan of action at the end
- Failure to demonstrate empathy while communicating
- Failure to apply knowledge of ethical principles and medical law to the context of the OSCE station

Practising with colleagues is most likely to be the mainstay of your practice in preparation for this station because you are unlikely to get many opportunities to discuss ethical issues with patients during your clinical attachments.

Generic points for all communication skills stations

Appropriate introduction
Confirms patient's name
Explains reason for consultation
Obtains consent
Systematic approach

Establishes rapport
Starts with two open questions and 1 minute of silence to allow patient to open up
Acknowledges and responds to patient's 'cues'
Explores and responds to ICE
Explores psychosocial factors
Uses a 'patient-centred' approach and works in partnership with patient
Identifies any 'hidden agenda' and addresses it appropriately
Involves the multidisciplinary team where appropriate
Remains non-judgemental and encourages a positive approach
Shows empathy
Uses simple and appropriate language, avoiding use of jargon
Listens carefully and uses non-verbal communication skills effectively, maintaining appropriate tone and eye contact
Checks patient's understanding at regular intervals
Non-verbal skills
Avoids technical jargon
Uses signposting appropriately
Devises a holistic management plan and addresses psychosocial issues as well as medical problems
Acknowledges any gaps in own knowledge and offers to discuss these areas with seniors
Gives patient a patient information leaflet
Offers contact details of support groups/patient associations if appropriate
Summarises
Invites questions
Organises follow-up

46 Breaking bad news

Checklist	P	MP	F
Introduces self and explains reason for consultation			
Identifies patient correctly			
Gains consent			
Ensures setting is private and dignified (bleep off, door closed)			
Establishes rapport			
(E – expectations) Establishes what patient is expecting to find out			
Establishes patient's understanding of the **sequence of events** leading to this consultation			
(I – ideas) Establishes patient's ideas of what the underlying cause of the symptoms might be			
Clarifies or confirms patient's understanding of the sequence of events			
(C – concerns) Establishes and acknowledges any concerns the patient has			
Signposts that bad news is going to be broken, using an appropriate 'warning shot'			
Breaks bad news in a gentle and empathetic manner			
Ensures that information given is accurate and unambiguous			
Uses a period of silence to allow patient to absorb the information			
Allows patient to express their emotions			
Acknowledges patient's emotions and the significance of the news			
Explains management strategy			
Acknowledges any gaps in own knowledge, and offers to seek advice from seniors/colleagues			
Encourages a **positive outlook**, highlighting any positive aspects of test/investigation results			
Manages uncertainty appropriately and empathetically			
Explores **psychosocial context** (who is at home, whether there is anyone to talk to, activities of daily living, work situation, etc.)			
Explores **psychosocial** situation and offer support: • Offer meeting with family/partner • Counselling • Social worker if the patient is elderly and has care needs			
Arranges **follow-up** appointment with specialist doctor/nurse/other member of the multidisciplinary team			
Safety net: asks patient to contact doctor if letter/ notification of appointment does not arrive			
Offers to help patient get home (call a taxi)			
Provides contact details			
Listens to patient and allows them to express their views without interruption			
Shows empathy			
Uses simple and appropriate language, avoids using jargon			
Listens carefully and uses non-verbal communication skills effectively, maintaining appropriate tone and eye contact			
Checks patient's understanding at regular intervals			
Invites questions			
Systematic approach			
Summarises			
Offers written information/patient information leaflets			
Offers contact details of support groups/patient associations if appropriate			

Summary of common conditions seen in OSCEs

Condition	Key issues to consider and discuss
Cancer	Stage and grade Any metastasis Chemotherapy, radiotherapy, surgery Macmillan team input
Diabetes	Insulin or not insulin Follow-up in primary or secondary care Detecting and preventing complications Can lead a completely normal life – there are many successful sportsmen with diabetes
Multiple sclerosis	Variability of prognosis Different types – relapsing/remitting, progressive
Leukaemia	Recent improvements in therapy and prognosis
HIV	See Chapter 51 on HIV There have been recent huge advances in treatment If adhere to HAART, could potentially have a normal lifestyle and life expectancy
Rheumatoid arthritis	Early treatment can prevent deformity and reduce or minimise debilitation
Emergency hysterectomy	Reasons for doing this as emergency – immediate threat to life

Hints and tips for the exam

This is one of the most common stations in all communication skills OSCEs at every level in medical school – and beyond in postgraduate exams. This is probably because it is a very common real-life scenario that almost all doctors will face, regardless of what speciality they work in.

SPIKES – an easy-to-remember generic structure

The tables above cover everything you need for a finals OSCE exam. In the early stages of revision, a quick and easy way of remembering the basics is to go through the SPIKES six-point framework. This was devised by Robert Buckman, a Canadian oncologist, who published his idea in the journal *Community Oncology*, since when it has been adapted, used and taught widely across the world. The mnemonic expands as follows:

- **S** – setting the scene: refers to the process of ensuring that the setting is appropriate, for example ensuring that the room is private, dignified and comfortable, that there will be no disturbances, etc.
- **P** – perception: refers to the patient's perception, i.e. eliciting the patient's understanding of what has happened so far, and why the investigation has been done.

- **I** – invitation: refers to the invitation given to patients to find out whether or not they want more information.
- **K** – knowledge: refers to the process of signposting and actually giving the patient the news.
- **E** – empathy.
- **S** – strategy and summary: refers to the closure, including a summary of what has happened and what the plan is.

Acknowledge lack of knowledge

You may not be familiar with the condition you are talking about – which is not a problem. But don't be tempted to confabulate and 'guesstimate'. Patients under such emotional duress will seek reassurance, sometimes even unrealistically – and naturally you may feel inclined to acquiesce with them. However, it is important that you give accurate information while still remaining positive and as optimistic as the situation allows.

How long do I have?

This is a common question, especially from patients who have been diagnosed with cancer. The honest answer is that we rarely know – so do not try to guess a time frame. Be honest and unambiguous, and explain gently and empathetically that although you cannot answer that question at the moment, further investigations (such as scans looking for metastases) will help to give a more accurate idea, and that, most importantly, the whole multidisciplinary team (including yourself) will try their absolute best to ensure the best possible outcome and to keep the patient comfortable and pain-free.

Don't bombard the patient with too much information

This station tests your ability to break bad news in a way that is structured, clear and empathetic. There will usually be relatively few marks for your technical medical knowledge of the illness – so do not spend too much time and effort trying to discuss minutiae. Keep the conversation simple, focused and clear.

Don't be too optimistic

The art of breaking bad news is to remain positive and empathetic, while also being realistic. Patients may be in denial, and it can be tempting to play along and agree that 'everything will be OK'. However, it is important to be truthful and ensure that you give the patient a realistic and honest account of what you know and understand.

To maintain a positive tone, first explain that there are specialist multidisciplinary teams with access to a vast array of investigations and therapeutics that can be utilised to their full potential, and second emphasise that everyone in the team will try their best and do absolutely everything within their means to help the patient in every way possible.

47 Explaining medication

Checklist	P	MP	F
Introduces self and explains reasons for consultation			
Identifies patient correctly			
Gains consent			
Establishes rapport			
Explains purpose of consultation			
(E – expectations) Establishes what patient is expecting to gain from the consultation			
(I – ideas) Establishes patient's understanding of situation and need for consultation, e.g. 'Can you fill me in on what has been happening so far?'			
Establishes sequence of events leading to this consultation.			
(C – concerns) Establishes and acknowledges any concerns the patient has			
Checks if the patient is currently taking any drugs or has any drug allergies			
Checks if there any contraindications to the drug			
Explains why the new drug is being started			
Explains in lay terms how the drug works			
Explains how the drug should be taken			
Explains how long the patient can expect to be on the drug			
Explains pre-treatment blood tests/other investigations required (if applicable)			
Explains common side effects of drugs			
Explains uncommon but serious or potentially life-threatening side effects of the drug			
Explains simple methods to avoid or counteract the side effects (if applicable – e.g. co-prescription of alendronate to prevent steroid-induced osteoporosis)			
Explains potential hazards of taking the drug (e.g. adrenal crisis if steroids are stopped suddenly)			
Gives specific important information (e.g. requirement to wear warfarin bracelet or hold steroid card)			

Explains how clinical condition and side effects will be monitored			
Provides effective safety net (e.g. for warfarin – need to seek attention if suffer a head injury; for steroids – need to seek attention if there is intercurrent illness)			
Acknowledges any gaps in knowledge, and offers to seek advice from seniors/colleagues			
Explores potential issues relating to drug compliance			
Devises practical feasible solutions with an agreed time frame to solve compliance/other issues (e.g. dosette box)			
Works in partnership with patient, exploring their ideas and preferences with respect to possible solutions, negotiating and compromising where necessary			
Asks if the patient has any specific concerns/questions about the new drug (e.g. 'Will I put on weight if I start steroids?')			
Responds positively and offers simple solutions for concerns (e.g. weight gain is a recognised side effect but can be countered by improving diet and taking more exercise)			
Advises patient to store medications out of reach of young children			
Explores psychosocial aspects: • Explores home situation (who patient lives with, activities of daily living, work) • Disruption to lifestyle as a result of medications			
Identifies and addresses any 'hidden agenda'			
Invites questions and checks patient's understanding regularly			
Communicates at an appropriate pace and shows empathy			
Offers leaflet/web-based information about the drug			
Arranges a follow-up appointment			
Actor's impression of overall consultation			

Summary of common medications seen in OSCEs

Drug	How does it work (in lay terms)?	Dosing regimen	Side effects	Hazards related to drug use	Safety netting, important advice	Monitoring	Other important information
Steroid (e.g. prednisolone)	Prevents immune system from attacking itself Reduces inflammation **Not** a pain-killer	Once daily tablet for 1–2 years for giant cell arteritis 7–10-day course after exacerbations of COPD 5-day course after asthma attacks	Peptic ulcer disease, heartburn Osteoporosis Weight gain and Cushingoid appearance Diabetes mellitus Hypertension Increased risk of infections Cataracts	Risk of adrenal crisis if stopped suddenly Increased risk of low-trauma fractures	Report new-onset heartburn, abdominal pain, impaired vision, polydipsia + polyuria Do **not** stop taking steroids suddenly; seek advice if there is intercurrent illness Alendronate is prescribed to counter bone thinning Increase exercise and reduce calorie intake to counter weight gain Consult GP before starting any new medication, especially aspirin	Oral glucose tolerance test Blood pressure DEXA scan Activity of underlying disease (e.g. ESR for giant cell arteritis)	Must carry steroid card at all times Avoid over-the-counter drugs, e.g. ibuprofen If smoker, advise cessation to decrease risk of osteoporosis
Warfarin	'Thins' blood and therefore prevents formation of clots that can block blood vessels	Dose titrated by International Normalised Ratio Heparin must be co-prescribed on the first 5 days because warfarin initially has a paradoxical pro-coagulant effect	Easy bruising Haemorrhage Rash Teratogenic Alopecia Gastrointestinal upset	Increased risk of intracranial haemorrhage with falls Interactions with alcohol, antibiotics and antiepileptic drugs	Report new-onset bleeding (e.g. haematuria, haematemesis, melaena) Report any head injury (even if minor) Consult medical practitioner before starting any new drug Do not take over-the-counter drugs, e.g. ibuprofen, without getting medical advice Seek immediate advice if you may be pregnant	International Normalised Ratio	Need to wear warfarin bracelet at all times Need to keep International Normalised Ratio booklet Need to attend appointments at local anticoagulation clinic Seek advice before planning pregnancy or breast-feeding while on warfarin

Methotrexate	Reduces activity of immune system and therefore reduces damage to body tissues Reduces inflammation **Not a painkiller**	Once weekly **Never** once daily Important to check dose carefully and seek prompt advice if there are any concerns about dose	Gastrointestinal upset Mouth ulcers Infections Rashes Hair thinning Bone marrow suppression leading to easy bruising Teratogenic Long term: increased risk of cirrhosis and pulmonary fibrosis	Men taking methotrexate should ensure their partners do not become pregnant while they are on treatment Women should seek immediate advice if they think they may be pregnant if they are taking methotrexate themselves or their partner is taking it Check the dose is correct before taking it	Report the following immediately: shortness of breath/decreased exercise tolerance, jaundice, fever or sore throat, bruising, continued gastrointestinal upset, shingles Inform medical practitioner you are taking methotrexate prior to surgery	**Before starting treatment:** full blood count, Us+Es, liver function tests, chest X-ray, Urine dipstick **During treatment:** Full blood count, Us+Es, liver function tests continued	Seek urgent medical help if you accidentally take an overdose or miss a dose Do not take if pregnant or breast-feeding Seek medical advice before taking any vaccinations. Live vaccines (yellow fever, MMR, rubella) are contraindicated Avoid alcohol as this precipitates liver damage Avoid unpasteurised milk Carry a monitoring booklet
Metformin	Increases sensitivity of tissues to insulin	Taken three times daily (a few minutes after meals)	Gastrointestinal upset Lactic acidosis Renal failure NB. **Not** hypoglycaemia	Precipitates renal failure if pre-existing kidney injury Precipitates lactic acidosis if tissue ischaemia (e.g. myocardial infarction)	Inform radiologist before any scan involving contrast Inform anaesthetist before surgery Seek medical attention if there are continued symptoms such as polydipsia/polyuria	Us+Es, HbA_{1c}	Continue to implement lifestyle modifications including increased exercise, reduced calorie intake, reduced salt intake, smoking/alcohol cessation
Statins	Reduce blood cholesterol and therefore reduce risk of myocardial infarction, stroke and peripheral vascular disease	Tablet taken last thing before going to bed	Jaundice Muscle damage		Seek immediate attention if jaundiced or with abdominal pain or muscle aches/weakness Call 999 if chest pain develops or notices any 'FAST' signs	Liver function tests Lipid profile	

NB. Asthma and post-myocardial infarction medication are covered in Chapters 49 and 54, respectively.

Hints and tips for the exam

This is a relatively difficult OSCE station because it tests the candidate in a number of domains:

• **Knowledge about commonly prescribed drugs:** You need a fairly detailed knowledge of the side effects, dosing regimens and potential hazards of the drugs outlined in the table above to be able to perform well in this station.

• **Communication skills:** You will be imparting a large volume of information in a small amount of time to a lay person. It is important to try to keep the station as interactive as possible – this is the best way to ensure you are only giving information that is relevant to the patient's needs. In some cases, however, actors will not guide you through the station by asking questions. In this case, it is important to stick to the generic structure whereby you explain the reason for the drug and its dosing regimen, and its side effects/hazards, and provide appropriate safety netting and monitoring.

• **Safety netting:** Make the patient aware of situations that may require emergency care. Stress the importance of having a low threshold for seeking medical help if they are concerned about their symptoms or any side effects of the drug.

• **Safe prescribing:** Although you are not required to write up a drug chart, this station tests several other aspects of safe prescribing. You should ask about **drug allergies** and check for **contraindications**.

• **Orchestrating an effective consultation:** No consultation is ever complete without exploring the patient's specific concerns. In the OSCE, you are almost guaranteed to be faced with an actor who does have a specific concern. You should ask about any specific concerns and respond positively by offering simple solutions where appropriate.

Potential variations at this station

• Completing a 'To take away' (TTA) form and explaining the medications to a patient.

• Explaining medications and conservative lifestyle measures to a patient.

Scenarios you may encounter at this station

• Mrs Smith was recently diagnosed with giant cell arteritis. She is now ready to be discharged from hospital. Your registrar has asked you to explain her new medication to her before she goes home. The medicine she has been started on is prednisolone 40 mg once daily.

• Mr Jones has been recovering on the ward from an acute exacerbation of COPD. He is being discharged home on a breakthrough course of oral prednisolone to be taken for 14 days. He has some questions about this.

• While recently recovering on the ward from an unrelated infection, Mrs Winters was found to be suffering from atrial fibrillation. A decision has been made to start her on warfarin. Your registrar has asked you to explain her new medication to her before she goes home.

• Mr. Arthur's blood cholesterol was recently found to be 7.5 mmol/L during routine screening at your GP practice. Secondary causes have been ruled out, and the senior GP feels he will benefit from taking simvastatin. He has invited Mr Arthur to the clinic today and has instructed you to explain simvastatin therapy to Mr Arthur.

• Mr Shaun has recently been diagnosed with rheumatoid arthritis and is now being started on methotrexate. Explain methotrexate therapy to him.

48 Explaining a procedure

Checklist	P	MP	F
Introduces self and explains reasons for consultation			
Identifies patient correctly			
Gains consent			
Ensures setting is private and dignified (bleep off, door closed)			
Establishes rapport			
Explains purpose for consultation, obtains consent			
(E – expectations) Establishes what patient is expecting to gain from the consultation			
(I – ideas) Establishes patient's current understanding of procedure/operation			
Establishes sequence of events leading to this consultation			
(C – concerns) Establishes and acknowledges any underlying concerns patient has about the procedure			
Establishes if the patient is currently on any medication that may need to be stopped/altered beforehand			
Explains why the procedure/operation is being proposed, without using jargon			
Explains what the procedure/surgery involves:			
• Duration			
• Location (e.g. designated procedure suite, outpatients clinic, theatre)			
• Pain/discomfort likely to be experienced			
• Use of sedation, anaesthesia or analgesia			
Explains common and serious risks and complications associated with procedure/surgery:			
• Immediate risks (e.g. pain, damage to local organs)			
• Short-term risks (e.g. risk of deep vein thrombosis/pulmonary embolism, wound infection)			
• Long-term risks (e.g. recurrence of disease)			
Explains consequences of not proceeding with proposed procedure/surgery:			
• Less invasive alternatives			
• Diagnostic delay			
• Complications of underlying disease associated with delay in diagnosis/treatment			
Outlines reasonable alternatives to the proposed procedure			
Explains what needs to be done before the procedure:			
• Recommended time of arrival at hospital			
• Instructions on eating/drinking the night before and/or on day of the procedure/surgery			
• Instructions regarding any special diet or medicines that need to be taken beforehand			
Explains what will happen after the procedure:			
• Length of hospital stay			
• Driving			
• Returning to work			
• Activities of daily living			
Explores psychosocial aspects and effects on patient's life that symptoms have had			
Identifies and addresses any 'hidden agenda'			
Works in partnership with patient, exploring their ideas and preferences with respect to possible solutions, negotiating and compromising where necessary			
Acknowledges any gaps in own knowledge and offers to seek advice from seniors/colleagues			
Provides appropriate safety netting giving clear advice about adverse symptoms to look out for			
Explains how the results will be disclosed			
Explores any specific concerns (e.g. risk of colonoscopy showing bowel cancer)			
Addresses concerns appropriately (does not give false reassurance)			
Invites further questions			
Closes consultation appropriately:			
• Ensures understanding			
• Invites questions			
• Offers written information			

Summary of common procedures/operations seen in OSCEs

Procedures

Procedure	Details	Risks	Benefits	Consequences of not going ahead	Alternatives	Pre-procedure	Post-procedure	Safety netting
Central line	Local anaesthetic over insertion site Lie flat with head tilted downwards looking away from side of insertion Needle inserted to guide a narrow tube Needle removed and tube taped to neck Sterile field	Discomfort Bleeding Infection Scarring Artery puncture Pneumothorax Nerve injury Arrhythmia	Monitoring Frequent replacement not required	Potentially fatal, depending on indication	Sometimes femoral line may be acceptable Often there is no alternative	Check International Normalised Ratio if on warfarin	Chest X-ray to check for correct placement	Breathing difficulty Palpitations/chest discomfort Fever Pain Red, hot, itchy skin over insertion site
Oesophago-gastro-duodenoscopy	Sedation Local anaesthetic spray on pharynx Suction of pharyngeal secretions Will be asked to swallow	Sore throat Amnesia for period of sedation Tube passed in to trachea (causing chest infection) Discomfort Extremely rarely: • Perforation • Cardiac arrest	Gold standard to diagnose upper gastrointestinal tract pathology	Diagnostic delay and uncertainty	Barium meal CT scan	Nil by mouth for 4 hours Stop antacid 2 weeks beforehand	Few hours of monitoring in recovery area until sedation has worn off Arrange to be picked up	Chest pain Haematemesis Vomiting Abdominal pain Difficulty swallowing Fever
Colonoscopy	Rectal examination beforehand Sedation Lie on one side but may be asked to turn	Perforation risk (very rare – would require emergency surgery) Infection Incomplete examination Allergic reaction to sedative drugs Discomfort Bloatedness	Gold standard for investigating colonic pathology Polyps can be removed	Diagnostic delay	CT scan of abdomen – does not necessarily give definitive diagnosis Barium enema Surgical exploration	Must take bowel preparation medication the day before the procedure Only clear fluids for 12 hours before procedure	Few hours of monitoring in recovery area until sedative wears off Arrange to be picked up	Abdominal pain Rectal bleeding Fever
Bronchoscopy	Sedation Local anaesthetic spray on pharynx Lying down Scope enters through nostril Breathing monitored and oxygenation provided	Pneumothorax Chest/throat infection Perforation Bleeding Allergic reaction to sedatives	Gold standard for diagnosing lung pathology	Possible diagnostic delay Possible diagnostic uncertainty despite other investigations	Imaging Aspiration guided by imaging	May need alteration to anticoagulant medication Nil by mouth for around 8 hours Lung function tests, blood tests Chest X-ray	Few hours of monitoring in recovery area until sedative wears off Arrange to be picked up	Breathing difficulty Fever Haemoptysis Haematemesis

Procedure	What it involves	Risks	Benefits	Consequences of not having	Alternative	Preparation	After	Warning symptoms to report
ERCP for gallstone removal	Sedation. Local anaesthetic spray on pharynx. Tube passed through mouth (patient asked to swallow) into duodenum and then turned into biliary tree. Dye injected to enable X-ray images. Cutting of sphincter, stenting of any blockage	Pancreatitis. Cholangitis. Perforation. Chest infection. Mortality <0.3%	Relief of gallstone-induced obstruction	Need for open surgery	Surgery under general anaesthesia	Nil by mouth for 12 hours. Blood test (liver function tests, platelets). Come to hospital the night before for prophylactic antibiotics (oral ciprofloxacin; NB. Ask about allergies)	Short hospital stay to monitor for potential complications	Abdominal pain. Vomiting. Fever. Rigors. Cough, breathing difficulty
Cardiac catheterisation for angiography	May be a day case or may have to stay in hospital overnight. Local anaesthetic applied over inner thigh. Femoral artery punctured and probe passed upwards to heart vessels. Dye injected to enable images of vessels to show up on X-ray. Stenting/balloon dilation may be performed	Bleeding, pain, infection at insertion site. Cardiac tamponade. Myocardial infarction. Anginal chest pain. Allergic reaction to contrast. Hot flushes due to contrast	Gold standard to image coronary arteries. Therapeutic – avoids open heart surgery	Medical management. Need for open heart surgery later on. Higher risk of acute coronary syndrome	Open heart surgery (in some cases). Continuing medical management	Establish allergies to iodine and seafood (contained in dye). Blood tests, ECG, chest X-ray. Nil by mouth for 6 hours beforehand. Changes to blood-thinning and diabetic medication	Blood tests. ECG. Monitoring in recovery area and on ward thereafter	Chest pain. Palpitations. Breathing difficulty. Light-headedness. Bleeding, pain, red, hot skin over inner thigh. Fever
CT head	Contrast injected into vein. Wheeled into a doughnut-shaped scanner. Duration about 20 minutes	Reaction to contrast ranging from nausea/flushing to anaphylaxis. Claustrophobia. High dose of radiation	Quicker than other scans. Accuracy	May be able to undergo a different mode of imaging	MRI scan	Alterations to drugs (e.g. metformin). Intravenous fluids to prevent contrast-induced nephropathy		Facial swelling. Breathing difficulty. Symptoms of hypoglycaemia (if diabetes mellitus)
Lumbar puncture	Performed to obtain a sample of the fluid around the brain and spinal cord. Patient on left lateral side with knees tucked in to chest. Local anaesthetic injected at site of lumbar puncture. Needle inserted between two vertebrae into fluid-filled space outside spinal cord. Duration 20–30 minutes	Discomfort when lumbar puncture needle manipulated to obtain sample. Pain and abnormal sensations down the legs (NB. Tell patient to warn doctor if this occurs). Infection. Bleeding. Headache afterwards (risk about one-third in the first 24 hours).	High diagnostic accuracy	Diagnostic uncertainty. Delay in commencing treatment	Imaging. Blood tests	CT head (? raised intracranial pressure). Blood tests (? clotting disorders)	Lie on back for a few hours. Pain-killers to prevent headache	Weakness/abnormal sensations of legs. Persistent headache. Fever. Photophobia. Drowsiness. Neck stiffness. Discomfort at lumbar puncture site

Operations

Operation	Details	Risks	Benefits	Consequences of not going ahead	Alternatives	Pre-procedure	Post-procedure	Safety netting
Elective inguinal hernia repair	Surgery performed under general anaesthesia Incision made in lower abdomen Hernia pushed back into abdomen and mesh used to secure it in place If laparoscopic method used, three small incisions are made	Damage to spermatic cord and nerves supplying male genitals	Avoid need for emergency surgery	Hernia can strangulate, necessitating emergency surgery	Conservative management, e.g. wearing special items of clothing to help push it back	Nil by mouth 12 hours preoperatively Alterations to medication for diabetes mellitus	Monitored overnight/over a few days on the ward for complications and recovery	Painful leg Breathing difficulty Wound site discharge after leaving hospital Fever
Appendicectomy	Surgery performed under general anaesthetic Keyhole surgery (with three incisions) or incision in lower abdomen	Damage to nearby nerves causing slightly increased chance of inguinal hernia Damage to reproductive organs in females Long term: adhesions causing bowel obstruction	Avoid need for emergency surgery, which carries higher risk	Symptoms unlikely to resolve with medical treatment alone	Medical treatment	Nil by mouth from time of diagnosis	Monitoring overnight or for a few days on ward Antibiotic prophylaxis	Painful leg Breathing difficulty Wound site discharge after leaving hospital Fever Long term: subfertility, symptoms of bowel obstruction
Laparoscopic cholecystectomy	Four incisions for laparoscopic removal of gallbladder Contrast injected into biliary tree and X-ray taken to ensure there are no remaining stones	Conversion to open operation (about 10%) Damage to liver and bowel Damage to local blood vessels, causing substantial bleed	Cures/prevents gallstones and biliary colic	Further episodes of cholecystitis, cholangitis, increased risk of gallbladder carcinoma in long term	Open surgery Medical therapy unlikely to be effective	Nil by mouth 12 hours preoperatively	Monitoring overnight or for a few days on ward Possible antibiotic prophylaxis Possible outpatient follow-up	Painful leg Breathing difficulty Wound site discharge after leaving hospital Fever
TURP	Spinal anaesthesia so no sensation below waist Tube inserted into urethra Hypertrophic prostate tissue cut away Irrigation	Total spinal anaesthesia leading to respiratory arrest Need for repeat TURP (approximately 10% in next 10 years) Haematuria (about 2 weeks) Prostatitis Post-TURP syndrome – potential for confusion, fitting, loss of consciousness Erectile dysfunction (about 10%) Impotence (<10%) Urethral stricture Blood-stained ejaculate Urinary incontinence (about 10%) Increased frequency for around 6 weeks postoperatively	Gold standard treatment for benign prostatic hypertrophy	Need for radical prostatectomy later on Side effects from medication	Medical treatment Radical prostatectomy	Nil by mouth 12 hours preoperatively	Catheter in situ Transfer to recovery area and then ward for monitoring (up to 1 week) Avoid driving and sexual intercourse for 2 weeks	Haematuria beyond 2 weeks Dysuria, fever, rigors Erectile dysfunction

Hints and tips for the exam

Clinical medical students are expected to have observed common procedures and operations in sufficient detail to be able to gain formal consent from patients, so you are more or less guaranteed to get at least one of these OSCE stations. Candidates are often worried about not knowing the minor details of all the common procedures – although this may be useful, there are seldom marks for stating every single benefit or complication of a procedure/operation. Hence, it is more productive to apply a generic framework to this type of station.

Pass/fail points

- **Explaining serious complications:** for example, the risk of oesophageal rupture following an oesophago-gastro-duodenoscopy
- **Safety netting:** warning the patient to call 999 if chest pain develops following oesophago-gastro-duodenoscopy (because this could signal oesophageal rupture)
- **Fulfilling the criteria to gain valid informed consent (according to the Mental Capacity Act 2005):**
  - Details of procedure
  - Reason for proposing procedure
  - Consequences of not going ahead with it
  - Risks and benefits
  - Alternatives
- **Careful communication is the key:**
  - Chunk and check.
  - **Do not** coerce the patient.
  - Objective language to describe frequency of complications. For example, 'Out of every thousand people having the procedure, on average one person will suffer . . . ' is better than saying 'The risk of . . . is extremely low.'
  - **Do not** give false reassurance. For example, do not tell the patient that a deep vein thrombosis is a 'minor' postoperative complication.

Other important points

- It is important to establish **what the patient wants to know** early on, **so ASK**. Allow the patient to ask questions freely so that they can guide you through the station. This way you will be scoring marks left, right and centre. If you simply regurgitate memorised information that the patient is not interested in knowing, you will not earn many marks.
- Have a logical structure. Complications can always be divided into those which are immediate, short term and long term, and those related to the procedure/surgery itself as opposed to the sedation/anaesthetic. Most of the procedures outlined here are carried out under sedation so you should remember the following items of information for the patient with regard to this:
  - Arrange to be picked up.
  - Have someone looking after you for 24 hours after the procedure.
  - Do not drive for 24 hours after the procedure.
  - Do not operate machinery or perform other potentially dangerous tasks for 24 hours after the procedure.
- Complications of general anaesthesia are as follows:
  - Damage to teeth/oropharynx during intubation
  - Allergic reactions to anaesthetic drugs
  - Weakness of limbs and difficulty weight-bearing postoperatively
  - Chest infection
  - Urinary retention leading to an increased chance of urinary tract infection
  - Catheterisation for a few hours or days postoperatively
- General postoperatively complications include:
  - Pain
  - Bleeding, poor healing and infection of the wound
  - Chest and urinary tract infections
  - Deep vein thrombosis and pulmonary embolism
  - Failure of surgery or a need for further surgery later
- Patients must be advised that they are unlikely to be able to return to work for at least 2 weeks following the operations described in this chapter.
- Remember the specific **serious and life-threatening complications** of common procedures and operations outlined in the table above.

49 Inhaler technique and asthma medication

Task (5 minutes): This is 18-year-old John, who has been diagnosed with asthma following an attack last week. He is being started on salbutamol and beclom- etasone inhalers. Advise him how to use these inhalers.

Checklist	P	MP	F
Introduces self and explains reasons for consultation			
Identifies patient correctly			
Gains consent			
Ensures setting is private and dignified (bleep off, door closed)			
Establishes rapport			
Explains purpose for consultation/obtains consent			
(E – expectations) Establishes what patient is expecting to gain from the consultation			
(I – Ideas) Establishes patient's understanding of situation and need for consultation, e.g. 'Can you fill me in on what has been happening so far?'			
Establishes sequence of events leading to this consultation			
(C – concerns) Establishes and acknowledges any concerns that patient has about their inhalers and/or asthma			
Establishes symptoms that led to the diagnosis of asthma			
Assesses prior knowledge and offers brief explanation of asthma without using jargon: • Relatively common disease affecting 5–8% of the population • Triggered by various stimuli including cold air, exercise, pollution, pollen and house dust mite droppings • Caused by narrowing of airways • Treated by medicine that reverses narrowing of airways			
Enquires about known drug allergies			
Explains inhaler technique without using jargon: • Shake inhaler • Remove cap • Exhale maximally • Form tight seal around mouth piece • Press canister and inhale simultaneously			

Checklist	P	MP	F
• Hold breath for 10–15 seconds (or as long as is comfortably possible) • Repeat this again • Demonstrate to the patient • Ask the patient to demonstrate before the end of the consultation • Offer written advice			
Explains salbutamol is a reliever: • Two puffs when symptoms of cough, shortness of breath or wheeze develop • Seek urgent medical help if no relief after four puffs • Side effects include tremor, headache and palpitations			

Explains beclometasone is a preventer:
• Used regularly irrespective of symptoms, e.g. two puffs twice a day
• Decreases likelihood of developing recurrent symptoms over the longer term
• Side effects:
  • Sore throat due to fungal infection: preventable by gargling with water after use
  • Rare to get side effects associated with oral steroid use
  • Advises patient that they may need to carry a 'steroid card' if the dose has to be increased			

Explains when emergency help should be sought: • Symptoms do not improve, or worsen, despite four puffs of the blue inhaler • Symptoms are severe, e.g. cannot talk in full sentences, lips become blue, becomes drowsy			
Explores specific concerns (e.g. perceived stigma caused by taking inhalers at school or in workplace)			
Shows empathy and offers simple solutions (e.g. school nurse can hold inhalers)			
Checks understanding and arranges follow-up			
Maintains rapport throughout consultation and closes appropriately			

Hints and tips for the exam

This is a relatively straightforward station. The vast majority of candidates will be able to explain asthma and inhaler technique to a patient, and most will be able to give basic information about dosing regimens and the side effects of medication. However, you will be expected to explore and address any specific concerns the patient has in order to secure a good score in this station. The key concepts that you should demonstrate in this station relate to the following:

• **Good communication skills:**
 • Do not overlook the importance of using phrases to **demonstrate empathy** at the start of the consultation because asthma is potentially a lifelong condition and can be particularly frustrating if it limits participation in sports or employment.
 • Remember to '**chunk and check**'. Check the patient's prior knowledge, provide information at an appropriate pace and check the patient's understanding afterwards. Ensure that you demonstrate inhaler use and check the patient's technique during the consultation.
 • In addition to the basics, the actor-patient is likely to have a **specific agenda**. Concerns about the side effects of steroids are quite common in OSCEs. This will only be revealed if the candidate specifically enquires about the patient's concerns. Candidates who explore the actor-patient's agenda are likely to be considered for a merit/distinction.
• **Safety netting:** Make the patient aware of situations that may require emergency care. Stress the importance of having a low threshold for seeking medical help if the patient is concerned about their symptoms. Failing to give advice about what to do if symptoms continue despite using salbutamol will be regarded as unsafe practice.
• **Safe prescribing:** Although you are not required to write up a drug chart, this station tests several other aspects of safe prescribing. You should ask about **drug allergies** and take a brief past medical history to ensure that it is safe for the patient to take the inhalers and that there are no contraindications to this. Ensure you have a sound knowledge of the **side effects** of asthma medication and can clearly explain the **roles** of salbutamol and beclometasone in symptom relief and prevention, respectively.

Potential variations at this station

• **Fill out a TTA form and explain inhaler technique to a patient who is ready for discharge after being admitted with a severe asthma attack for the first time.** In addition to explaining inhaler technique, this scenario also tests your ability to prescribe on a drug chart, complete a discharge summary and explain post-discharge asthma care.
• **Explain use of inhalers with a spacer device.** You must communicate the following information to the patient:
 • The inhaler is plugged in at one end. A tight seal is formed around the mouth piece at the other end. One puff should be delivered into the spacer at a time, and the patient should breath in and out deeply several times.
 • Once a week, the spacer should be washed by immersion in water (or soap solution) followed by drip-drying. It should not be scrubbed or dried by rubbing. It should be replaced every 6–12 months.
 • Spacer devices increase ease of inhaler use by removing the need for precise coordination between pressing the canister and inhaling.
 • Spacer devices increase the amount of drug delivered into the airway and decrease the amount deposited on the back of the throat. They are therefore more effective, and patients are less likely to suffer from local side effects such as a sore throat.
• **Explain how to use a peak flow meter and a salbutamol inhaler to this patient recently diagnosed with asthma by his GP.** In addition to inhaler technique, you must communicate the following concepts to the patient without using jargon:
 • **Instructions:**
  • Stand up.
  • Ensure the pointer is at zero, and hold the meter horizontally at the sides without occluding the pointer.
  • Inhale maximally and form a tight seal around the mouth piece.
  • Exhale as quickly as possible.
  • Record the number the pointer is pointing to.
  • Replace the pointer to zero and repeat the procedure three times, taking the highest reading.
 • Don't forget to demonstrate the procedure to the patient and check their technique.
 • Peak flow meters assist in diagnosing asthma and monitoring response to treatment.
 • Peak flow should be recorded in the morning, at night and when symptoms are experienced. The values should be entered in a peak flow diary.
 • A diurnal variation of greater than 20% on three or more days of the week supports a diagnosis of asthma.
 • The existence of significant diurnal variation despite treatment may be an indication for stepping up treatment.

50 Exploring reasons for non-compliance

Checklist	P	MP	F
Introduces self and explains reason for consultation			
Identifies patient correctly			
Gains consent			
Establishes rapport			
(E – expectations) Establishes reason for patient's attendance			
Establishes patient's ideas of what the underlying cause of the symptoms might be			
Clarifies or confirms patient's understanding of the sequence of events			
(C – concerns) Establishes and acknowledges any concerns the patient has			
(I – ideas) Explores patient's understanding of the condition and their health beliefs			
Explores patient's understanding of medication and the following aspects: • Purpose of medication • How it works • Benefits of compliance • Consequences of non-compliance • Fears of medication, adverse effects and/or the condition itself **(C – concerns)**			
Explores all aspects of the pathway of the patient's usage chronologically, and identifies problems: • Obtaining medication (travel to chemist) • Paying for prescription • Understanding regimen (dose, frequency, duration) • Administering medication (swallowing, etc.) • Adverse effects • Monitoring			
Psychosocial aspects • Explores home situation (who patient lives with, activities of daily living, work) • Disruption to lifestyle as a result of the medication • Stigma/fears about being stigmatised			

Identifies and addresses any **'hidden agenda'**			
Explores and addresses each problem identified in a logical and non-judgemental manner			
Works in partnership with the patient, exploring their ideas and preferences with respect to possible solutions, negotiating and compromising where necessary			
Devises practical feasible solutions with an agreed time frame			
Acknowledges any gaps in own knowledge and offers to seek advice from seniors/colleagues			
Encourages **positive outlook**, highlighting advantages of compliance			
Arranges follow-up appointment to monitor patient's progress			
Safety net: asks patient to contact doctor if there are any problems			
Listens to patient and allows them to express their views without interruption			
Shows empathy			
Uses simple and appropriate language, avoids using jargon			
Uses non-verbal communication skills effectively and maintains appropriate tone and eye contact			
Checks patient understanding at regular intervals			
Invites questions			
Systematic approach			
Summarises			
Offers written information/patient information leaflets			
Offers contact details of support groups/patient associations if appropriate			

Summary of common conditions in OSCEs

Condition	Key issues to consider and discuss
Statins Antihypertensive agents	Lack of obvious physical improvement Side effects (such as muscular pains with statins, ankle swelling with amlodipine)
Insulin	Phobia to needles Stigma – use of needles may look similar to illicit drug abuse to general public Inconvenience of using needle and apparatus if busy at work and during social activities (e.g. at cinema) Lack of obvious physical improvement
Inhalers	Lack of understanding about mechanism of action and the different roles of preventers versus relievers
Warfarin	Monitoring (with regular International Normalised Ratio) may be perceived to be arduous Lack of understanding about need for prevention
Steroids	Misperception of steroid (confusion with anabolic steroids used by sportsmen) Side effects (e.g. weight gain, bruising)
Antiepileptic agents	Lack of understanding about the need for prevention Lack of obvious physical improvement
Immunosuppressive medication	Side effects (e.g. gum hypertrophy with ciclosporin)
Tuberculosis medications	Duration of course Lack of understanding of public health issues and seriousness of disease

Hints and tips for the exam

This is a common scenario in OSCEs as it assesses a broad understanding of psychosocial issues and the ability of candidates to think laterally and devise practical solutions that can be implemented in real life.

Solutions

The checklist above should help you establish the underlying cause of the patient's non-compliance. The key to getting into the upper echelons of the pass mark and into the merit range is to devise a practical and realistic solution that both the patient and examiner find convincing. Here are some possible solutions that could be applied to any scenario.

Obtaining the prescription

Elderly patients may have mobility problems that make it difficult for them to physically travel to their local pharmacist – possible issues could range from going up and down flights of stairs, to arranging transportation. Practical solutions may involve simple measures, like utilising help from **friends and family** to help out. **Social services** may be able to organise carers to do this, who could liaise with pharmacists. **Third-sector** organisations, for example charities such as Age UK, may also

be useful and have significant experience of helping elderly patients in such situations.

If you are thinking of broader, more long-term solutions (and have time remaining at your station!), you could even consider discussing ways to improve the patient's mobility in general – for example, through physiotherapy or occupational therapy. This would not only help the patient obtain their medication, but also improve their life in general.

Pharmacists could also help by organizing **deliveries** to patients' homes. Some pharmacies are even involved in **batch prescribing**, in which GPs write prescriptions for 6 months and pharmacies then dispense to patients on a monthly basis.

Paying for prescriptions

The cost of a single prescription item at the time of publishing is about £7.40. This is significant for patients on a low income and may well prove to be a deterrent.

There are, however, various ways of minimising this, for example **Prescription Payment Certificates,** which allow patients to pay for a 'bulk' of prescriptions for a year at a cheaper cost than the sum of individual prescriptions. Various patient groups are also exempt from prescription charges, such as those with certain conditions (e.g. thyroid problems), certain age groups (e.g. the under 16s and over 60s). A detailed list of exempted groups can be found on this official NHS website (www.nhsbsa.nhs.uk/792.aspx).

You could also consider ways to help patients with their general financial situation, such as asking **social workers** to help those with chaotic routines and difficult lifestyles. **Benefit advisors** often see patients in GP surgeries and could help patients obtain benefits they do not know they are entitled to.

Medication regimens (dose, frequency, times, duration)

Some medication regimens are easy to understand and remember – such as taking one aspirin a day. Other more complex regimens may, however, be quite difficult to fathom, especially for elderly patients and those with cognitive impairment, who are ironically usually taking multiple medications with more complex regimens. Patients may simply not know about the correct regimen, or may have difficulty remembering to take all their medications at the right time – patient education is always a good place to start.

As with the other problems, try simpler solutions first. Basic measures such as posters on walls and doors may be all that is needed – the more technologically astute could utilise reminders on their mobile phones. Again, **friends and family** may be able to help, and social services could organise **carers**. Pharmacists could provide **dosette boxes** or **blister packs**, which divide the medications into little slots or boxes according to the day and time they are to be taken.

Again, thinking more laterally, you may find that you have uncovered a larger underlying problem. This may be an early presenting sign of dementia or an underlying social or psychiatric problem – investigating and managing this could help the patient's life and health in a much bigger way.

Administering medication

Some tablets may be difficult to swallow, or may be of a size or taste that deters patients from taking them. Most medications can be prescribed in **soluble or liquid suspension** forms, and several are available in **modified-release** form, involving taking fewer tablets that then slowly release the medication over a longer duration of time (e.g. 12 or 24 hours).

Needles

The injection of medications such as insulin is often associated with more specific problems, such as the **stigma associated with using needles** (similar to illicit drug users) and needle phobias. The answer may lie in simple **educational** measures – such as offering to speak to a patient's employer to help educate the staff about the patient's condition, or to find a separate room for the patient where they can administer their injections. **Needle phobias** may need specific treatment such as cognitive-behavioural therapy or counselling. More basic issues include the availability of **sharps disposal bins**. Changing the regimen could often be useful – for example, consider long-acting, slow-release insulin preparations rather than those which are short-acting.

Above all, remember to show empathy and provide reassurance – needle phobia and the stigma associated with injection can be very demoralising.

Work through and devise solutions for each problem individually

To ensure that your answer at this station is well structured, make a list of all the problems and find solutions for each one separately. Without this, you may well find that you lose track of the problems and merely have a helpful 'chat' rather than devise workable practical solutions.

Directly observed therapy

In this approach, the patient's medication is supervised by either a pharmacist or sometimes a community nurse. It is used rarely when compliance is absolutely essential – such as with tuberculosis.

Be 'patient-centred'

This is a perfect station to show your 'patient-centredness'. If your patient is difficult, use the opportunity to **negotiate and compromise**, and devise a solution that both you and the patient agree with.

51 Counselling for an HIV test

Checklist	P	MP	F
Introduces self and explains reasons for consultation			
Identifies patient correctly (uses at least two identifiers)			
Gains consent			
Ensures that setting is private and dignified (bleep off, door closed)			
Establishes rapport			
Explains purpose for consultation, obtains consent			
(E – expectations) Establishes patient's reason for attending			
(I – ideas) Establishes patient's understanding of situation and need for pre HIV test discussion, and if patient has ever had an HIV test before			
(I – ideas) Establishes patient's understanding of HIV and what it is: • Destroys immune system • Makes sufferers susceptible to bacteria/viruses • If not treated, can lead to AIDS			
Establishes sequence of events leading to this consultation			
(C – concerns) Establishes and acknowledges any underlying concerns that patient may have about the HIV test and explores possible sociocultural impact of being stigmatised			
Mentions confidentiality (separate notes from medical notes if is a genitourinary medicine clinic, insurance company, GP)			
• Has the patient ever been tested before (when? result?)			
Explains why patient needs HIV test			
Risk assessment – mentions risk factors:			
• Other sexually transmitted infections (increases risk of HIV-positive status and HIV transmission)			
• Partner known to be HIV-positive			
• Men who has sex with men (MSM), especially high-risk sex acts such as unprotected anal intercourse			
• Bisexual partner (if female)			
• Partner from high-risk country (e.g. sub-Saharan Africa and Caribbean)			
• Intravenous drug user			
• Blood transfusion abroad or before 1985 in UK			
• Is patient a sex worker or has patient had contact with a sex worker?			
Assess patient's knowledge of HIV, AIDS and transmission (sex, vertical transmission, blood, needles)			
• Most HIV-positive patients are asymptomatic			
• One-third of those HIV-positive in the UK are unaware of their status			
Patient's perception of own risk and expectation of result (responds appropriately)			
Benefits of testing			
• If positive:			
• Treatment available			
• Normal life expectancy with proper antiretroviral treatment			
• Able to have children (HAART and sperm-washing) but not able to breast-feed			
• Explains difference between HIV and AIDS			
• Reduction of further transmission			
• Counselling available if needed			
• If negative:			
• Can end a period of not knowing			
Basics of testing:			
• Point of care test (POCT): low risk. Not used for West African contacts due to insensitivity to HIV-2			
• Antigen/antibody blood test: high risk and also used to confirm reactive POCT			
• Explains window period clearly (3 months) and checks patient's understanding			
• Emphasises need for follow-up testing in 3 months			

• Asks when last exposure was (<72 hours + high risk – may give post-exposure prophylaxis. May be mentioned earlier)			
• Arrangements for how result will be given (usually given in person)			
Asks whether patient has support if they are found to be HIV-positive and who they would they disclose to			
Explores how patient may feel or react if HIV test is positive			
Remains empathetic and non-judgemental throughout the consultation			
Mentions documentation of discussion			
Gives patient information leaflets			
Discusses importance of avoiding spreading HIV • Condoms/safe sex			
Discusses need to test for other sexually transmitted disease			
Explores **psychosocial** aspects • Explores home situation (who patient lives with, activities of daily living, work) • Disruption to lifestyle as a result of the situation			

Identifies and addresses any '**hidden agenda**'			
Works in partnership with patient, exploring their ideas and preferences with respect to possible solutions to any issues/problems, negotiating and compromising where necessary			
Obtains informed consent for test (written consent is usually unnecessary)			
If patient is unsure after discussion, gives them time to consider and return			
If patient refuses, tries to carefully explore the reasons why. May be misinformed (e.g. criminal prosecution, insurance). The reasons for refusing a test should be documented			
Summarises and checks understanding			
Offers to answer any questions the patient has			
Acknowledges any gaps in own knowledge, and offers to seek advice from seniors/colleagues			

Hints and tips for the exam

This is a sensitive station. A patient waiting to have a HIV test will be understandably apprehensive and anxious. Part of this anxiety will relate to who will have access to the result of the test and or even know that the patient is having the test. Build a strong rapport early by stating the confidential nature of your discussion with the patient, as well as the fact that you will need their permission before any disclosure (something that is implicit in other OSCE stations). Do not start detailing the finer points of confidentiality with regard to positive results and serious harm unless asked specifically. It is, however, important to mention safe sexual practices while a patient's status is unknown.

Clarity is key in this station. You will be explaining the testing while also taking a brief history to ascertain the patient's risk. Asking the patient at regular (and natural) intervals whether they have understood you is important.

Try to use generalised statements and questions to assess the risk of HIV as well as the patient's level of knowledge. This will make the history more conversational and sound less accusatory. For example:

• 'Certain risk factors increase a person's chance of contracting HIV. Are you aware of any?'
• 'That's right. Also . . . can increase the likelihood.'
• 'How do you feel about your risk? Would any of these factors apply to you?'

Also ask about the patient's own perceptions of the disease and be prepared to politely correct any incorrect preconceived notions such as HIV being a disease solely of the homosexual population.

In some medical schools, one hurdle students are expected to navigate relates to the use of terms such as 'homosexual'. Refrain from using this, and ask directly about whether the patient has ever had sex with a man or whether their partner has (i.e. a man who has sex with another man).

A difficult area of the station is explaining the practicalities of the test, especially the window period. Practise this and have a memorised statement that is short and clear, such as: 'All HIV tests have a "window period" of 3 months. This means that if a person was exposed to HIV in the previous 3 months, the test may not pick this up, and they should come again for re-testing.' Note that this means the individual should have two tests separated in time.

Marks will be awarded for assessing the patient's expectations of the result and how they will cope. Who will they disclose to? Do they have adequate support at home? Would they benefit from seeing a counsellor? You may also mention the Terrence Higgins Trust, which provides support and information regarding HIV and AIDs.

A common difficulty among students is explaining the difference between HIV and AIDS. Make sure you have memorised a clear statement such as:
• 'HIV is an virus infection that damages the protective cells in the body, weakening the immune system.' (Note the lack of the word 'your')
• 'AIDS is a result of untreated long-standing HIV infection. When the immune system is very weak, the body cannot defend itself against other infections.'
• 'The test detects the HIV virus and not AIDS.'
Results can usually be available with a few minutes for the POCT or up to 2 weeks for the blood test. Results are usually given in person if the patient is deemed high risk. Low-risk patients can be phoned, texted or sent a letter.

The patient can, of course, decline the test (after all your hard work!). Although this is unlikely in the OSCE, be prepared for this and aim to explore their reasons for this and gently persuade of the benefits – but do not try to force them.

The point of the OSCE is to determine first and foremost whether you will be a safe junior doctor. Akin to this is good documentation. Remember to mention to the patient (and the examiner) that you would document everything discussed today.

Potential variations at this station
• **You may have to talk to a HIV-positive patient who is having unprotected sex and does not wish to disclose to their partner.**
  • This variation requires you to assess the risk to the partner of contracting HIV as a result of unsafe sexual practices.
  • You will also need to explore the patient's reasons for not telling their partner, as well as their awareness of the risk of transmission.
  • You may be asked what will happen if they refuse to disclose their status to their partner. Here you will have to clearly explain the boundaries of doctor–patient confidentiality.
    • Say particularly that you would have to disclose in the interests of the partner to prevent transmission.

• The patient would be notified prior to disclosure.
• Only as much information as is needed will be disclosed.
• It is worth mentioning that a doctor dealing with such a case should seek advice from their medical defence union on how to deal with it.
• Remember to ask at regular intervals if the patient understands.
• Allow them to make a decision in their own time. But remember to advise them to practise safe sex to prevent transmission in the interim.
• If the situation arises where both parties are HIV-positive, this still does not remove the need for protection as they may have different serotypes (HIV-1 and HIV-2). This also increases the risk of resistance to HAART (if partners have different resistant strains) and subsequently makes it more likely that treatment will fail.
• **You may have to counsel a pregnant woman about an HIV antenatal test.**
  • Use the phrase 'routine test' as this will ease conversation.
  • Knowing the mother is HIV-positive will mean:
    • Caesarean section
    • Prompt antiretroviral treatment for the baby after delivery
    • Advice regarding breast-feeding

Questions you could be asked

You may be asked questions related to the following topics:
• Confidentiality: when can it be broken?
• Insurance policies and HIV:
  • Taking a test does not have to be declared.
  • A negative test does not have to be declared to an insurance company.
  • A positive test should be declared, but the original policy is usually continued or 'honoured' by the insurance company.
• Antiretroviral therapy and side effects.
• What other illnesses would prompt you to offer a HIV test?

52 Post mortem consent

Checklist	P	MP	F
Introduces self			
Identifies relative correctly			
Identifies patient correctly			
Confirms patient's relationship to relative and checks that relative is the next of kin			
Establishes rapport			
Ensures that setting is private and dignified (bleep off, door closed)			
Offers condolences and shows empathy			
Establishes what the relatives already know			
Explains reason for consultation			
Explains reasons for post mortem: • If mandatory – to establish cause of death if unknown • Educational and research purposes			
Establishes relative's understanding of what a post mortem is and how it is done			
Explores relatives' 'ICE' regarding cause of death and post mortem: • Ideas: What were the relatives expecting to happen to the body? • Concerns: What concerns do the relatives have about the post mortem and/or the patient's cause of death • Expectations: What are the relatives' expectations from a post mortem?			
Allows relatives some time for reflection and asks if they would like to ask any questions at this point			
Explains post mortem procedure			
• Usually done as soon as possible, depending on availability of pathologist • Procedure will be performed by pathologist • Will be carried out in the hospital mortuary • A midline cut will be made for examination of internal organs and also the back of the head • Internal organs will be removed and returned once the procedure has been completed • Specimens may be taken for further investigation if deemed necessary • Emphasises that body will not be disfigured and will be treated with the utmost respect and dignity			

• Photographs may be taken if necessary and appropriate (at the discretion of the pathologist • The procedure takes approximately 3–4 hours • Once the procedure is complete, the body will be closed up and ready for burial or cremation			
Emphasises that organs will only be retained if and after the relative consents in writing			
Explores possibility of limited post mortem if relative not happy with full post mortem			
Allows relative to gather their thoughts and invites questions			
Enquires about preference of body, i.e. burial or cremation			
Emphasises that funeral will not be delayed			
Summarises back to relative			
Offers to answer any questions relative may have			
Acknowledges any gaps in own knowledge, and offers to seek advice from seniors/colleagues			
Identifies and addresses any 'hidden agenda'			
Asks for approval of the post mortem and gains written consent if appropriate			
Is empathetic throughout the consultation			
Explores psychosocial situation and offers support: • Offers meeting with family/partner • Who is at home? • Counselling			
Arranges follow-up appointment with specialist doctor, nurse or other member of the multidisciplinary team if any further discussion/ clarification is required			
Offers patient information leaflets			
Offers details of bereavement officer and counselling services			
Offers details of chaplaincy/religious services			
Offers to help relative get home (call taxi)			
Provides contact details			
Listens to relative and allows them to express their views without interruption			
Shows empathy			

Hints and tips for the exam

This is a difficult station – the topic of discussion is a very sensitive one that is potentially difficult to understand. Discussing a post mortem with someone who is already shocked and distressed having lost a loved one just makes it more difficult.

Keep your explanation clear and simple

Don't dig yourself into a hole trying to explain every single nook and cranny of an aspect of the post mortem that the patient is having difficulty in understanding. You can always offer to arrange a meeting between the relative and a pathologist, or give them written information – or even revisit the issue later when the relative may be more settled.

Empathy is essential (again)!

This may be the last station you undertake, and you may be exhausted and totally fed up with the OSCE – if this shows during a cardiovascular examination or cannulation station, the examiner will probably show some understanding. However, a post mortem is a very sensitive and potentially emotive issue, and you must ensure, regardless of other factors, that you are as empathetic and polite as possible.

What if the relative refuses a mandatory post mortem?

Mandatory post mortems have to be carried out by law, with or without the relative's consent. This may be difficult to explain, especially in a way that comes across empathetically. It may help if you explain that it is not your decision, but a legal requirement that everyone involved in must abide by. You could also stress the reasons for it being done (e.g. if the cause of death is suspicious), and the advantages of obtaining the information from it, especially with respect to helping the grieving family have some sort of psychological closure.

Referring a death to a coroner

The coroner will decide whether a post mortem is necessary. Although any deaths *can* be discussed or referred to a coroner for their opinion, in some circumstances it is legally mandatory to do so:
- If the cause of death has not been identified
- If the patient was not seen by a doctor in the 2 weeks preceding death
- If the death occurred within 24 hours of the patient being admitted to hospital
- If the death occurred after a termination of pregnancy or after delivery
- If the death was violent, suspicious, accidental or possibly resulting from poisoning
- If the death was due to a medical/surgical complication
- If the death was from a condition resulting from/associated with the patient's occupation (e.g. mesothelioma in patients who have worked with asbestos)
- If the death was the result of an accident
- If the death took place in prison or police custody

Questions you could be asked

Q. When might you have to report a death to a coroner?
Q. What is the procedure for a post mortem?
A. The answers to these questions can be found in the text.

53 Explaining a DNAR (Do Not Attempt Resuscitation) decision

Checklist	P	MP	F
Introduces self and explains reasons for consultation			
Identifies patient correctly			
Gains consent			
Ensures that setting is private and dignified (bleep off, door closed)			
Establishes rapport			
(E – expectations) Establishes what patient is expecting to find out			
(I – ideas) Establishes patient's ideas of the **sequence of events** leading to this consultation.			
Clarifies or confirms patient's understanding of the sequence of events			
(C – concerns) Establishes and acknowledges any concerns that the patient has			
Signposts that would like to discuss a direction and strategy for the patient's future management			
Explains what treatment is being given now			
Explains that patient's condition is critical and may deteriorate, possibly resulting in a cardiac arrest			
Explains that a decision is to be made on whether or not the patient is suitable for resuscitation			
Ascertains patient's views			
Offers to include family/relatives or next of kin in discussion			
Explains that resuscitation may not be appropriate in someone with their medical condition			

Suitable explanation for inappropriateness of resuscitation			
Explains that patient is still for full treatment except resuscitation and that you will continue to try your best for them			
Explains that the resuscitation order will be reviewed if the patient's condition improves			
Intention to inform other multidisciplinary staff involved in the patient's care			
Intention to complete a DNAR form, but awareness that it must be signed by a consultant			
Provides contact details			
Listens to patient and allows them to express their views without interruption			
Shows empathy			
Uses simple and appropriate language, avoids using jargon			
Listens carefully and uses non-verbal communication skills effectively, maintaining appropriate tone and eye contact			
Checks patient's understanding at regular intervals			
Invites questions			
Systematic approach			
Summarises			
Offers written information/patient information leaflets			
Offers contact details of support groups/patient associations if appropriate			

Hints and tips for the exam

This is a challenging station, but if you keep it simple, you will get most of the marks. It is highly unlikely that you will face this task alone in your early postgraduate years, as the decision-making and discussion with patient and family should be handled by the most senior doctor available on the team, and this is almost always the consultant.

When to discuss resuscitation status with patients

If cardiorespiratory arrest is not expected to occur, it is not necessary to have this discussion with the patient unless they wish to do so.

If a decision is taken on clinical grounds that the patient is inappropriate for resuscitation, discussion with the patient is not always required. In some circumstances, it may cause more distress than benefit, for example with end-stage terminal disease in which death is imminently expected. Such decisions should be made on an individual basis.

Some patients will not want to have this discussion, while others may request a second opinion. In either case, the patient's choices must be respected.

Patients who lack capacity may have made a living will, or have appointed an attorney, deputy or guardian in order to make their wishes known. The family may also know what the patient is likely to have wanted. While the patient's wishes should be respected, they can only refuse resuscitation. They cannot demand treatment that, on clinical grounds, is deemed inappropriate (i.e. if they are made 'not for resuscitation' for sound clinical reasons, they cannot demand to be· resuscitated).

When is resuscitation inappropriate?

It is difficult to give a generalised answer to this question. In general, patients should be resuscitated unless:
• The outcome is unlikely to be successful, or it is very unlikely that the heart could be restarted and breathing sustained for any period of time
• A patient with full mental capacity refuses
• Successful resuscitation may result in a very poor quality of life for the patient that may prolong their distress or suffering

If in doubt about a patient's resuscitation status when arriving at a cardiac arrest, you **must** commence cardiopulmonary resuscitation, as this can always be stopped later if the patient is not for resuscitation.

Reviewing a resuscitation status

Once a decision is made, it is **not** carved in stone. Patients sometimes improve, and the prognosis then changes. In such circumstances, the resuscitation order should be reconsidered, although often, even after an improvement, the original DNAR order is still deemed most appropriate.

Many hospitals use a brightly coloured DNAR form that, once completed, is attached to the front of the patient's notes, so that it can easily be found and will stand out in what are often large, thick bundles of notes.

Summary of key points

• You must practise this station many times before the OSCE. It is easy marks, a large proportion of which are related to communication skills, but these can be affected by the general anxiety associated with the OSCE exam. It may be wise to have a few rehearsed phrases up your sleeve that can be used to good effect without having to think about them in the heat of the moment.

• Many such stations will give you a scenario involving a patient who has a chronic illness in its latter stages. You may be asked to explain a resuscitation status to the patient or their relative, or discuss their views with them.

• Do not resuscitate does **not** mean stop treating. It does have some associated implications, for example that such a patient would be unsuitable for invasive ventilation .or haemofiltration, but current medical management should continue. This **must** be communicated to the patient at some point in the discussion, so that they are reassured you are not just giving up on them.

• Ensure the patient knows about their condition and how they are being treated at present, for example that their pneumonia is severe but they are receiving antibiotics, fluids, etc.

• Go on to explain that they may deteriorate and if, in this deterioration, the heart were to stop, the medical team would need to decide whether or not cardiopulmonary resuscitation would be in the patient's best interest.

• Sometimes the actor-patient will ask further questions about whether or not they can refute this decision, whether the decision can be altered, etc. This may be set up to assess your knowledge of the ethics surrounding this issue, or it may be to test your communication skills in terms of how you would answer such questions. In addition, such questions may also serve as prompts to get the required information out of you, so do not get put off or fooled by questions, reactions or comments from the actor.

• A significant number of marks are given for communication skills – eye contact, empathy, etc. – as dealing with such complex situations can be a significant communication (as well as clinical) challenge.

• You must tell the examiner that you would afterwards document the discussion in the notes, ensure a DNAR form had been filled, and communicate the decision to all the team members involved in patient care.

• Demonstrate your awareness that a consultant/senior doctor must make the final decision, if your scenario has not already told you so.

54 Explaining post-myocardial infarction medication

Task: Mr Jones recently suffered a myocardial infarction (MI). He has recovered well on CCU and is now ready to be discharged home. Your registrar has told you to explain the medications on his TTA before he leaves. The medications are as follows:

- Aspirin (75 mg once daily)
- Bisoprolol (5 mg)
- Enalapril (5 mg)
- Simvastatin (40 mg)
- GTN spray (as required)

Checklist	P	MP	F
Introduces self and explains reasons for consultation			
Identifies patient correctly			
Gains consent			
Ensures that setting is private and dignified (bleep off, door closed)			
Establishes rapport			
Explains purpose of consultation			
(E – expectations) Establishes what patient is expecting to gain from the consultation			
(I – ideas) Establishes patient's understanding of situation and need for consultation, e.g. 'Can you fill me in on what has been happening so far?'			
Establishes sequence of events leading to this consultation			
(C – concerns) Establishes and acknowledges any concerns that patient has about medications			
Asks patient about preadmission medication			
Checks if patient has existing knowledge about discharge medications			
Explains each drug separately			
Explains each drug systematically, including reason for use, dosing regimen, side effects, safety netting and length of time the patient can expect to be taking it			
• Aspirin:			
• Must be taken daily			
• Works by 'thinning' the blood, thus reducing clot formation			
• Inform doctor if experiencing heartburn, vomiting or black stools			
• Metoprolol:			
• Must be taken daily			
• Works by reducing chances of subsequent MI			
• Inform doctor if have cold peripheries, erectile dysfunction or sleep disturbance			
• Enalapril:			
• Must be taken daily			
• Works by reducing blood pressure and assisting recovery of heart muscle, therefore reducing risk of subsequent MI			
• Inform doctor if develop dry cough, shortness of breath or facial swelling			
• Advises patient that blood tests will be performed to monitor kidney function			
• Simvastatin:			
• Must be taken every night before going to bed			
• Works by reducing blood cholesterol, thus reducing chance of subsequent MI			
• Inform doctor if develop muscle pains or jaundice			
• Advises patient that blood test will be performed to check liver function			
• GTN spray:			
• To be taken only if angina develops			
• Must stop all activity and rest if pain arises; call 999 if pain not relieved within 5 minutes or pain is of a different nature from usual angina chest pain			
• Inform doctor if frequency of use or time taken for pain relief is increasing			
• Side effects involve headache, facial flushing and postural dizziness			
Explains that all drugs are likely to be required lifelong			

Demonstrates knowledge of common drug interactions and contraindications if appropriate to the scenario				Suggests simple solutions (e.g. meeting with a specialist nurse to check technique) with agreed time frame			
Explores potential difficulties with compliance and offers simple solutions (such as use of a dossette box)				Explores **psychosocial** aspects: • Explores home situation (who patient lives with, activities of daily living, work) • Potential disruption to lifestyle as a result of medications and MI			
Acknowledges any gaps in own knowledge, and offers to seek advice from seniors/colleagues				Identifies and addresses any '**hidden agenda**'			
Explores specific concerns (e.g. difficulty spraying GTN under the tongue)				Offers follow-up appointment to monitor for side effects			
Explores and addresses any problems identified in a logical and non-judgemental manner				Invites questions and checks patient's understanding regularly			
Demonstrates effective safety netting for each drug				Maintains rapport and communicates empathetically			
Works in partnership with patient, exploring their ideas and preferences with respect to possible solutions, negotiating and compromising where necessary				Appropriate close with plan for follow-up appointment			

Hints and tips for the exam

This is a relatively difficult OSCE stations because it tests a number of different skills:

• **Knowledge:** A basic working knowledge (at the very least) of the drugs used in secondary prevention of MI is required.

• **Communication skills:** The station is designed to test the candidate's ability to impart a relatively **large volume of potentially complicated information** over a short period of time **in lay terms**. You must provide information in a way that is understandable and regularly invite questions from the patient. This will only come by practising this station with colleagues and taking opportunities to explain medications to patients on the ward who are about to be discharged.

• **Safety/prescribing skills:** All medications are potentially dangerous so you must:
  • Check that it is safe for the patient to be taking the drugs prescribed on the TTA (i.e. there are **no adverse interactions or contraindications**)
  • Provide appropriate **safety netting** (i.e. clearly explain what the major side effects are and how these may be manifest)

• **Orchestrating a successful consultation:** No consultation is ever complete without addressing the patient's specific concerns. In the OSCE, you are guaranteed to be faced with an actor-patient who has a specific agenda. You must ask about any **specific concerns** and address these in a positive manner by offering simple and appropriate solutions.

Special points to remember for this station
Do:
• Check the patient's prior knowledge. This will ensure that you do not waste time giving the patient information they already have.
• Ask the patient if they feel ready to go home. This is important not only to demonstrate empathy, but also to ensure safety – if patients do not feel safe to go home, their concerns must be addressed before discharge.
• Explain each drug separately. If you explain 'the drugs' as a whole, there is more potential for confusion over why the drugs have been prescribed and how they should be taken.
• Ensure there are no contraindications to any of the drugs.
• Provide effective safety netting. Without this, your explanation is likely to be deemed unsafe.
• Ask if there are any particular concerns.
• Respond positively to concerns raised by the patient.
• Offer a follow-up appointment.
• Invite questions throughout the consultation and at the end.

Don't:
• Don't assume the patient already has information without checking with them.
• Don't lecture to the patient without pauses to check for concerns or questions.
• Don't hurriedly offload as much information as possible if you find yourself pushed for time. A better approach is to acknowledge the time constraints and

respond to this by offering to arrange a follow-up appointment.
• Don't spend a lot of time providing information regarding general lifestyle changes and other aspects of secondary prevention of MI unless this is specifically stated in the instructions.
• Don't ignore cues provided by the patient. Act positively on these to help guide the consultation.
• Don't ignore specific concerns raised by the patient.

Scenarios you may encounter at this station

• **Provide general advice in addition to explaining medication for the secondary prevention for MI.** You are likely to be given more time (e.g. a **10-minute station**) if this variation of the station is used in the exam. 'General advice' includes information regarding several aspects of lifestyle and post-MI review.
  • Lifestyle:
  i. Discuss current dietary habits, and encourage a Mediterranean diet with low saturated fat intake and increased intake of fruit and vegetables.
  ii. Encourage alcohol intake within limits and to avoid binge drinking.
  iii. Encourage/provide support for smoking cessation.
  iv. Encourage 20–30 minutes of physical activity per day to the point of slight breathlessness/sweating and advise a step-by-step increase in activity.
  v. Assess stress levels and offer stress management.
  vi. Advice resumption of sexual activity a minimum of 4 weeks following uncomplicated recovery from MI.
  vii. Include patients in a cardiac rehabilitation programme.
  viii. Advise the patient to take at least 2 months away from work and to review and reassess their occupation to consider workplace modifications to minimise their risk of MI.
  • The patient should avoid air travel for 2–3 weeks (if there are no complications), in line with NICE (2007) guidelines.
  • Review:
  i. 6 weeks post-MI for a review of symptom recurrence
  ii. 3 months post-MI for a review of blood lipid levels
• **Complete a TTA for a patient being discharged after an MI and explain the medications to the patient.** NB. This is also likely to be tested in two linked 5-minute stations.

Reference

National Institute for Health and Clinical Excellence (2007) MI: secondary prevention. Available from: www.nice.org.uk/nicemedia/live/11008/30497/30497.pdf (accessed June 2012).

55 Dealing with an angry patient

Checklist	P	MP	F
Introduces self and explains reason for consultation			
Identifies patient correctly			
Gains consent			
Attempts to establish rapport and to converse calmly with the patient			
(E – expectations) Establishes reason for patient's attendance and what they are expecting from the consultation			
Establishes chronological sequence of events leading to the complaint			
Gives patient opportunity to express and release their anger			
(I – ideas) Identifies and explores reasons for patient's anger			
Acknowledges patient's anger in a non-judgemental and empathetic manner, negotiating and compromising where necessary			
Apologises to patient and accepts their grievance if appropriate			
Tries to diffuse situation, explaining that the intention is to help the patient			
Does not react personally to any negative personal remarks			
Avoids apportioning blame to any individual or department			
If appropriate, explains their own version of events to help the patient's understanding of the situation			
Devises a practical solution to the patient's problems, working in partnership with the patient			
Reassures the patient that concrete steps will be taken to prevent such occurrences in future, including a significant event analysis if appropriate			
Emphasises that the process will be transparent and efficient			
Offers to organise a meeting for the patient with members of the team involved in the situation in question			

Checklist	P	MP	F
Explains complaints procedure and offers to help patient if they wish to make a complaint, giving a time frame for the response: • Hospital: patient advice and liaison centre service • GP: practice manager			
Psychosocial aspects: • Assesses impact of situation on patient's home and social and work life • Offers to help reduce this impact if possible			
Identifies underlying (C) concerns/fears			
Acknowledges and addresses patient's fears/concerns empathetically and offers help and reassurance			
Acknowledges any gaps in own knowledge and offers to seek advice from seniors/colleagues			
Arranges follow-up appointment/phone call to inform patient of progress made on solving the problem			
Safety net: asks patient to contact doctor if they have any problems			
Ensures that own safety is not compromised, and takes necessary measures, calling for help or pressing panic alarm if necessary			
Shows empathy and adopts a calm conciliatory tone			
Uses simple and appropriate language, avoids using jargon			
Listens carefully and uses non-verbal communication skills effectively, maintaining eye contact			
Checks patient's understanding at regular intervals			
Invites questions			
Systematic approach			
Summarises			
Offers written information/patient information leaflets			
Offers contact details of support groups/patient associations if appropriate			

Summary of common conditions seen in OSCEs

Cause of anger	Key issues to consider and discuss
Missed diagnosis Misdiagnosis Incorrect treatment	Patient safety is paramount – ensure there is a swift and definitive follow-up plan in place to establish the diagnosis and start treatment of the condition Ensure you set specific time frames for follow-up
Long waiting times for elective procedure/surgery	Try to explain the reason for waiting lists and waiting times, and the basic issues surrounding resource allocation and rationing Emphasise that emergencies, 'urgent' and serious cases are dealt with promptly
Lack of information/ communication	Offer to be the main point/source of communication yourself Ensure you set specific time frames for follow-up
Rudeness on the part of staff members	Emphasise that rudeness (in general) is never acceptable Plan to speak to the member of staff in question to explore their views or version of events
Unrealistic/unreasonable expectations	Empathise unreservedly with the patient Try to avoid colluding with the patient Explain your perspective and try to give patient some insight
Hidden agenda	This could be anything – such as a devious agenda to have time off work, or underlying financial or relationship problems, or even just normal anxiety because of their diagnosis Once you identify the 'hidden agenda', try to help the patient and devise a plan of action to manage it
Psychiatric problems	Remain calm and collected

Hints and tips for the exam

This a difficult station, both in real life and even more so in the OSCE setting. Unfortunately, it is also very common.

Control yourself

This is the most important tip. Don't let the situation overwhelm you, don't become defensive, and above all don't get angry. Remaining calm will show the examiner that you are can cope with difficult situations under pressure – and it will also help the patient to calm down. Don't feel pressurised to respond to everything the patient says – don't hesitate to remain silent and give the patient time and space to express his emotions.

Be aware of your own emotions

Most of us would find it difficult not to get annoyed or angry when faced with a patient who is aggressive or rude, and this may inadvertently start to show in your expression and behaviour. If you feel angry or fed up, try to actively work against it and suppress your annoyance – at least until the end of the station!

Apologise

This is often all the patient wants, and may be enough to pacify them. Saying sorry does not mean that you are taking liability or accepting blame for the issue – rather, it is an expression of regret for the situation that the patient finds themself in.

Don't blame your colleagues

It could be tempting to collude with an angry patient and join them in their condemnation of a colleague or another department. Resist this at all costs. Be empathetic towards the patient, and if appropriate reassure the patient that their anger is understandable and that you would also feel angry in the same position. But rather than blame colleagues, convince the patient that you will do everything to find out where the fault (if one exists) lies, and that you will investigate and address it with the person in question. Always put the emphasis on helping the patient, and ensuring that any error or untoward incident does not recur.

Know the complaints procedures

As a finalist, it is unlikely that you will be expected to know complaints procedures in any great detail. However, a basic understanding will not only make you sound convincing to the patient, but will also highlight how well informed you are for the examiner.

Hospital: patient advice and liaison service

Every hospital has a patient advice and liaison service department, and this should generally be the patient's first port of call for any complaints. They will be able to help with the patient's complaint and escalate it to the most appropriate agency or member of staff. Other than this, they can also provide information on how different departments within the NHS work and who the patient can approach for independent intervention, as well as providing details of support groups.

GP: practice manager

If the scenario lies within the GP setting, the first port of call should be the practice manager, who should always respond to the patient within 48 hours of receiving the complaint.

If the patient wanted to complain at a higher level independently of the GP practice or hospital, they could contact either the primary care trust or the NHS Ombudsman – although this is usually reserved for intractable or very serious complaints.

Significant event analysis

A common motive for patient complaints is to prevent other patients suffering the same fate as them. Hence, it is important to be able to reassure the patient that you are taking concrete steps and reviewing relevant guidelines and policies. The first step towards this in both hospitals and GP surgeries is to mark the event as a 'significant event' – this could be any incident where a patient has been harmed or had potential to be harmed. Every GP surgery and hospital holds significant event analysis meetings as part of clinical governance on a regular basis (usually once every 1–2 months) to review these cases. The whole multidisciplinary team is involved, and the aim is to learn from mistakes and to institute measures to prevent them in future – usually in the form of policy and protocol changes.

Stay safe

There will of course never be a true risk to your safety in the OSCE setting, although your examiners may create a simulated scenario where there is a risk. Observing the following precautions will demonstrate to your examiners that you are prepared for such an emergency:

• Sit as close to the door as possible.
• Keep the door open if possible.
• Ensure you know where the 'panic' button or alarm is – and use it if necessary.
• Put any objects that could pose a risk to your safety out of the patient's reach.
• Shout for help if things get out of hand!

56 Carrying out a handover

Checklist	P	MP	F
Introduces self, including name and grade			
Requests to speak to the appropriate team (e.g. respiratory team if handing over a patient with an acute exacerbation of COPD)			
Asks name of colleague			
Explains reason for call (e.g. 'Can I hand over a patient to you?')			
Explains **S**ituation:			
• States name and age of patient			
• States date and reason for patient being brought to medical attention			
• Makes a subjective comment on condition of patient (e.g. 'Mrs Winters was admitted with a fall and currently seems very unwell')			
• States urgency of referral correctly and is able to give a reason for this			
Explains **B**ackground:			
• States relevant points in patient's history			
• States relevant examination findings			
•Provides baseline observations and other objective indicators of patient's condition, e.g. pulse rate, blood pressure, respiratory rate, oxygen saturation, Glasgow Coma Scale score (if appropriate)			
• States results of preliminary bedside and blood tests that are relevant			

Explains **A**ssessment of patient's current situation:			
• Comments on haemodynamic stability (if appropriate)			
•States working diagnosis			
•Explains other current problems that need to be addressed			
Makes a **R**ecommendation with regard to further patient care:			
• Explains treatment required and further investigations that need to be requested			
•Outlines any anticipated complications			
•States conditions/deterioration that will warrant a senior review			
• Checks colleague understands plan and asks if any alterations or additions are advised			
Invites questions from colleague and answers appropriately			
At end of conversation, confirms handover can be made and recommended management plan implemented			
Provides colleague with appropriate contact details and encourages contact to be made if the need arises			
Communicates politely and maintains rapport throughout conversation			

Summary of common conditions seen in OSCEs

Make sure you know common/important **referral criteria outlined by NICE** (2005).

Suspected cancer	Age of patient	Criteria for urgent referral	Criteria for immediate referral	Team to refer to
Lower gastrointestinal tract	Any age	Right lower abdominal mass		Colorectal surgeons
		Palpable mass on rectal examination		
		Unexplained iron deficiency anaemia		
		Haemoglobin <11 g/100 mL		
		Non-menstruating women with iron deficiency anaemia and haemoglobin <10 g/100 mL		
	40–59	Rectal bleeding + change in bowel habit towards looser stools for more than 6 weeks		
	60+	Rectal bleeding for over 6 weeks		
		Change in bowel habit towards looser stools for more than 6 weeks		
Upper gastrointestinal tract	Any age	Dysphagia, chronic gastrointestinal bleeding, weight loss, persistent vomiting, iron deficiency anaemia, epigastric mass, suspicious barium meal result		Upper gastrointestinal surgeons
	55+	Unexplained and persistent recent-onset dyspepsia		
Lung	Any age	Suspicious chest X-ray (including pleural effusion and slowly resolving consolidation)	Superior vena cava obstruction	Chest physicians
		Asbestos exposure + recent-onset chest pain/shortness of breath/unexplained systemic upset/suspicious chest X-ray	Stridor	
		Haemoptysis		
		>3 weeks of: chest pain, shoulder pain, weight loss, chest signs, hoarseness, clubbing, cervical/supraclavicular lymphadenopathy, cough, suspected metastases, change in symptoms of chronic underlying respiratory disease		Radiologist for urgent chest X-ray
	40+	Persistent haemoptysis in smoker/ex-smoker		Chest physicians
Urological	Any age	Painless macroscopic haematuria		Urologist
		Abdominal mass identified clinically or radiologically that is thought to arise from urological tract		
		Swelling/mass in body of testis		
		Signs of penile cancer		
		Elevated age-specific prostate-specific antigen		
		Hard, irregular prostate		
	40+	Recurrent/persistent urinary tract infection + haematuria		
	50+	Unexplained microscopic haematuria		

Hints and tips for the exam

Performing a handover using the widely accepted and universally recognised 'SBAR' – **situation, background, assessment, recommendation** – framework is an OSCE station that is increasingly being tested in finals. This station requires a systematic approach and tests your abilities in several different areas:

• **Knowledge:** You will usually be given a significant amount of background information about the patient you are handing over in the station. However, you will usually be instructed to **formulate your own management plan** based on your **interpretation of the clinical information** you are given. This requires skill in data interpretation as well as factual knowledge of how common conditions are managed.

• **Communication:** Your ability to communicate effectively with a colleague is being tested. Remember that this is different from communicating with a patient because you will be required to use medical 'jargon'. If you **follow the SBAR framework**, you will find it easier to impart meaningful information in a precise manner. Like all communication skill stations, do NOT forget to check whether your **colleague has any questions**. In addition, it is also important to remember to discuss whether your colleague **agrees with the management plan and has any additions to make**.

• **Safety:** Your ability to **gauge the urgency** of a clinical situation is being tested. Beware that the actor to whom you are handing over may have been instructed to deliberately avoid taking an urgent handover. If this is the case, **do not panic** or backtrack – this situation is deliberately being simulated to test your ability to justify why you think a situation is urgent.

You will get several opportunities on all your clinical attachments to observer handovers being performed:

• **Attend the morning handover meeting before the ward round:** Listen carefully to how the night on-call team communicate information about new admissions to your team members. Attending the evening handover will serve the same purpose. Close to your exams, it may be worthwhile noting down some of the patients' clinical details and practising handing these over to each other with your colleagues. You can then check how closely your recommendation matches the management plan implemented by the team.

• **Look out for opportunities during GP attachments:** Patients are commonly referred to secondary care by GPs, and you can benefit from observing your tutors do this. Some tutors may also allow you to practise referring patients by telephone yourself under supervision, so take such opportunities when they present.

• **Arrange to shadow the acute team on-call radiologist at your teaching hospital:** You will be able to observe several patients being referred to the radiology department for urgent imaging. Focus particularly on how the referring doctors justify why their patients urgently require imaging.

• **Practise with your colleagues in your study groups:** You can formulate scenarios among yourselves, or use the ones you have observed during your attachments, to test each other.

Questions you could be asked

Q. Write a referral letter based on clinical information provided in the OSCE scenario (5 minutes).

Q. Take a history and then hand the patient over to the appropriate team by telephone.

Q. Double station: Take a history and then hand the patient over to the appropriate team by writing a referral letter.

The marking schedule for a **referral letter** is likely to be very similar to that of a referral. You should remember to **write legibly**. Remember to give information about **allergies to contrast, metallic prostheses** (e.g. metallic heart valves) and drugs such as **metformin** when **referring a patient for imaging**.zxz

Reference

National Institute for Health and Clinical Excellence (2005) Referral guidelines for suspected cancer. Available from: www.nice.org.uk/nicemedia/live/10968/29813/29813.pdf (accessed June 2012).

Part 4: Procedures

Top tips

Do:

- **Prepare well** (see below).
- **Know the steps of the procedure well:** You will have only a few minutes (usually 5) to a perform the procedure and answer questions on it.
- Practise! Visit your medical school's clinical skills centre or teaching room and use the manikins or equipment there to practise and rehearse how you would do the procedure if it came up in the exam. Use the mark schemes provided and have a friend watch and time you.
- **Ask for help with your learning if you are unsure:** Many people will be able to show you a procedure if you are unfamiliar with it. Do not be shy or too proud to seek help before the exam if you do not know it, as it is better to make mistakes before the exam than in it.
- **Be as comprehensive and as thorough as possible in the short time you have:** Say as many points as you can when asked a question, and cover as many details of the procedure as you can. It is often a good idea to talk while you are doing the procedure, and sometimes the specific instructions of the station may ask you to do this.

Don't:

- **Don't panic!:** The majority of the procedures will be carried out on manikins, so you do not need to worry about hurting a patient. However, you must treat the manikin as you would a real patient.
- **Don't worry!:** In the exam, the manikin may not be perfect, so even though your intravenous cannula may go into the manikin's vein, you may not get any blood back. This may be the manikin rather than your technique, and the examiner is likely to know this. Even if you are penalised for it, it would be only a mark, and it must not play on your mind.
- **Don't think about the station you have just done:** It is rare to pass every single station! If you feel that one station may not have gone well, do not let it play on your mind. You get marks for lots of things, and you may have got more than you think. Also, this will hinder your chance of doing well on the next station. You must put it behind you and move on.
- **Don't overcomplicate simple procedures** . . . keep simple things simple!

Preparation

With any procedure in general, preparation is the key. Preparation should be of:

- The patient
- The environment
- The equipment

The patient

- Confirm the patient's identity.
- Explain the procedure, including why it is being done and the risk of any complications.
- Ensure there are no contraindications to the procedure or to any drug being given, including allergies.
- Appropriately position and expose the patient in order to access the relevant site for your procedure.

The environment

- Ensure adequate privacy and lighting.
- Ensure there is a sharps bin with you.
- Ensure you have an assistant who can help you, or who you can call on for help when things go wrong.
- Ensure you are doing the procedure in an appropriate setting.

The equipment

- Ensure you have all the equipment you are going to need.
- Lay it out in an easily accessible manner – it is often helpful to place it in the order you are going to use it.
- Where drugs are involved, check the prescription, dose and timing, and check the ampoule with a colleague, including the drug name, dose and expiry date.

OSCEs for Medical Finals, First Edition. Hamed Khan, Iqbal Khan, Akhil Gupta, Nazmul Hussain, and Sathiji Nageshwaran.
© 2013 John Wiley & Sons, Ltd. Published 2013 by John Wiley & Sons, Ltd.

• Ensure you have a drawing up needle and a separate injection needle if required.

Generic points for most procedures stations

Understands the task from the scenario that is given

Introduces self to the patient/actor

Obtains consent

Washes hands and wears gloves as appropriate

Is methodical in approach

Makes it very clear to the examiner what is doing, so that each step gets noticed

Cleans up after the procedure and disposes of any sharps

Thanks patient

Appears confident

57 Urinary catheterisation

Checklist	P	MP	F
Appropriate introduction to patient and informed consent obtained			
Ensures privacy and good lighting			
Prepares the following sterile equipment with aseptic technique: • Sterile catheter pack • Kidney dish/collecting dish • Sterile towel and cotton swabs/gauze • Sterile gloves • Antiseptic solution, poured into a pot from sterile pack • Foley catheter (10–16 F) of appropriate size • Lubricant gel • Catheter bag • 10 mL 1% lidocaine lubricant gel (usually in pre-filled sterile syringe) • 10 mL 0.9% saline (usually in pre-filled sterile syringe)			
Adequate exposure: ideally umbilicus to knees			
Positions the patient, lying supine: • Males: legs extended, flat • Females: hips and knees flexed, legs apart			
Washes hands and dons sterile gloves			
Establishes sterile field by placing sterile towel/sheet: • Males: around the penis • Females: around the labia			
Uses one hand used to hold the penis or labia, other hand being kept clean			
Retracts foreskin/parts labia and cleans appropriately			
Inserts 1% lidocaine gel into urethra			
Occludes urethral meatus for 3–5 minutes			
Lubricates tip of catheter and places kidney dish/collecting dish between patient's legs			
Gently inserts catheter into urethra, to the hilt			
Does not use force, handles resistance appropriately and watches for urine			
Fills balloon with sterile water			
Gently retracts catheter until resistance is felt			
Attaches appropriate catheter drainage system			
Replaces foreskin			
Covers patient, ensuring patient's comfort and dignity			
Records residual volume			
Sends residual urine sample for report on catheter specimen of urine and urine Dipstix testing			
Ensures good communication with patient throughout			

Summary of key points for OSCEs

Know the relevant anatomy

It is vital that you understand the anatomy very well, or else you may find yourself in the embarrassing situation of catheterising the wrong meatus, both in the exam as well as in real life! It is obvious where the urethra is in males, but to the unfamiliar candidate it is sometimes unclear on a female manikin where the catheter should go. Figure 57.1 illustrates the anatomy of the female genitalia.

Indications and contraindications

Indications	Contraindications
Monitoring urine output, e.g. fluid resuscitation, fluid balance measurements, sepsis, etc.	Patient refusal
Relieving urinary retention	Urethral trauma
Urinary incontinence	Active urinary tract infection
Immobility, e.g. low Glasgow Coma Scale score, coma, lower limb fractures, cerebrovascular accidents, postoperatively, etc.	
Cystograms and other urology investigations	

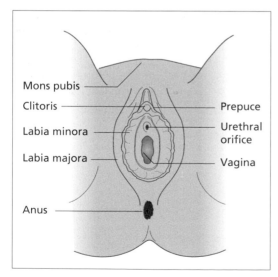

Figure 57.1 Anatomy of the female genitalia – many students and junior doctors have been embarrassed by catheterising the incorrect meatus.

Potential complications

Early complications	Late complications
Pain or discomfort on insertion	Paraphimosis if foreskin is not replaced
Local tissue trauma, e.g. premature inflation of the balloon, causing prostatic or urethral trauma	Urethral stricture formation
Bleeding	Creation of false passage
Urinary tract infection	
Blockage of catheter	

Hints and tips for the exam

Equipment

• A sterile catheter pack is often available, containing a kidney dish, cotton gauze, a pot for saline or cleaning solution, and sometimes sterile gloves. It is advisable to know what your clinical skills centre uses as this is likely to be the same set you will get in the exam.

• If the pack does not contain cleaning solution, you may need an assistant to pour some cleaning solution into your pot as you will be sterile.

• The lidocaine local anaesthetic comes as a gel, often in a prepacked 10 mL syringe that is not normally included in the catheter pack.

• The catheter itself should come with saline to fill the balloon in a prepacked syringe. Note that you will need to use sterile saline and a sterile syringe.

• The balloon capacity will be indicated on the inflation port.

• As the OSCE station may last only 5 minutes, the set you need will have sometimes already have been opened and prepared for you. In such circumstances, tell the examiner that you would like to make sure that this is a completely sterile set.

Technique

• The procedure will be carried out on a manikin, so you may be expected to say, for example, that you would introduce yourself to the patient and obtain informed consent, etc. Alternatively, there may be an actor with whom you may have to interact.

• If you are asked to catheterise a member of the opposite gender, always offer a CHAPERONE.

• It is vital that you know the anatomy.

• Take full aseptic precautions – one of the most common causes of acquiring a urinary tract infection is urinary tract instrumentation. Some hospitals suggest you give a dose of prophylactic antibiotic after insertion of the catheter. Ensure you know your medical school's policy.

• Cleaning technique is important and must be clearly demonstrated to the examiner. In males retract the foreskin, and in females part the labia. Cotton gauze must be soaked in your cleaning solution and applied generously in such a way that you start at the urethra and clean away from it. Ensure you clean the area well at least three or four times.

• In males, after insertion of the local anaesthetic lidocaine gel, hold the shaft of the penis vertically and occlude the meatus in order to prevent the local anaesthetic coming out.

• Don two pairs of sterile gloves at the start, and remove the outer pair once the initial cleaning and handling has been completed.

• Generously apply lubricant gel to the catheter tip.

• **Do not force** the catheter! If resistance is met, try and gently manoeuvre past it. In males, hold the penis vertically and then try to advance the catheter further.

• Try not to touch the actual catheter itself. It usually comes in a plastic wrapper so try to open the wrapper and shuffle the tip of the catheter into the urethra.

• Try not to handle any lubricant gel with the same hand as the catheter as this can make it slippery and difficult to handle.

• Never force the balloon full – the process should not be difficult. If it is, and the patient complains of pain, the balloon is probably in the urethra and should be advanced further. It is to avoid this situation that it is advisable to advance the catheter to its hilt.

• Ensure urine flows back. If not, check that the catheter is far enough in and flush it with saline to ensure it is not blocked, for example by lubricant gel.

After catheterisation
• Attach the catheter bag.
• Record the residual volume

• Send a urine sample for analysis, including microbiology as this should be a sterile sample.

• It is important to say that you would provide instructions to the nursing staff, such as to take an hourly urine record or complete a fluid input–output chart, etc. according to the scenario you are given.

• In a catheterised patient who is not hypovolaemic, low urine output may be the result of a blocked catheter. Hence, the catheter should always be flushed to check.

• It is important, at the end of the procedure, to mention the importance of patient comfort.

• Express your intention to document the procedure in the notes.

Types of catheter
This station assumes the use of indwelling Foley catheters, distinguished by the presence of a balloon at the tip that keeps them in place. There are many other catheter types (e.g. the Robinson catheter, which does not have a balloon) but these are beyond the scope of this book.

Foley catheters are usually made of silicone rubber or natural rubber, and are sized in French units (F). The larger the number, the larger the catheter size so, for example, 16 F is larger than 10 F. You should use the smallest suitable size for your patient. Catheters used for males are longer than those for females as the male urethra (typically 20 cm long) is longer than the female urethra (typically 6–7 cm long).

Generally, there are two-way or three-way catheters, depending on the number of ports that are present. There is always a passage open at both ends for drainage of urine. The two-way catheters also have a port with a one-way valve that allows balloon inflation. Three-way catheters have an additional port for bladder irrigation, which is separate from the port for drainage.

58 Insertion of nasogastric tube

Checklist	P	MP	F
Appropriate introduction to the patient and informed consent obtained			
Adequate positioning, patient sitting upright, head supported by a pillow			
Checks the indication for nasogastric (NG) tube and excludes contraindications			
Prepares equipment: • NG tube to be inserted • Lubricating gel • Spigot or bag for NG tube • Bowl for collecting secretions, gastric content or vomit • Glass of water with straw • Adhesive tape			
Washes hands			
Dons non-sterile gloves and apron			
Measures length of insertion of NG tube: distance from tip of nose, to tragus of ear, to a point immediately inferior to xiphisternum			
Lubricates distal part of NG tube with gel			
Stands facing the patient, on the same side as the nostril to be used			
Gives patient a glass of water			
Gently inserts NG tube into nostril, a few centimetres at a time, aiming towards the occiput (i.e. backwards) *There are no marks for aiming cranially (upwards)*			
Asks patient to swallow sip of water when they feel the tip of the NG in the oropharynx			
Continues to insert tube, coordinating with patient's swallowing			
Inserts tube to previously measured length			
Attaches drainage bag/spigot			
Uses adhesive tape to fix NG tube securely to nose			
Appropriate disposal of waste			
Cleans hands appropriately			
Asks for a chest X-ray before the tube is used			
Ensures patient's comfort			

Summary of key points for OSCEs

Indications and contraindications for NG tube insertion

Indications	Contraindications
Gastric emptying, e.g. bowel obstruction, ileus	Patient refusal
Enteral nutrition	Basal skull fracture or other facial trauma
Gastric lavage or aspiration after poisoning or drug overdose	Recent nasal surgery
Administration of medication	Oesophageal strictures
Administration of contrast for radiological investigation	Known oesophageal varices
Upper gastrointestinal bleed:	Caution in unconscious patients, and in patients with coagulopathy
• Evaluation (e.g. presence, volume, etc.)	
• Sengstaken–Blakemore tubes help in controlling variceal bleeds	
Identifying oesophagus and/or stomach on chest X-ray	Alkaline ingestion

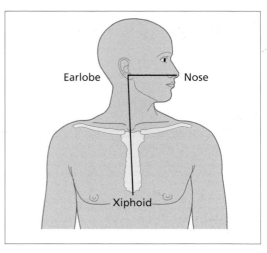

Figure 58.1 How to measure the required length of insertion of an NG tube. The tube is measured by placing the tip at the tip of the patient's nose, and measuring the length from the tip of the nose, to the ear lobe/tragus and then to the sternum

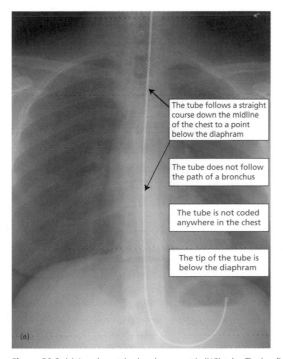

The tube follows a straight course down the midline of the chest to a point below the diaphram

The tube does not follow the path of a bronchus

The tube is not coded anywhere in the chest

The tip of the tube is below the diaphram

(a)

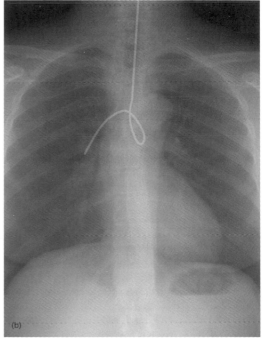

(b)

Figure 58.2 (a) An adequately placed nasogastric (NG) tube. The key finding is that the tip of the NG tube is visible below the diaphragm. Although this X-ray clearly demonstrates the entire NG tube, often only the tip is radio-opaque. (b) A NG tube that has gone into the patient's lung so must be withdrawn and reinserted. Reproduced courtesy of Pennsylvania Patient Safety Authority

Potential complications of NG tube insertion

These include:
- Bleeding (e.g. oesophageal, major epistaxis)
- Pain or discomfort during insertion
- Gag reflex:
  - Caused by the presence of the tube in the oropharynx
  - This may cause vomiting
  - Aspiration of vomitus
- Misplacement, for example:
  - Coiling in the nose or oropharynx ᾽
  - Passing into the trachea (if the patient coughs)
  - Passing too far into the duodenum
  - Entering the cranial cavity
- Local tissue necrosis
- Oesophageal/gastric perforation
- Failure

Hints and tips for the exam

- You will be performing the procedure on a manikin, so it is prudent to tell the examiner that you would introduce yourself to the patient, obtain informed consent, etc.
- If there is an actor present, speak to them as you would a patient.
- Prior to inserting the tube, it is often helpful to briefly examine the nose to check for a deviated septum in order to determine which nostril is more suitable to use.
- It is vital to give the patient good clear instructions.

Technique

- Be very gentle in your approach to the patient.
- Aim to pass the tube along the floor of the nasal cavity, in a posterior direction. **Do not** aim superiorly as you will meet obstruction at the cribriform plate. With facial trauma, it is not difficult to push the NG tube through into the cranium.
- There are different types of NG tube of different sizes. Typically, 16–18 F is appropriate for an adult, whereas in children the necessary size varies with age.
- Use a cold NG tube. Colder tubes are less pliable and are therefore more likely to keep their curvature for longer. This makes them easier to direct, and reduces the chance of their curling in the wrong place.
  - Ask for a cold NG tube, fresh from the fridge.
  - If cold tubes are not available, placing the distal part in ice for a few minutes or spraying it with cold spray/cryogesic will help.

- Lubricate the NG tube very, very generously! This is vital to ensure easy passage.
- If resistance is met, the tube should **not** be forced but should be withdrawn and redirected.
- If you are unable to pass the tube through one nostril, try the other.
- When the tip of the tube reaches the oropharynx, it is helpful to ask the patient to swallow. By coordinating insertion of the tube with the patient's swallowing, you maximise your chance of correct placement, as the swallowing action should help to steer the tube to the oesophagus.
  - Some patients can swallow without anything in their mouth.
  - Many patients prefer to swallow with a sip of water as this then becomes similar to swallowing a pill.
- If the patient gags (they then cannot swallow) or coughs, stop the insertion, withdraw the tube and start again.
- Insert the tube to the length you measured before insertion. If you forget to measure this length, insert to 30–40 cm, and confirm placement on a chest X-ray.
  - To measure the required length, ask patient to hold their head straight. Hold the tip of the NG tube at the tip of the nose, run it past the tragus of the ear and down to just below the xiphisternum, and read off the length on the calibration markings on the NG tube itself.
- Fix the tube securely with adhesive tape. To minimise pressure necrosis around the tube insertion point, it is advisable to apply a skin ointment/aqueous cream before fixing the tube with tape.
- The use of lidocaine gel for the nose, and benzocaine or lidocaine spray for the throat, can help to minimise discomfort, but their use for this purpose is uncommon.
- In some situations, for example gastric decompression, it is advisable to attach suction (with a Yankauer suction catheter) or aspirate with a 50 mL syringe after insertion.
- Attachment to a drainage bag or spigot minimises the spreading of gastric secretions.

Methods of confirming placement

There are several, but only a chest X-ray is considered confirmatory:
- **Chest X-ray:** Essentially, you must ensure that the tip of the NG tube is lying below the diaphragm and not in the bronchial tree.

• **NG aspiration:** Aspirate a few millilitres of fluid from the NG tube and test its pH with litmus paper. A pH <5 is highly suggestive of gastric contents, but this may be inaccurate if the patient is on medication such as omeprazole, ranitidine or other antacids.

• **Air injection:** Injection of 20–30 mL of air into the NG tube while auscultating over the stomach with your stethoscope is also suggestive of correct placement, but this method is unreliable.

59 Venepuncture/phlebotomy

Checklist	P	MP	F
Appropriate introduction to the patient and informed consent obtained			
Confirms the indication for venepuncture			
Prepares equipment: • Needle of appropriate size (21 G green or 23 G blue) • Syringe or Vacutainer • Alcohol swab • Tourniquet • Blood collection bottles • Sharps bin • Cotton wool			
Positions the patient			
Adequately exposes the limb, removing any tight clothing			
Applies a tourniquet proximal to the elbow			
Palpates for a suitable vein at an appropriate site			
Cleans the area with alcohol swab and does **not** touch this area again			
Washes hands and dons a clean pair of gloves			
Attaches the needle to the syringe and unsheaths it			
Pulls the skin taut from 1–2 mm distal to the puncture site			
Warns patient there will be a sharp scratch			
Inserts the needle into the vein at an adequate angle (until flashback is seen if applicable)			
Applies good technique for obtaining blood from the vein with a Vacutainer or syringe			
Loosens the tourniquet before withdrawing the needle			
Applies pressure to the puncture site with cotton wool as the needle is withdrawn			
Applies a plaster over the puncture site			
Safe disposal of sharps			
Washes hands after procedure			
Correct labelling of blood samples			

Hints and tips for the exam

This is a simple procedure, and it is important to keep it simple in the OSCE. It is one that you will probably have done many times before on real patients, and if this station is given to you in the exam, it is no less than a gift.

Venepuncture in general

• Common sites for venepuncture include the antecubital fossa, forearm and dorsum of the hand. It is likely that you will get a manikin model of an upper limb, with a very prominent vein.

• If blood is taken downstream of an intravenous cannula through which fluid is running, it is very likely that the results obtained will be of doubtful significance.

Technique

• As the manikin may have been used several times before, you will be able to see where it has previously been punctured, but it may not necessarily give you a blood sample. This may well be due to some fault in the manikin rather than in your technique, so a demonstration of your safe technique is more important than actually obtaining a blood sample.

• If you are presented with an actor from whom you are asked to obtain consent or explain what you are doing, it is vital to be polite and courteous.

• A sharps bin should always accompany you to the bedside, to enable the immediate and safe disposal of sharps.

• When positioning the patient, it is best to ensure their comfort by, for example, placing a pillow under their arm.

• In is important to ensure good stability of the needle and to keep it steady and still while actually taking the blood sample.

• The collected blood should be promptly placed in the appropriate bottles and immediately labelled in order to reduce the risk of errors.

• Good hand hygiene should be demonstrated clearly before and after the procedure.

• Needles should **never** be resheathed.

• A Vacutainer reduces the risk of needlestick injury. If using a needle and syringe, discard the needle, and remove the tops from the blood sample bottles, allowing you to place blood in the blood bottle without the need for sharps. Blood should be first placed in a coagulation and full blood count sample bottle, as these tests cannot be done on a clotted sample.

• Prolonged tourniquet application should be avoided due to discomfort, but specifically in patients with, for example, peripheral vascular disease, Raynaud's phenomenon, hypocalcaemia, etc.

60 Intramuscular injection

Checklist	P	MP	F
Appropriate introduction to the patient and informed consent obtained			
Confirms the indication for injection			
Checks the prescription on the drug chart			
Ensures there are no allergies or contraindications			
Washes hands and wears clean gloves			
Prepares equipment: • Alcohol wipe or other skin preparation • Syringe (2 mL or 5 mL) • 21 G needle (usually green) to draw up medication • 23 G needle (usually blue) to inject medication • Cotton wool/gauze with tape • Sharps bin			
Checks the drug, dose and expiry date with a colleague or nurse			
Draws up the drug with the 21 G green needle and expels any air bubbles			
Replaces the 21 G green needle with a 23 G blue needle on the syringe			

Positions the patient appropriately to access the chosen site			
Cleans the site with the alcohol swab and leaves to dry for 30 seconds			
Tenses the skin to make it taut			
Introduces the needle into the muscle layer, perpendicular to the skin and muscle			
Aspirates first to ensure that a blood vessel has not been punctured			
Injects the medication slowly			
Withdraws the needle, applying mild pressure with cotton wool/gauze			
Disposes of sharps immediately and washes hands			
Observes patient and vital signs for a few minutes			
Records signature and time on the drug chart			
Thanks patient, ensures comfort and offers to answer any questions			

Summary of key points for OSCEs

Sites that can be used are the:
- Deltoid muscle
- Lateral thigh muscle (vastus lateralis)
- Gluteus muscle and the upper outer quadrant of the buttock, in order to avoid the sciatic nerve

Table of drugs that can be administered via the intramuscular route

Conditions	Indication for injection	Example of drug
Pain	Analgesia	Morphine, tramadol, pethidine, diclofenac, ketoprofen
Nausea and vomiting	Antiemetic	Ondansetron, cyclizine, metoclopramide
Psychosis	Antipsychotic	Haloperidol, olanzapine
Infection	Antibiotic	Co-amoxiclav
Cardiac arrest		Adrenaline (epinephrine), atropine
Anaphylaxis	Rapid drug administration if intravenous access difficult	Adrenaline, chlorpheniramine

Hints and tips for the exam

- Always **aspirate before injecting**. The importance of this cannot be overemphasised as inadvertent intravascular injection may be fatal.
- In the event of aspirating blood, abandon the procedure, apply pressure and try again at a different site with a fresh set of equipment.
- Never resheath a needle. As you change your needle, immediately dispose of it in the sharps bin, ensuring the examiner sees you do this.
- Always have a sharps bin with you to minimise any risk of injury.
- It is very likely that you will receive a manikin or a slab of modified sponge on which to perform the procedure. There may, however, be an actor-patient present from whom you may be asked to obtain consent. If not, it is wise to tell the examiner that these are the steps you would take prior to performing your injection.
- If you do get an actor-patient, being polite and courteous and using a suitable introduction will get you some marks before you even start the procedure.
- Ensure the examiner sees that you would wash your hands before and after the procedure.

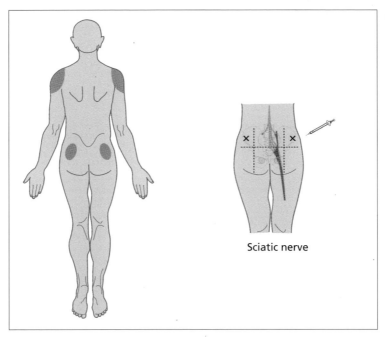

Sciatic nerve

Figure 60.1 Suitable sites for intramuscular injection: the deltoids and the upper outer quadrant of the buttock (as this position avoids the path of the sciatic nerve)

Questions you could be asked

Q. What are the indications for intramuscular injection?

A. The intramuscular route may be the only tolerated, available or possible way of administering a particular medication. See the text above for examples.

Q. List some contraindications to intramuscular injection.

A. These may include patient refusal, allergy to the medication you are going to inject, thrombocytopenia, coagulopathy or the patient taking anticoagulant medication.

Q. What complications may arise from an intramuscular injection?

A. These can be classified broadly into local and general complications. Local complications include pain at the injection site, localised swelling, haematoma formation from local bleeding, damage to surrounding structures, for example adjacent nerves, introduction of air and bruising. General complications include introduction of infection, intravascular injection, anaphylaxis or reaction to the drug injected, and injection of the wrong dose or volume of the drug.

Q. What if your patient has anatomy that is difficult to discern, for example if they are obese?

A. If the patient is obese, longer needles can be used. If you feel you are unhappy performing a procedure on a patient, ask for senior help before attempting it. Intramuscular injections are relatively safe to perform, even if the anatomy is difficult.

61 Intravenous cannulation

Checklist	P	MP	F
Suitable introduction to the patient and informed consent obtained			
Confirms the indication for the intravenous cannula			
Prepares equipment: • Intravenous cannula of appropriate size • Alcohol swab • Tourniquet • 0.9% saline to flush with a 5 mL or 10 mL syringe • Sharps bin • Cannula dressing • Cotton wool/gauze with tape			
Positions the patient			
Adequately exposes the limb, removing any tight clothing			
Applies a tourniquet proximal to the elbow			
Palpates for a suitable vein at an appropriate site, noting its depth, length and course			
Cleans the area with alcohol swab and does **not** touch this area again			
Washes hands and wears a pair of clean gloves			

Selects a cannula of suitable size			
Inspects to ensure the cannula is not defective or broken, and loosens the needle from the plastic covering			
Pulls the skin taut from 1–2 mm distal to the puncture site			
Warns the patient just before insertion that there will be a sharp scratch			
Inserts the cannula at an angle of approximately 20 degrees until flashback is seen in the flashback chamber			
Advances the needle and cannula a further 2–3 mm to ensure the tip is in the vein			
Withdraws the needle at the same time as advancing the cannula			
Appropriately disposes of the sharp and puts the cap on the cannula			
Flushes the cannula with 0.9% saline			
Applies the cannula dressing as appropriate			
Washes hands, reassures patient and answers any questions			

Summary of key points for OSCEs

Sites for intravenous cannulation

In practice, intravenous cannulation can be performed wherever a suitable vein can be found. This may mean using a vein in the lower limb or foot. In infants, sometimes even the scalp is cannulated.

In general, one should start by looking as distally as possible and working proximally. The antecubital fossa is a very tempting place to go but really should be a last resort because in situations where a good intravenous access may be needed, such as unexpected emergencies, this acts as a site of easy intravenous cannulation.

Where you SHOULD site a cannula	Where you should NOT site a cannula
Non-dominant hand or forearm	Joints, e.g. antecubital fossa, as this is more likely to be painful, especially when the patient bends their arm
Consider the dominant hand if the non-dominant one has no suitable vein	Arms that have an arteriovenous fistula
Can consider lower limb if upper limbs are difficult	Arms on the side from which axillary lymph nodes have been removed, e.g. patients who have had a mastectomy with lymph node clearance
Largest, longest, straightest vein palpable	Veins that are thrombosed or sore from multiple previous unsuccessful attempts

Indications for and contraindications to cannulation

Indications	Contraindications
Administration of drugs and intravenous fluids	Patient refusal
Administration of blood and blood products	Arteriovenous fistula (look elsewhere)
Emergencies, acute illness, resuscitation	Caution with the length of time the tourniquet is applied in patients with vascular insufficiency or hypocalcaemia
Preparation for theatre or anaesthesia, e.g. nil by mouth	

Potential complications of intravenous cannulation

Possible complications may include:
- Bleeding and haematoma formation
- Pain, both on insertion and afterwards
- Failure to cannulate
- Subcutaneous administration of fluids and drugs (i.e. 'tissuing')
- Infection, cellulitis, bruising
- Air embolism

Hints and tips for the exam

Technique

- You will be performing this procedure on a manikin. This may be mechanically more difficult than cannulating a real patient as the manikin's rubbery skin is usually thicker and more tough than real skin, and the vein is often harder. As it may have been used several times before, do not be disheartened if you do not get a flashback in the flashback chamber. In real life, it will frequently require more than one attempt to site a suitable cannula. It is far more important to show the examiner your technique. If it is likely that the manikin is the problem, the examiner may say to just pretend you did get a flashback and move on.
- Don't forget to mention at the end of the station that you would inform the nurse looking after the patient that there is a new cannula in place they can use.
- Check the cannula before you use it and loosen the needle from the plastic cover before starting.
- When advancing the cannula over the needle, it is important that this is done slowly and carefully.
- Flush the cannula with normal saline soon after insertion or else the blood will clot in it.
- Mention how you would position the patient, for example placing a pillow under the arm to stabilise the arm.
- There may be an actor-patient present from whom you may be asked to obtain consent. If not, it is wise to tell the examiner that these are the steps you would take prior to performing your injection.
- If you do get an actor-patient, being polite and courteous with a suitable introduction will get you some marks before you even start the procedure.

Safety

- **Never** resheath a needle. Immediately dispose of it in a sharps bin, and ensure the examiner sees you do this.
- Always have a sharps bin with you.
- It is important that you know what to do should you get a needlestick injury, according to your local

hospital protocol (and also because the examiner may ask you!):

• Stop the procedure you are doing.
• Wash the injured part under a running tap with warm water, encouraging bleeding.
• Inform the occupational health department and arrange an urgent visit for post-exposure prophylaxis.
• Discuss what has happened with the patient and obtain their consent to test for transmissible viruses such as hepatitis C, hepatitis B and HIV.
• A colleague should take the patient's blood and yours for the appropriate blood tests.
• If an injury happens at 3 am with a high-risk patient, there are still local protocols you can follow, usually receiving post-exposure prophylaxis from A&E. Arrange a visit to the occupational health department the following day.
• Ensure the examiner sees that you would wash your hands before and after the procedure.

Cannula care

The site of cannula insertion should be inspected every day, and the cannula should ideally be removed after 72 hours. Before replacing it, consider whether or not a cannula is still needed. If a new cannula is required, secure it first before removing the old one.

If there is evidence of occlusion, 'tissuing' or surrounding pain, redness or inflammation, the cannula should be removed before 72 hours have elapsed. If it seems to be blocked, try to flush it gently with normal saline. Remove the dressing gently and check to see that the cannula is not kinked, as is often the case. In patients who are confused or likely to pull the cannula out, it is wise to additionally dress the cannula with a bandage.

Cannula flow rates

This is something it is wise to know about in case you get asked at the end of the station, as it is can gain you easy marks.

As you know, cannulas come in different colours and sizes. The rate of fluid flow through a cannula is calculated in laboratory conditions, using a fluid bag of distilled water at 22°C, pressurised at 10 kPa, through tubing of internal diameter 4 mm and length 110 cm.

Intravenous cannulas are sized by *standard wire gauge*. In this system, the larger the gauge size, the smaller the cannula. Which colour represents a particular size varies by manufacturer, and there is no internationally accepted colour scheme. In the UK, one common colour scheme is shown in the table.

Colour	Gauge	Estimated flow rate (mL/min)
Blue	22	20–40
Pink	20	40–80
Green	18	75–120
White	17	100–140
Grey	16	130–220
Orange	14	250–360

So, if there is a well-running 14 G cannula, you can give a 1 L bag of fluid in under 4 minutes, which is actually quicker than can be given via a central access.

62 Intravenous drug administration

Checklist	P	MP	F
Appropriate introduction to the patient and informed consent obtained			
Confirms indication for administration of the drug			
Checks prescription on the drug chart, including: • Patient identity, with wrist band • Dose • Time to be given • Route of administration • Appropriate prescription If is in doubt regarding dose or frequency, consults the *BNF*			
Ensures there are no allergies or contraindications to the drug			
Ascertains whether patient has appropriate intravenous access			
Washes hands and wears clean gloves			
Checks the drug, dose and expiry date with a colleague or nurse			
Checks the administration fluid into which drug is to be mixed with a nurse or colleague			
Checks the manufacturer's instructions regarding the preparation and administration of the drug(s)			
Draws up into a syringe/fluid bag the appropriate amount of drug in a suitable volume of fluid, as per the manufacturer's instructions			
Appropriately labels the drug			
Draws up a saline flush			
Positions the patient comfortably			
Cleans the injection port of the cannula site with an alcohol-based or chlorhexidine-based wipe			
Gently injects 5–10 mL saline flush to ensure the cannula is patent			
Ensures air is expelled from the drug preparation: • If a syringe, tap it to remove air bubbles • If a giving set, ensure the line is run through			
Gives drug by injection or fluid giving set as per instructions over the appropriate amount of time			
Observes patient and vital signs for a few minutes			
Records signature and time on the drug chart			
Thanks patient, ensures comfort and offers to answer any questions			

Summary of key points for OSCEs

Types of drug administration

You will sometimes be asked to give a drug intravenously to a patient who does *not* have an intravenous cannula. In such situations, you may say that you would either insert one first or give the drug by injection directly into the vein.

In addition, drugs come in different preparations. Some will come as liquids that can be given as they are. These are usually drawn up into a syringe and injected slowly. Other drugs (whether powders or liquids) will need to be reconstituted into a certain volume of fluid before injection.

Some drugs will be given as a bolus injection. Others (e.g. insulin for sliding-scale infusion) may be given via syringe driver. Some are placed in a given volume of intravenous fluid and infused over a particular time interval. A volumetric pump is often used for precision and accuracy.

Remember that the essential principles do not change whatever the manner of drug administration.

Essentially, safety is the key to this station. Checking you have the correct patient and their drug chart, and ensuring that there are no allergies/contraindications to the drug, will provide the majority of the marks.

Hints and tips for the exam

• This is a simple procedure, so keep it simple.
• Emphasise that you would check the drug, etc., and that you would check the prescription with the *BNF*.

• Priority is given to safety.
• Ensure that you flush the intravenous cannula with normal saline before and after drug administration.
• Always say you would monitor the patient for a few minutes after administration of the drug.
• Ensure that you document the event on the drug chart.
• Note that two appropriate healthcare staff (i.e. doctors and/or nurses) are required to check the drug.
• You must ensure adequacy of the intravenous access. There are certain drugs that should be given only via a large central vein and not peripherally. Examples include inotropes, concentrated KCl solutions and total parenteral nutrition.

Risks of intravenous drug administration

There are a few risks of intravenous drug administration, including the following:
• Phlebitis, for example from irritant drugs
• Extravasation into the surrounding tissues
• Intra-arterial injection
• Pain on injection
• Introduction of infection
• Emboli, for example air embolism
• Anaphylaxis, a reaction or hypersensitivity to the drug
• Dosing errors
• Errors in the rate of administration. For example, if gentamicin is given too quickly, its plasma concentration may rise above its therapeutic window and give rise to ototoxicity.

63 Arterial blood gas analysis

Task: You are the medical ward cover FY1 on call. The nurses have bleeped you to see a 23-year-old man complaining of difficulty breathing who has saturations of 91% on 15 L/min oxygen. They inform you that his other observations are stable and that he is alert. He was admitted from A&E this morning with severe lobar pneumonia. *Please perform an ABG on the manikin provided. You will then be shown the result by the examiner. Please interpret this and answer the examiner's questions regarding further management.*

Checklist	P	MP	F
Appropriate introduction and verbal consent obtained			
Checks identity of the patient using wristband/medical notes			
Collects appropriate equipment			
• Needle			
• Arterial blood gas (ABG) syringe			
• Soft swab and tape			
• Sterile wipes			
• Sharps bin			
Sterilises skin			
Enquires about patient preference regarding which hand to use			
Repositions patient appropriately			
Performs Allen's test			
Warns patient there will be a sharp scratch			
Inserts needle at an appropriate angle			
Gets flashback on first attempt			
Waits for syringe to fill syringe or fills syringe manually			
Removes needle and disposes of it in sharps bin			
Puts cap on syringe			
Applies firm pressure over artery and tapes swab down to stop bleeding			
Mentions need to get the sample tested promptly			
Thanks patient			
Interpretation of ABG shown by examiner: pH 7.44, P_{O_2} 7.9 kPa, P_{CO_2} 3.5 kPa, lactate 3.5 mmol/L, HCO_3 25 mmol/L, BE −1.8 mmol/L			

When asked: Is able to name two or three hospital locations where ABG processing machines are available (e.g. ITU, HDU, A&E, obstetrics/labour ward)			
Mentions the need to accurately enter the patient's details into the interpretation machine			
Asks how many litres of oxygen the patient is receiving (examiner replies '15 L per minute' *if* the candidate asks)			
Correctly interprets P_{O_2}			
Correctly interprets P_{CO_2} and acid–base status			
Correctly interprets base excess and bicarbonate			
Calculates and comments on anion gap (if interpreting metabolic acidosis)			
Correctly interprets lactate			
Makes appropriate comments regarding any other abnormalities (e.g. haemoglobin, sodium, potassium, glucose, calcium)			
Correctly interprets overall picture (e.g. refractory type 1 respiratory failure)			
Requests results from previous ABGs			
Comments on possible causes of the observed ABG abnormalities (type 1 respiratory failure secondary to severe pneumonia)			
Correctly identifies further steps in management:			
• Sits patient up			
• Informs ITU with a view to start CPAP			
• Considers complications and alternative diagnoses, e.g. adult respiratory distress syndrome or pulmonary embolism in addition to pneumonia			
• Considers changing antibiotics			
Identifies importance of further ABGs to monitor progress			

Performing an ABG and being able to interpret the results is a hugely important skill, especially for the FY1 on call who has been bleeped to review a sick patient on the ward. However, unlike venepuncture and cannulation, it is massively underpractised by the vast majority of medical students approaching finals.

Hints and tips for the exam

Practise on actual patients

Although you will be provided with a manikin arm in the OSCE, it is wise to practise the ABG on real patients because it is a vital skill for an FY1 to have. The best way to do this is to meet the FY1 on the respiratory or acute medicine firm after the ward round and ask them which patients will be requiring an ABG. Other opportunities may arise if you take time to shadow the on-call medical FY1.

Do not forget to perform Allen's test

You risk failing the entire station if you do not perform this simple test, so make sure you always perform it when you practise so that it becomes second nature.

Allen's test is used to check that both the ulnar and radial arteries are intact. This is important because an ABG can theoretically damage the radial artery and cause haematoma formation that compresses the artery and compromises blood flow. If this were to happen, the ulnar artery would have to be intact to supply blood to the hand and prevent ischaemic tissue damage. Carry out the test as follows:

1. Elevate the hand.
2. Occlude the ulnar **and** radial artery by applying firm pressure until the hand becomes pale.
3. Release pressure from the ulnar artery.
4. Check whether the hand goes red.
5. If it does, the ulnar artery is intact and it is safe to perform an ABG on the radial artery.

Know how to calculate the anion gap if presented with metabolic acidosis

• This is calculated using the formula (values in mmol/L): $K + Na - HCO_3 - Cl$.
• The normal anion gap is 10–18 mmol/L.
• The anion gap is important because the causes of metabolic acidosis with an increased and a normal anion gap differ significantly (see the table).

Always ask about results from previous ABGs and mention you would like to perform further ABGs after starting management

Interpreting ABG results is much easier if you have a series of results from different stages of a patient's illness. Furthermore, it is necessary to monitor the response to treatment.

Summary of common conditions seen in OSCEs

	Abnormalities on ABG	Causes	Important investigations	Management
Type 1 respiratory failure	Po_2 <8 kPa Pco_2 (normal or low)	Obstructive airway disease (asthma, COPD) Pulmonary oedema Pulmonary embolism Lower respiratory tract infection	Peak expiratory flow rate Chest X-ray CT pulmonary angiogram or V/Q scan	High-flow oxygen CPAP if resistant to oxygen therapy Treat underlying cause, e.g. antibiotics, anticoagulation, bronchodilators
Type 2 respiratory failure	Po_2 <8 kPa Pco_2 >6.5 kPa pH is normal if compensated, <7.35 if uncompensated	COPD Respiratory muscle weakness (e.g. Guillain–Barré syndrome) Head injury Opiate or benzodiazepine overdose	Chest X-ray CT of the head Urine toxicology screen Nerve conduction studies	BIPAP (if conscious) Invasive ventilation (**if** Glasgow Coma Scale score <8) Treat underlying cause, e.g. with naloxone or plasma exchange
Respiratory acidosis	Pco_2 >6 kPa pH <7.35 kPa HCO_3 may be >30 mmol/L (and BE >+2 mmol/L) if compensated	Life-threatening asthma Excessive oxygen therapy in a 'blue bloater' Head injury Opiate or benzodiazepine overdose	Peak expiratory flow rate Chest X-ray Urine toxicology	BIPIAP (or invasive ventilation if lack of response to BIPAP) Bronchodilators
Respiratory alkalosis	Pco_2 <4.7 kPa pH >7.45 HCO_3 may be <24 mmol/L (and BE <−2 mmol/L) if compensated	Hyperventilation Early stages of salicylate toxicity	Blood salicylate levels Ask about other symptoms of anxiety	Simple hyperventilation: rebreathe into a brown paper bag Salicylate overdose: activated charcoal, correction of metabolic derangement, intravenous rehydration, dialysis

Metabolic acidosis	pH <7.35 HCO$_3$ <24 mmol/L, BE <−2 mmol/L	Normal anion gap	Diarrhoea Road traffic accident	Abdominal X-ray	Fluid and electrolyte support Antimicrobial agents
		Raised anion gap	Ketoacidosis Lactic acidosis Late stages of salicylate toxicity Paracetamol overdose Renal failure	Capillary blood glucose Toxicology screen	Fluid resuscitation Insulin sliding scale N-Acetylcysteine Dialysis
Metabolic alkalosis	pH >7.45, HCO$_3$ > 30 mmol/L, BE >+2 mmol/L		Vomiting Nasogastric intubation Pyloric stenosis Primary or secondary hyperaldosteronism Diuretics Hypercalcaemia	Abdominal X-ray Bloods: Us+Es, bone profile, liver function tests, plasma brain natriuretic peptide, renin–aldosterone ratio Echocardiogram (NB. cardiac failure can cause secondary hyperaldosteronism)	Treat underlying cause
High lactate	Lactate >2 mmol/L		Systemic inflammatory response syndrome Severe sepsis Bowel perforation Ischaemic bowel Disseminated intravascular coagulation Chronic hypoxia (e.g. 'blue bloater' COPD) Liver failure Dehydration	Bloods: full blood count, C-reactive protein level, liver function tests, clotting screen Blood cultures Amylase Erect chest X-ray and abdominal X-ray CT abdomen	

Potential variations at this station

• Interpretation of an ABG, followed by 'SBAR' (situation, background, assessment, recommendation) referral to ITU for ventilatory support.
• Interpretation of an ABG, followed by examiner questions on further management.

Questions you may be asked

Q. What are the indications for CPAP and BIPAP?
A. Indications for CPAP include type 1 respiratory failure refractory to high-flow supplementary oxygen. Indications for BIPAP are:

• Type 2 respiratory failure secondary to obstructive sleep apnoea, neuromuscular disease for chest deformities
• Decompensated COPD with CO_2 retention causing acidosis (pH 7.25–7.35)
• Weaning off endotracheal intubation

Q. Briefly explain how CPAP and BIPAP work.
A. CPAP works by:

• Positive airway pressure throughout the respiratory cycle
• Splinting the alveoli open during expiration, thus preventing premature closure/collapse of the alveoli
• Increasing the time and surface area available for ventilation, therefore increasing gas exchange and oxygenation of the blood

BIPAP works by:

• Providing positive pressure throughout the respiratory cycle

• Pressure being more positive during inspiration than expiration
• High positive pressures during inspiration splinting the alveoli open and thus increasing oxygenation
• Lower positive pressures during expiration increasing minute ventilation so that more air (and hence CO_2) is exhaled per unit time

Q. How do you calculate the oxygen delivery to tissues?
A. Oxygen delivery (mL O_2/min) = Cardiac output (L/min) x [Hb] (g/L) x 1.31 (mL O_2/g Hb) × Sao_2

Q. What are the potential complications of an ABG?
A. • Haematoma formation (can cause compression of the artery and compromise blood flow)
  • Damage to local structures
  • False aneurysm formation
  • Failure to get blood despite multiple attempts

Q. How can lactic acidosis be classified?
A. Type A lactic acidosis is caused by tissue hypoperfusion (e.g. systemic inflammatory response syndrome, hypoxia, severe anaemia)

Type B lactic acidosis has three subtypes:
• Drugs (e.g. metformin, paracetamol overdose)
• Tumours (e.g. lymphoma)
• Inborn errors of metabolism (e.g. glucose 6-phosphate deficiency)

64 Measuring peak expiratory flow rate

Checklist	P	MP	F
Appropriate introduction to patient			
Explains procedure and obtains informed consent			
Washes hands			
Prepares equipment: • Peak flow meter • Clean disposable mouth piece			
Checks the peak flow meter, ensuring the dial is not stuck			
Explains the technique and checks the patient's understanding			
Demonstration by performing the technique first			
Positions the patient – standing upright			
Sets the dial to zero			
Ensures the peak flow meter is held horizontally and the dial is not obstructed, e.g. by fingers			

Checklist	P	MP	F
Patient takes a deep breath in to vital capacity			
Patient forms airtight seal around mouth piece			
Patient exhales as fast and as hard as possible			
Records result			
Resets dial to 0 and then repeats procedure twice			
Records the best of three readings in the notes and/or patient's peak flow diary			
Thanks patient, reassures them and answers any questions			
Discards mouth piece and washes hands			
Consultation conducted in a professional manner with appropriate use of language and avoidance of medical jargon			
Satisfactory interpretation of result			

Summary of key points for OSCEs

Peak flow rate is measured using a simple peak flow meter that consists of a long cylindrical tube and a disposable mouth piece (Figure 64.1). As the patient exhales into the mouth piece, a piston is forced along the long axis of the peak flow meter. This is connected to a pointer that moves along the upper surface to give a reading on a calibrated scale.

Uses of peak flow measurement

Peak flow measurement is useful in the diagnosis and monitoring of obstructive airway disease.

Diagnosis

Peak flow can be used to diagnose asthma by demonstrating 'reversibility'. Following administration of a bronchodilator, for example via a salbutamol nebuliser or inhaler, an improvement of over 15% in peak flow rate indicates that the airway obstruction has a reversible component, in keeping with asthma.

If there is no convincing reversibility, the diagnosis is unlikely to be asthma but may well be chronic obstructive pulmonary disease (COPD). However, there are also patients with COPD or emphysema who demonstrate a degree of reversibility, so the differentiation in diagnosis between COPD or asthma is not always clear.

Monitoring

The trend in peak flow rate is more important than the actual value. Recording serial peak flow readings provides objective evidence of progress or response to treatment of the airway obstruction. In addition, diurnal variation is often seen in asthma, with early morning dips in the peak flow values. Patients will often keep a peak flow diary, which can be used to demonstrate this. If measurements are taken daily for monitoring purposes, they should be taken at the same time each day.

Interpretation of the result

The best reading of three is taken so that the patient's best effort is what is documented. This will often be the second reading. The greatest reading is compared either with the patient's own best known reading or with a standardised chart that predicts what it should be according to height and gender (Figure 64.2). 'Normal' is considered to be a reading that is at least 80% of the predicted or best known value.

The peak expiratory flow rate (PEFR), expressed as a percentage of the best or predicted value, is a useful tool in establishing the severity of an asthma attack.

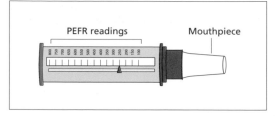

Figure 64.1 A typical bedside peak flow meter, similar to ones you are likely to be given in the exam

PEFR expressed as % of best or predicted value	Severity of asthma attack
80+	Normal
50–75+	Moderate
33–50	Severe
<33	Life-threatening

Limitations of peak flow measurement

Although peak flow measurement is a simple, inexpensive and easily performed technique, there are several drawbacks to its use, which must be considered:
- It depends significantly on the patient's technique, cooperation and effort, so clear instructions, demonstration and encouragement are required. If patients do not put in their best possible effort, the results may not give a true reflection of their current respiratory state.
- The technique measures the PEFR but gives no indication of other markers of lung function, for example volume measurements.
- It does **not** assess the calibre of the smaller airways.
- It is unsuitable for use in children below 5 years of age as the airway resistance encountered in using a peak flow meter is too high, and it may be difficult to explain the technique to a small child and get their cooperation.

Spirometry

You will probably not be asked to demonstrate this in the exam, but you may be asked to interpret spirometry graphs as part of the station on PEFR.

Spirometry is performed in the laboratory by specially trained technical staff. Essentially, the patient exhales with maximum possible force through a mouth piece as rapidly as possible for as long as possible, *after a maximum inspiration*. This can be difficult and exhausting for patients, especially those with obstructive airway diseases since they have prolonged expiratory phases. The spirometer then produces a graph as shown in Figure 64.3.

Two key measurements are made with this technique:

• **Forced vital capacity** (FVC): the maximum volume of air that can be forcefully exhaled after a maximum inspiration

• **Forced expiratory volume in 1 second** (FEV₁): the volume of air that is exhaled in the first second of the FVC measurement

Together, these values help to decide whether the patient has a restrictive or an obstructive lung pathol-ogy. There are, once again, charts that give predicted values for FVC and FEV_1. However, the ratio of FEV_1 to FVC is important:

• In normal lungs, the FEV_1/FVC ratio is about 75%.
• If the FEV_1/FVC ratio is <75%, the disease is likely to be obstructive.
• If the FEV_1/FVC ratio is >75%, the disorder is likely to be restrictive, or the lungs are normal.

	Obstructive lung disease	Restrictive lung disease
Examples	Asthma, chronic obstructive pulmonary disease	Intrinsic: pulmonary fibrosis, sarcoidosis, interstitial lung disease Extrinsic: • Non-muscular chest disorders, e.g. kyphosis, rheumatoid arthritis, obesity • Neuromuscular disorders, e.g. myasthenia gravis, Guillain–Barré syndrome
FVC	Reduced	Reduced
FEV_1	Reduced significantly more than FVC	Reduced almost in proportion to FVC
FEV_1/FVC ratio	<75%	>75%

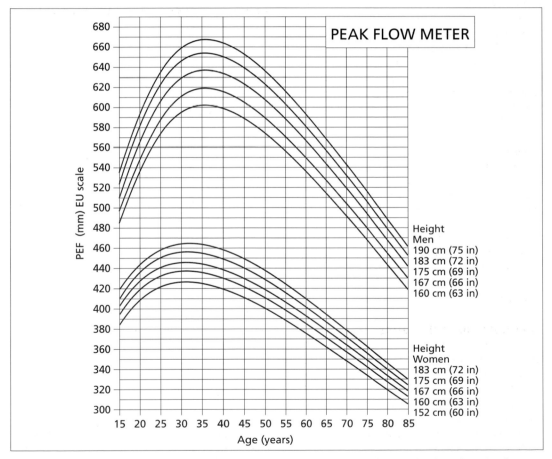

Figure 64.2 Peak expiratory flow rates for males and females – normal values. The graphs demonstrate predicted peak flow values for healthy males and females of different ages and weights. You only need to learn a few typical values for the exam, as well as how to interpret the graph. Adapted by Clement Clarke for use with EN13826/EU scale peak flow meters from Nunn AJ, Gregg I, *Br Med J* 1898;298:1068–70

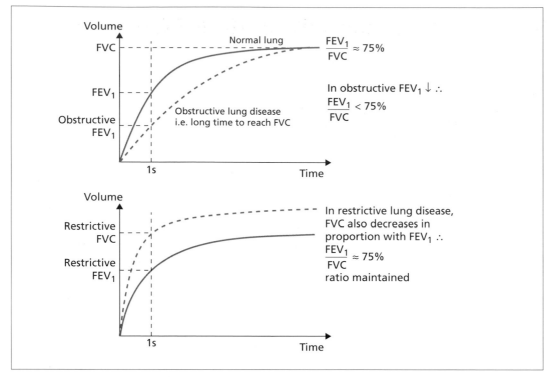

Figure 64.3 Spirometry graphs for obstructive and restrictive lung disease. The graphs demonstrate the spirometry graphs you can expect to see for patients with obstructive and restrictive lung diseases, and show how the FEV_1/FVC ratio changes

Hints and tips

Technique

• Practise! It is important that you practise how you are going to explain the technique to the patient so that you do not waste vital minutes in the exam in trying to do so. It may be something along the lines of:

Please stand up. Hold this tube horizontally. Take a deep breath in, as deep as you possibly can. Then form a good seal around this mouth piece and blow into it as hard and as fast as you possibly can. I will then take a reading from the dial on top, so it is important that you hold the tube from the sides and not above and below. Let me show you . . . .

• You must make sure that you check the peak flow meter, making sure that it is patent, and that the dial is set to zero between readings and is able to move freely.

• Demonstrate to the examiner that you clean your hands between attempts.

• It is important to be professional and courteous to the patient-actor throughout, and this alone will get you a few marks.

Interpretation

• You should familiarise yourself with the charts that compare predicted values with actual values, as well as learn a few typical values. The patient or actor in the exam is going to be reasonably well in order to carry out up to three peak flows for the entire OSCE cohort in your sitting. However, they may be told not to give their full effort, and hence give lower peak flow readings than are true.

• The examiner may give you the graph shown in Figure 64.3 and ask you to interpret your results and say how they compare with the predicted value.

Questions you could be asked

These are likely to be based on the following topics:

• Interpretation of the result based on predicted value charts

• Problems and shortcomings of peak flow measurement

• Reversibility

• Interpretation of spirometry graphs and FEV_1/FVC ratios

65 Performing and interpreting ECGs

Task (5 minutes): Demonstrate how you would record a 12-lead ECG on this manikin and interpret the ECG traces presented by the examiner.

Checklist	P	MP	F
Appropriate introduction and confirms identity of patient using wrist band			
Briefly explains the procedure			
Requests patient to remain as still and silent as possible during recording			
Correctly attaches the limb leads			
Correctly attaches the chest leads: • V1 – 4th intercostal space, right sternal border • V2 – 4th intercostal space, left sternal border • V3 – Half way between V2 and V4 • V4 – 5th intercostal space, midclavicular line • V5 – 5th intercostal space, left anterior axillary line • V6 – 6th intercostal space, left anterior axillary line			
Explains that stickers will be left on the chest in case a further trace is needed in the near future and thanks patient			
Checks for correct calibration of the ECG (25 mm/s, 1 cm/mV)			

States intention to write indication for ECG on the recording			
Reports on following aspects of the trace:			
• Heart rate			
• Rhythm			
• Axis			
• P wave, QRS wave, T wave			
• PR interval			
• ST segment			
• Other abnormal waveforms, e.g. J waves, U waves, pathological Q waves			
Offers appropriate differential/ correct diagnosis			
Offers appropriate management plan: • Recognises the need for resuscitation with respect to airway, breathing and circulation (if appropriate) • Discusses further management (if appropriate)			

Summary of common ECGs seen in OSCEs

Disease/abnormality	Characteristic ECG features	Specific points in management
ST segment elevation MI	ST elevation: (leads 2, 3, aVF – inferior; V1–V4 – anteroseptal; V4–V6, 1, aVL – anterolateral) Tall T waves in acute setting Pathological Q waves (>0.04s wide and >2mm deep) LBBB (of new onset)	Percutaneous coronary intervention is treatment of choice Thrombolysis if • ST elevation >1 mm in two or more limb leads, or >2mm in two or more chest leads • New LBBB Streptokinase for non-anterior MI Tenecteplase if anterior MI, systolic blood pressure <100mmHg, new LBBB, previous use of streptokinase Alteplase if previous adverse reaction to streptokinase
Non-ST segment elevation MI	ST depression Inverted T waves	Aspirin (300mg) + clopidogrel (300mg) + low molecular weight heparin Nitrates, beta-blockers, ACE inhibitors, lipid management Consider glycoprotein 2b/3a inhibitors
Posterior infarct	Tall R waves and ST depression in leads V1–V2	See ST segment elevation MI
Ventricular fibrillation	Characteristic broad complex tachycardia that should be instantly recognised No clear QRS complexes Rate >120/min	See Chapter 69 on ALS
Ventricular tachycardia	Positive QRS concordance in chest leads Left axis deviation Rate >100/min Fusion and capture beats Atrioventricular dissociation Polymorphic QRS complexes with constantly changing axis in torsade de pointes	If no pulse, follow ALS protocol If patient has a pulse, check for adverse signs (systolic blood pressure <90mmHg, chest pain, heart failure, heart rate >150/min) If pulse is present, sedate and administer DC shock If pulse is absent, correct underlying causes, try chemical cardioversion (amiodarone/lidocaine) and then give DC shock
Supraventricular tachycardia	Rate >100/min QRS <120ms Rhythm regular	Vagal manoeuvres Adenosine 6mg followed by 12mg and 12mg (into a central vein) Rate control if no adverse signs (esmolol, digoxin, verapamil, amiodarone) Sedation and synchronised shock if adverse signs
Atrial fibrillation	Irregular baseline Irregularly irregular rhythm Rate may be >100/min (or <100/min if on rate-controlling drugs) No P waves	Refer to NICE (2006) guidelines

Heart block	First degree: prolonged PR interval	Correct underlying causes (e.g. hypothyroidism), stop precipitating drugs (e.g. beta-blockers, digoxin, calcium channel blockers) No treatment if rate >40/min and asymptomatic If rate <40/min or symptomatic, give atropine, or pace if this is not effective
	Second degree (Mobitz type I/Wenckebach): PR gets progressively longer over a few beats and then a QRS wave is dropped. The PR interval following the dropped QRS beat is shorter Second degree (Mobitz type II): PR interval is uniform but some P waves are not followed by a QRS. Is 2:1 if QRS is dropped after every third P wave, and 3:1 if QRS is dropped after every fourth P wave	Mobitz type II has a higher rate of progression to third-degree heart block and therefore usually requires pacing Mobitz type I requires treatment only if symptomatic
	Third degree (complete): dissociation between P wave rate and QRS rate	All patients require pacing
Trifascicular block	RBBB + left axis deviation	Pacing
Wolff–Parkinson–White syndrome	Short PR interval Wide QRS with slurred upstroke	See supraventricular tachycardia Ablation
Hyperkalaemia	Tall tented T waves, wide QRS complexes, small P waves Ventricular fibrillation	Arrest protocol if ventricular fibrillation 10mL 10% calcium gluconate intravenously over 2 minutes (preferably into a large vein) 50mL 50% glucose with 10U of rapid-acting insulin over 30 minutes. Monitor BM readings 5mg salbutamol via nebuliser Calcium resonium Dialysis if potassium remains persistently high
Hypokalaemia	ST elevation, T wave inversion Prolonged QT interval Flattened T wave, may be followed by U wave Long PR interval	ALS protocol if patient is in cardiac arrest Correct underlying cause (vomiting, diuretics, Cushing's syndrome, Conn's syndrome) Oral potassium if K > 2.5 mmol/L and asymptomatic Intravenous potassium if K < 2.5 mmol/L or symptomatic
Hypothermia	Osborne J waves (positive deflection at junction of QRS wave and ST segment) May be confused with bundle branch block or ST elevation but identification enabled by: • Shorter duration of positive deflection • Present in all (or most) chest and limb leads • Coexisting bradycardia	Slow rewarming aiming for increase in temperature of approximately 0.5°C per hour. Hot drinks, warm intravenous infusion Antibiotic prophylaxis against pneumonia in patients aged over 65 Monitor rectal temperature, urine output, blood pressure, pulse and respiratory rate at least half-hourly NB. Falling blood pressure is the first sign of overrapid rewarming, which can cause ventricular and atrial fibrillation Review patient's social situation before discharge

(Continued)

Disease/abnormality	Characteristic ECG features	Specific points in management
Acute pericarditis	Widespread concave ST segment elevation	Analgesia (e.g. ibuprofen) Colchicine, steroids Treat underlying cause (e.g. dialysis if uraemia, antineoplastic agents if malignancy, etc.)
Possible pulmonary embolism	Sinus tachycardia RBBB Deep S wave in lead 1 + Q wave in lead 3 + inverted T wave in lead 3 (although this picture is uncommon in practice)	Thrombolysis if massive pulmonary embolism or patient haemodynamically unstable Intravenous low molecular weight heparin Start warfarin once systolic blood pressure >90mmHg Heparin + warfarin for 5 days. Stop heparin once INR >2 6 weeks' warfarin if cause is remediable; if no remedial cause, 3–6 months' warfarin Search for underlying causes
Pacemaker	Spikes before P and QRS waves If there are spikes without QRS complexes, pacemaker is likely to be dislodged	
Dextrocardia	Poor R wave progression in leads V1–V6 Inverted P, QRS and T waves in lead 1	
Cardiac tamponade	Low-voltage QRS complexes Tachycardia Electrical alternans	See Chapter 69 on ALS

ALS, advanced life support; INR, International Normalised Ratio; LBBB, left bundle branch block; MI, myocardial infarction; RBBB, right bundle branch block

Hints and tips for the exam

The mark sheet for this station appears brief, but do not be deceived because it is testing several key areas of your knowledge. This station effectively has three parts:
- **Setting up the ECG:** You either know how to do this or you don't! Make sure you practise this a few times so that you can get it out of the way quickly in the exam before you take on the harder task of interpreting the traces.
- **Interpreting findings from a 12-lead ECG:**
  - You may be provided with brief history and/or examination findings related to the ECG. If so, it would be wise to quickly formulate a list of differential diagnoses in your head before starting to report the ECG. Regardless of this, make sure you clearly point out any glaring abnormality (if present) at the beginning. For example, if there is obvious ST elevation in leads 2, 3 and aVF, you can start by saying, 'On initial analysis, there is ST elevation in 2, 3 and aVF. Upon review . . . ' – and then go through the whole trace systematically.
  - Traces of ventricular tachycardia and ventricular fibrillation require spot diagnosis so make sure you are able to identify them instantaneously. You will not be expected to adopt a systematic approach to recognise these traces.
  - You will probably be asked to interpret more than one trace, in which case one of them may be of a less common condition, such as dextrocardia. Although you are unlikely to fail if you are unable to diagnose something as rare as dextrocardia from the ECG trace, it would be wise to use the systematic approach of interpreting an ECG and offering a reasonable differential diagnosis and further investigations at the end.
- **Management of common medical emergencies:** The traces you will be shown in the exam are likely to relate to commonly encountered medical emergencies such as acute coronary syndrome, arrhythmias and serious electrolyte disturbances. You must remember the need to resuscitate an acutely ill patient with respect to ABC (covered in detail in other stations) before proceeding to further specific steps in management outlined in the table above.

Potential variations at this station

- An ECG spot diagnosis of a 'shockable' rhythm followed by the advanced life support management protocol.

- Interpreting results from an arterial blood gas (ABG) analysis followed by an ECG from the same patient. For example, you might be shown an ABG of type 1 respiratory failure, which may be followed by an ECG showing sinus tachycardia. You might then be asked for the most important differential diagnosis (which in this case is pulmonary embolism).
- Interpreting a chest X-ray followed by an ECG from the same patient. For example, you may be shown a chest X-ray with diffuse reticulonodular shadowing followed by an ECG with right-heart strain pattern and then be asked the most important differential diagnosis (in this case cor pulmonale secondary to fibrotic lung disease).
- An ECG followed by viva questions, for example the causes of hypokalaemia or hyperkalaemia.

Questions you could be asked

Q. Where is the isoelectric point?
A. The point at which the P wave begins to rise on the ECG.
Q. What are the posterior chest leads?
A. Leads V7–V9 (useful if a posterior infarct is suspected).
You may also be given the following ECGs or ECG-related scenarios to interpret:
- Chest X-ray, for example cardiomegaly, + related ECG
- ABG, for example of type 1 respiratory failure, + ECG reflecting pulmonary embolism; type 2 respiratory failure + right heart strain ECG showing cor pulmonale; lactic acidosis/ increased troponin + ST segment elevation
- ECG + advanced life support
- ECG + viva (e.g. causes of hyperkalaemia)
- ECG + focused history (e.g. to rule out contraindications to thrombolysis)

Reference

National Institute for Health and Clinical Excellence (2006) Atrial fibrillation: the management of atrial fibrillation. Available from: www.nice.org.uk/nicemedia/live/10982/30054/30054.pdf (accessed June 2012).

66 Scrubbing up in theatre

Checklist	P	MP	F
Wears surgical scrubs, shoes and theatre cap			
Applies a mask over the nose and mouth			
With sterile technique, opens an appropriately sized surgical gown			
With sterile technique, opens sterile gloves			
Is bare below the elbows, removing watches, rings, etc.			
Opens a sterile sponge/brush and leaves to one side			
Turns on tap, adjusting water temperature			
Wets hands and forearms, but only allows water to flow proximally from hands down to elbows			
Uses only one scrub solution (not more), and operates dispenser using elbows and **not** hands			
Initial pre-scrub wash: lather formed from hands to above elbows and then rinsed off			

	P	MP	F
Uses brush and/or nail file to scrub below each of the nails for 30 seconds per hand			
Scrubs between each of the fingers, and between forefinger and thumb			
Scrubs both dorsal and palmar surfaces of fingers			
Scrubs palms, dorsum of hands and wrists			
Washes from hands to elbows, always keeping hands elevated above elbows			
Does not shake water off after washing			
Dries hands with sterile towels, starting with hands and then working back to elbows			
Gown applied appropriately			
Sterile gloves applied satisfactorily			
Asks for an assistant to tie gown from behind			

Summary of key points for OSCEs

Scrubbing up effectively in theatre is vital in preventing the transmission of infection both to the patient and from the patient to the staff. In order to pass this station successfully, practice is important. The best people to show you how to scrub up are probably friendly and enthusiastic operating department practitioners – but remember to ask them nicely! Many hospitals and operating departments have their own scrub policies, and becoming familiar with them will make you more efficient in the exam.

Hints and tips for the exam

About scrubbing up in general

The examiners may ask you some basic facts about scrubbing up, which are worth knowing:
• Scrubbing for the first case of the day should take you 4–5 minutes, and you must clean your nails with the brush or nail file.
• Once you have scrubbed, this is thought to be effective for approximately 2 hours.
• If the patient is a high-risk case (in terms of transmissible infections), for example is an intravenous drug user or is known to be HIV-positive, one should double-glove, and the eyes should be protected either with goggles or a mask with a visor.

Technique

• Even before scrubbing, you must say that you would don appropriate surgical scrubs, shoes and a theatre or operating hat.
• Your nose and mouth should be covered by a mask that fits snugly over the contour of your face. Most standard disposable surgical masks can be adjusted to achieve a good fit.
• Being bare below the elbows is vital, and, accordingly, all apparel below the elbows must be removed.
• At all times, you must ensure that water and scrub solution run back from your hand to your elbow and never the other way, in order to make sure your hands remain sterile.
• There will be often be a choice of a chlorhexidine-based or an iodine-based solution. You must only ever use one scrub solution at a time – never more than one.
• Scrubbing solution is applied using one elbow to depress the dispenser. Never use your hands or they will cease to be sterile.
• If at any time you have become unsterile, everything must be discarded and the whole procedure commenced from the beginning.
• The initial phase is a pre-scrub wash in which the scrub solution is lathered up as high as a point just proximal to the elbow and then rinsed off.
• Do not dry your hands by shaking the water off. Just let it drip off, and then wipe your hands with sterile towels.

Equipment

• It is important that all the surgical apparel is opened using a sterile technique.
• The brush and sponge are used to clean under the nails. Nowadays, they often come as a single piece. Read the package as some makes are impregnated with a scrubbing solution, whereas others are not. The brush should not be used on the skin as it may cause breaks in the skin as well as disrupting the normal skin flora.
• The gown must be handled with care. Once the hands are dry after scrubbing, the gown must be picked up by what will be its inside and allowed to unfold itself down without touching the floor or any unsterile surface. The ends of the sleeves cover as far as the palms of your hands.
• You may be asked to demonstrate how you would open and wear the gown and the gloves using a sterile technique.
• The gloves are worn without touching their outsides. They significantly overlap the ends of the gown's sleeves. It is worth practising with sterile gloves so that you become efficient at wearing them before the exam.

67 Suturing

Checklist	P	MP	F
Appropriate introduction to the patient and informed consent obtained			
Asks patient whether they have any allergies, e.g. to local anaesthetic			
Checks that suturing the wound would be appropriate, including: • Presence of Infection or contamination • Presence of foreign body • Neurovascular state of skin • Location of wound • Wound not more than 24 hours old			
Adequate exposure and good lighting			
Prepares equipment: • Sterile drape • Sterile suture pack (forceps, needle holder, gauze, pot for cleaning solution, scissors) • Wound cleaning solution, poured into the pot • Appropriate local anaesthetic • 10 mL syringe with 21 G (green) needle and 25 G (orange) needle • Suitable size and type of suture • Sterile gloves			
Washes hands and dons sterile gloves			
Cleans the area with cleaning solution, and applies sterile drape to create a sterile field			
Draws up local anaesthetic with 21 G needle			

	P	MP	F
Infiltrates wound area appropriately with local anaesthetic using 25 G needle			
Places suture needle in needle holder two-thirds of its length away from its tip			
Raises skin edge on one side of wound with forceps			
Inserts needle perpendicular to skin 5 mm from the wound edge, and gently pulls through with needle holder			
Raises opposite skin edge with forceps, and passes needle through directly opposite to insertion point, from dermis upwards, emerging 5 mm from wound edge			
Ties three knots, clockwise–anticlockwise–clockwise, and cuts to leave approximately 1 cm of thread on wound			
Pulls knot to sit to one side of wound, not directly above it			
Ensures skin edges appose but do **not** overlie each other, and are not under tension			
Continues in a similar fashion to close wound			
Applies appropriate dressing			
Enquires about tetanus status			
Thanks patient and disposes safely of sharps			

Summary of key points for OSCEs

Indications and contraindications

Indications	Contraindications
Wound closure	Patient refusal
Fixing drains in place, e.g. chest drains, drains sited intraoperatively	Foreign matter in the wound, including glass, dirt, etc.
Repair of deep structures, e.g. tendons	Infected wound
	Large wound whose ends cannot be suitably apposed without significant tension

There are some situations where alternative wound closure methods would be more appropriate. For example, glue may be used on facial wounds or for children; Steri-Strips may provide a useful and less painful alternative.

Certain wounds may need specialist referral (e.g. to a plastics centre), and simple closure methods are inappropriate.

Types of suture

Choosing the appropriate suture material is important. Suture material can be broadly classified as absorbable or non-absorbable.

Type of material	Absorbable	Non-absorbable
Properties	Dissolve	Remain *in situ* until removed
Examples	Monocryl Vicryl Polydiaxonone (PDS)	Nylon Silk Prolene
Removal required?	No	Yes, timing depends on site
Suitable sites	Lips, mouth, tongue, viscera	Limbs, face, neck, abdominal/ chest wall

Suture needles come in a variety of shapes, including circular, semi-circular, three-eighths of a circle, five-eighths of a circle, straight, compound curved, half curved, etc. You do not need a detailed knowledge of these differences for the exam, but it is likely that you will get a curved needle to use and be asked to demonstrate that you can close a wound without actually touching the needle with your hands, i.e. using only forceps and a needle holder.

Sutures also come in different sizes: the larger the number, the smaller the suture. Hence, a 5/0 suture is larger than a 6/0 suture. The following table provides some guidance, but there may be local protocols in your hospital or medical school.

Site	Suture and size	Time to removal
Scalp	Non-absorbable 3/0	7 days
Face	Non-absorbable 5/0–6/0	4–5 days
Chest wall	Non-absorbable 3/0	10 days
Limbs and hands	Non-absorbable 4/0–5/0	10 days
Lips/tongue/mouth	Absorbable 6/0	n/a

Choice of local anaesthetic

Lidocaine is the first choice of local anaesthetic agent as it has a reasonably quick onset and relatively short duration of action. The alternative is bupivacaine (Marcaine), which has a longer onset of action but is more dangerous in terms of toxicity.

Some local anaesthetic preparations contain adrenaline (epinephrine). The aim of this is to cause local vasoconstriction, hence limiting blood flow to the area and resulting in a reduced absorption of the local anaesthetic. This prolongs the action of the local anaesthetic agent. However, when applying the solution to the extremities or to areas that do not have a notable collateral circulation, you must **not** use a solution containing adrenaline as vasoconstriction may cause necrosis of distal tissues.

The maximum safe dose of local anaesthetic depends on a patient's body weight. For lidocaine it is 3 mg/kg, and with adrenaline it is 5 mg/kg as its absorption is less. For bupivacaine it is 2 mg/kg. One may give as much local anaesthetic as required as long as it does not exceed these maximum doses.

If a larger volume is required to cover a wider area, a greater volume of a more dilute concentration is sufficient to achieve the same effect. If no dilute preparations are available, dilute your local anaesthetic with saline to the desired volume.

Local anaesthetic does not work as effectively in infected tissue.

Suturing technique

The following should be considered:

• Local anaesthetic infiltration, from around the perimeter of the wound inwards, including corners and angles

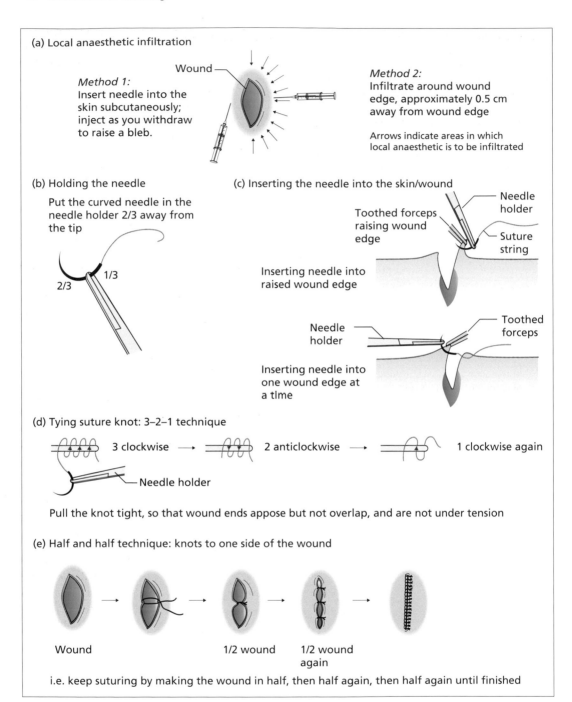

(a) Local anaesthetic infiltration

Wound

Method 1:
Insert needle into the skin subcutaneously; inject as you withdraw to raise a bleb.

Method 2:
Infiltrate around wound edge, approximately 0.5 cm away from wound edge

Arrows indicate areas in which local anaesthetic is to be infiltrated

(b) Holding the needle

Put the curved needle in the needle holder 2/3 away from the tip

2/3   1/3

(c) Inserting the needle into the skin/wound

Toothed forceps raising wound edge

Needle holder

Suture string

Inserting needle into raised wound edge

Needle holder

Toothed forceps

Inserting needle into one wound edge at a tIme

(d) Tying suture knot: 3–2–1 technique

3 clockwise → 2 anticlockwise → 1 clockwise again

Needle holder

Pull the knot tight, so that wound ends appose but not overlap, and are not under tension

(e) Half and half technique: knots to one side of the wound

Wound   1/2 wound   1/2 wound
                              again

i.e. keep suturing by making the wound in half, then half again, then half again until finished

Figure 67.1 One technique to suture a simple skin wound

- Position of the suture needle in the needle holder
- Half and half suture technique
- Tying the suture knot

This station is written to demonstrate one method of suturing. There are, however, other techniques that, for example, do not start in the middle of the wound and that advocate tying the knot differently. There are still other methods that allow you to use your hands to handle the suture needle. It is important that you check with your own medical school syllabus or clinical skills centre what techniques they suggest and follow them, as this will be what you face in your exam.

Tetanus

In the UK, tetanus prophylaxis is given monthly for 3 months from 2 months of age, with boosters at 4 years and 14 years of age. The need for prophylaxis depends on the nature of the injury and the patient's immunisation status. After these five doses, one is considered to have lifelong immunity.

Human anti-tetanus immunoglobulin (HATI) should be given instead if the patient has a history of severe reactions to tetanus vaccine.

Examples of tetanus-prone wounds include:
- Those contaminated with soil or manure
- Those harbouring infection or with a wound more than 6 hours old
- Puncture wounds, for example from nails or bites

Immunisation status	Prophylaxis required
Full course of five injections, or booster within the last 10 years	Clean wounds need no prophylaxis HATI can be given for tetanus-prone wounds contaminated with manure
Partial course, or booster more than 10 years ago	Tetanus booster should be given to all wounds HATI should additionally be given for tetanus-prone wounds
Unknown status, or non-immunised	Start tetanus course for all wounds If tetanus prone, additionally give HATI

Hints and tips for the exam

- You will be asked to suture a slab of sponge or fake skin. A piece of chicken is sometimes used. In either case, the principle is the same.
- The wound is typically straight and just 1–2 cm long.
- In a 5-minute station, it is unlikely that you will be asked to close the entire wound but instead to perhaps produce one or two sutures.
- You must say you would position the patient comfortably. This is often supine or semi-reclined, with the part to be sutured well supported.
- Show the examiner your aseptic technique.
- You may need an assistant in preparing your equipment, for example to pour the cleaning solution into your pot, but it is likely that, in 5-minute stations, this will already be set up for you, and you will just need to check that everything is there.
- Clean and wash the wound thoroughly before closure. If there is dirt or foreign matter, say that you would thoroughly irrigate the wound.
- The wound should be cleaned with sterile solution before local anaesthetic is given.
- Be generous with the amount of local anaesthetic because if the patient feels pain, they will tense their muscles and this can interfere with wound closure. However, take care that your local anaesthetic does not distort the wound edges.
- Infiltration of local anaesthetic should be from the outside inwards; do **not** forget the very edges and angles of the wound.
- Leave 1 cm of thread so that suture removal is easier.
- Do not leave the knot in the middle of the wound.
- Ensure there is no tension in opposing edges, and that the knot is not so tight as to cause pressure on the skin that it is holding.
- Document the number of sutures you have inserted so that, on removal, it can be ensured that all the stitches are out.
- **Practise** in your clinical skills centre as suturing without handling the suture needle is a difficult task until you have done it many times.
- Always mention tetanus.

68 Basic life support

Checklist	P	MP	F
Ensures safety of self			
Ensures safety of patient			
Adequate positioning of patient			
Checks for response			
Shouts for help			
Opens airway with manoeuvres			
Immobilises cervical spine if appropriate			
Adequate inspection and clearance of the airway			
Looks, listens and feels for breathing for 10 seconds			
Calls 999 or puts out cardiac arrest call appropriately			
Communicates location and situation well to the receiver			
Commences chest compressions at a rate of approximately 100/min			
Chest compression technique is adequate			
Stops after 30 chest compressions and gives two rescue breaths			
Adequate ventilation			
Continues cycle in a 30:2 ratio			
Knows to continue until return of spontaneous circulation, appropriate help arrives or becomes exhausted			
Puts patient in recovery position when return of spontaneous circulation occurs			
Frequently reassesses the patient			
Basic life support performed in confident manner			

Summary of key points for OSCEs

This situation may arise in the OSCE as either an out-of-hospital or an in-hospital situation, but in any case, until help arrives, the basic life support (BLS) technique is the same. The 'help' awaited will either be the emergency medical services outside the hospital or the cardiac arrest team in hospital.

There will be a manikin on whom you will be asked to perform the technique. This may be a simulation station, in which the dummy will be able to talk, or you may be demonstrating on a lifeless (sometimes limbless) manikin. It is important to know what equipment your clinical skills centre has and to familiarise yourself with it, as it is highly likely that this will be what appears in the exam.

BLS sometimes occurs as part of another scenario in which you have been called to see a sick patient and they suddenly become unresponsive. This is why frequent reassessment of the patient in any such scenario is important. The moment there is any doubt, start checking for the patient's response and begin BLS if necessary.

Note that, in the same station, BLS may then progress to advanced life support (ALS) when the necessary help arrives. ALS follows on from BLS, and is covered in the next station.

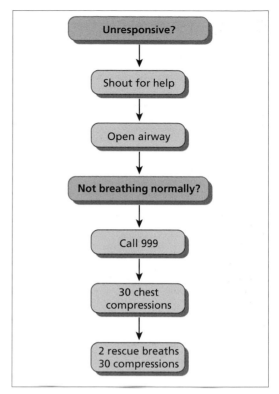

Figure 68.1 The Adult Basic Life Support Algorithm. Reproduced with kind permission of the Resuscitation Council (UK)

Hints and tips for the exam

• You **must** learn the Resuscitation Council (UK) guidelines and follow them to the letter. This should easily secure you a pass in this station.
• Always ensure your own safety first. Do not start BLS in the middle of a busy road for example, and ensure you have easy access to the patient without risking your own comfort.
• The patient's safety is paramount. Move the patient to a place of safety before you begin BLS.
• The ideal patient position for BLS is supine. If the patient arrests in a chair, they should be gently laid down with help, and space cleared around them in order for the resuscitation team to be able to reach the patient.
• Some situations require cervical spine immobilisation, which means that you must not carry out a head tilt in your airway manoeuvres. Cervical spine immobilisation is required in the following situations:
  • Known or suspected neck trauma
  • Drowning situations
  • Unknown or uncertain mechanism in cases of injury

• In any such station, your very first step is to *confirm cardiac arrest*:
  • Check for a response by gently shaking/stimulating the patient, and shouting 'Are you all right?'
  • Look, listen and feel for breathing for 10 seconds:
    • Open the airway with head tilt, chin lift, jaw thrust, as illustrated in Figure 68.2.
    • Place your face near the mouth, looking at the chest, and listen for sounds of breathing while feeling for warm breath on your cheek and observing the chest wall (Figure 68.3).
• You should then shout for help.
• If help arrives, they should be instructed to contact 999 or the cardiac arrest team:
  • The communication here must be clear.
  • It must be emphasised that the patient is **not** breathing, is unresponsive or has arrested, and your location must be clearly described.
  • If no help is available, you must call for help yourself prior to commencing BLS.
• As always, take an ABC approach.

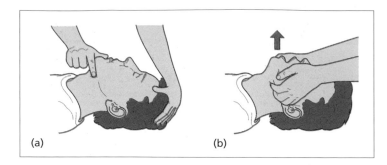

(a)   (b)

Figure 68.2 Manoeuvres to open the patient's airway. Head tilt and chin lift are usually sufficient. Jaw thrust is performed by placing your fingers behind the angle of the patient's mandible and applying firm upward pressure

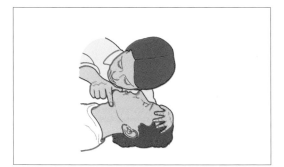

Figure 68.3 How to look, listen and feel for breathing. While listening for breath sounds, you should simultaneously observe for chest movement and feel for breath on your cheek. Ensure the patient's airway is open while you do this!

• When you open the airway, check for things that may obstruct the airway, for example blood, vomit, loose teeth or poor-fitting dentures. Turn the head to one side and scoop any obstructions out with your finger:
  • Do **not** do this with the head in neutral position or the debris may be pushed back into the pharynx.
  • Leave well-fitting dentures in place as they will help to maintain airway contour and make ventilation easier.
• Do good chest compressions at a rate of approximately 100/min:
  • The emphasis now is on good quality chest compressions, and in a BLS station you will get marks for this!
  • Place the palm of one hand on the lower third of the sternum (Figure 68.4).
  • Place your other hand on top of the first, and interlock the fingers. The pressure needs to be on the sternum and not the ribs, so your fingers should be away from the chest wall.

• The chest should be depressed to a depth that is approximately one-third of its anteroposterior dimension, or about 4–5 cm.
• The rate should be at approximately 100/min.
• Count out loud while you do this, so that the examiner knows you know how many to do.
• After 30 chest compressions, give 2 ventilations:
  • Open the airway adequately and remove any obstructions.
  • Form a good seal around the patient's mouth.
  • Inflate their chest for approximately 1 second.
  • Between breaths, maintain an open airway.
  • Watch for chest movement; if the chest wall does not move, your ventilation has been ineffective.
  • In hospital, you should use a self-inflating bag-valve-mask (e.g. Ambu-bag) rather than your mouth for ventilation (Figure 68.5). This should always be a two-person technique as you obtain a better seal between the mask and the patient's mouth.
  • **Do not** waste time if you have been unsuccessful in giving two good ventilations. There should be **two** attempts at effective ventilation, but no more. Instead, immediately recommence chest compressions. The Resuscitation Council (UK) suggests that continuous chest compressions with minimal interruption are associated with a better outcome.
• Continue in a 30:2 fashion until:
  • There is a return of spontaneous circulation
  • You are exhausted
  • Help arrives – in which case, continue CPR until the help takes over
• Following return of spontaneous circulation, put the patient in the recovery position, as pictured in Figure 68.6.
• BLS is a simple but essential skill.
• If you are unpractised, it will show in the exam.
• You must go your clinical skills centre, familiarise yourself with the exam manikins if possible, and practise.

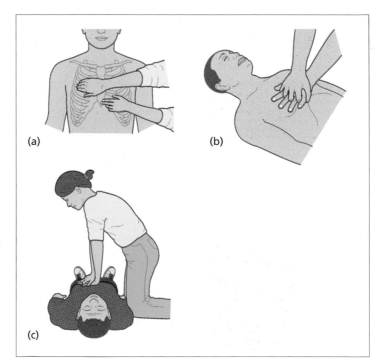

Figure 68.4 The correct method for chest compression. Your palm should be placed on the lower third of the patient's sternum, one hand over the other with the fingers interlocked. You should be positioned such that your arms are completely vertical above the patient's chest. The movement should be generated by your upper body, not your arms; aim to depress the patient's thorax by a depth of approximately one-third of its thickness

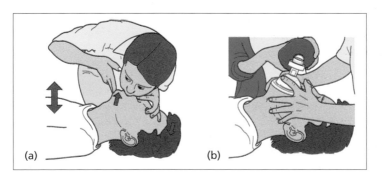

Figure 68.5 Mouth to mouth resuscitation is no longer necessary for bystander CPR. However, if it is to be performed, form a good seal with the patient's mouth and pinch their nose while delivering a breath. In hospital, use a two-person technique to ventilate the patient with a bag and mask; it takes two hands to form a good seal between the mask and the patient's face, so another person is required to squeeze the bag

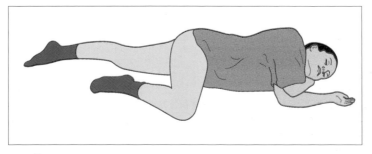

Figure 68.6 The recovery position

69 Advanced life support

Checklist	P	MP	F
Takes a safe approach			
Calls for help			
Checks for signs of life for 10 seconds			
Calls cardiac arrest team			
Gives 30 chest compressions at rate of 100/min			
Commences assisted ventilation with bag and mask			
Good two-person bag mask ventilation technique			
Continues uninterrupted CPR when the arrest team arrive			
Appropriately applies defibrillator pads			
Stops CPR **only** to assess rhythm			
Correctly diagnoses rhythm			
Safely administers shock of appropriate energy if indicated			
Immediately continues CPR for 2 minutes			

During 2 minutes of CPR, must express intention to: • Obtain a definitive airway, allowing uninterrupted chest compressions • Secure intravenous access and send off basic bloods, including a gas (venous/arterial)			
Uses adrenaline (epinephrine) appropriately			
Uses atropine appropriately			
Reassesses situation after 2 minutes and continues down the appropriate algorithm			
Looks for and considers all reversible causes of the arrest, arriving at the most likely			
Takes steps to correct the cause, while continuing CPR			
Good, effective, communication to team members throughout			

Summary of key points for OSCEs

The algorithm
The key to doing well in this station is following the Resuscitation Council (UK) algorithms to the letter. For advanced life support (ALS), this is included in Figure 69.1.

Reversible causes
Any resuscitation effort should not stop until and unless all reversible causes have been excluded. These can be broadly classified into 'the 4Hs and the 4 Ts'.

H	T
Hypoxia	Tamponade
Hypovolaemia	Tension pneumothorax
Hypo/hyperkalaemia or other metabolic cause	Thromboembolism
Hypothermia	Toxins

You are likely to be given a scenario, and that should allow you to establish the most likely cause. For example, if you are told that your patient has been rescued from submersion in a river, the most likely

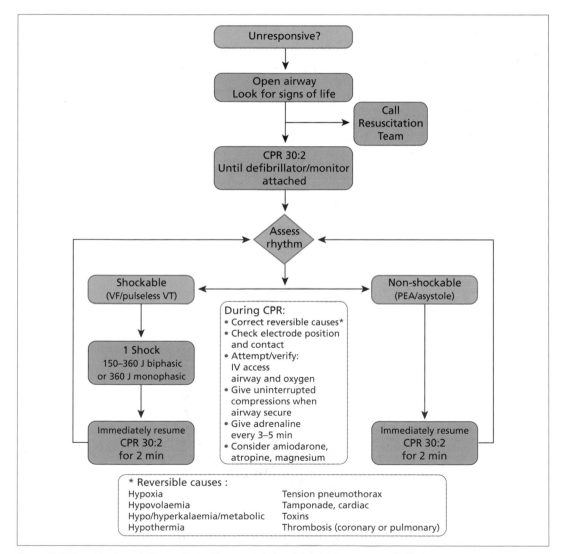

Figure 69.1 The adult Advanced Life Support Algorithm. PEA, pulseless electrical activity; VF, ventricular fibrillation; VT, ventricular tachycardia. Reproduced with kind permission of the Resuscitation Council (UK)

causes are hypothermia or hypoxia. If you then get further details, such as that the patient had consumed unknown pills before jumping in the river, 'toxins' becomes a possible cause. Suppose your patient had been thrown into the river by means of a road traffic accident as the cyclist hit by a car. This would lead to suspicion of tamponade, tension pneumothorax and hypovolaemia (as for any other trauma scenario) in addition to all the above.

In each case, the key is to begin good quality CPR and work through each of these possible causes. It should be reiterated that resuscitation should not stop until each of them has been addressed.

Cardiac arrest rhythms

Figure 69.2 illustrates the cardiac arrest rhythms you will encounter. Learn what they look like. It is highly likely that you will be asked to recognise them in the exam.

Defibrillation

The ventricular fibrillation/ventricular tachycardia (VF/VT) side of the algorithm is the side that is 'shock-able' and associated with a better outcome (although a good outcome post-cardiac arrest is rare).

Good defibrillation needs good technique. Applying the defibrillation pads in such a manner that the maximum possible voltage reaches the myocardium through thoracic wall tissues is vital. This means applying pads in a position of maximum contact, and using gel-based pads to reduce the impedance of the chest wall to the voltage delivered. In older machines, paddles and gel pads came as separate pieces. More modern machines use disposable self-adhesive paddles, with gel included.

Getting good access to the chest wall may mean cutting off the patient's shirt/blouse, jacket, etc. All medication patches should be removed as these will explode when shock is delivered. Oxygen must be taken away at the time of the shock. It is prudent to check that no member of the resuscitation team is touching the patient or the bed before delivering the current. A 'visual sweep' (i.e. looking around the bed to ensure nobody is touching any part of it) must be exaggerated in the exam to show the examiner that you know how to defibrillate safely.

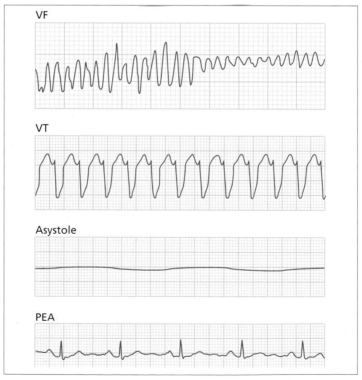

Figure 69.2 The following ECG rhythm strips demonstrate the shockable and non-shockable rhythms of a cardiac arrest: ventricular fibrillation (VF), ventricular tachycardia (VT), asystole and pulseless electrical activity (PEA)

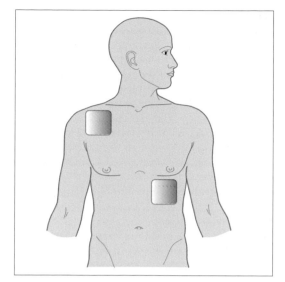

Figure 69.3 The diagram illustrates where on the thorax the defibrillation paddles should be placed. One should be placed to the right of the sternum under the clavicle, the other should be placed in the left mid-axillary line

Correct placement of the paddles is illustrated in Figure 69.3. One paddle is placed to the right of the sternum, below the clavicle, the other in the left mid-axillary line in the V6 position. If the patient has a permanent pacemaker, the paddles must be placed at least 15 cm away from any part of it or it may malfunction, or burn and cause tissue damage.

Most defibrillators are self-explanatory. If you look closely enough, most modern machines indicate what buttons to push in order by numbering them 1, 2, 3. Hence, do not panic if you find an unfamiliar machine confronting you in the exam. Some of the newer machines automatically analyse the rhythm for you, and these are found in public places to allow even the lay public to deliver defibrillation. In the exam, you may or may not get such machines, and you should take the time to familiarise yourself with the machines in your local place of work, or where the exam is to be held.

Selecting the correct energy value is important for good effective resuscitation. Most defibrillators are biphasic as this is less damaging to the tissues. A smaller amount of energy is required because the current travels in two directions, thereby traversing the myocardium twice. The initial setting for biphasic defibrillators is usually 150–200 J for the initial shock, and then 150–360 J for all subsequent shocks. Older monophasic defibrillators may be present as well, and these are usually set at 360 J for all shocks.

Following defibrillation, you must **immediately** recommence CPR, the emphasis being on good quality chest compressions. There is often a delay in getting an ECG trace, and the initial cardiac cycles after defibrillation may not be associated with a pulse. Reassess only after 2 minutes of CPR.

CPR

The strong emphasis is on good quality CPR. Early attainment of a definitive airway and continuous uninterrupted chest compressions are vital. The latest Resuscitation Council (UK) guidelines (2010) suggest that chest compression should continue even during charging of the defibrillation paddles, and halt for as little a time as possible to deliver assess the rhythm and deliver the shock.

The non-shockable side of the algorithm

If the initial rhythm is pulseless electrical activity (PEA), also termed electromechanical dissociation, or asystole, no shock is required. Uninterrupted CPR should continue, and the patient should be reassessed every 2 minutes.

In many cardiac arrest situations, you will switch cycles between algorithms, some cycles being shockable, others being non-shockable.

Key drugs

Adrenaline 1 mg intravenously should be given every 3–5 minutes, i.e. every other cycle after two cycles have been completed. It usually comes in a prepacked 10 mL syringe, with a strength of 1:10,000; 1 mg adrenaline is equivalent to all 10 mL of this preparation.

Atropine 3 mg intravenously should be given once only, if there is PEA with a heart rate of <60/min or asystole.

If patient has hyperkalaemia, hypocalcaemia or hypermagnesaemia, **10 mL 10% calcium chloride** over 10 minutes may be helpful.

Amiodarone could be considered for VF or pulseless VT.

In torsade des pointes, **magnesium sulphate** is important.

Hints and tips for the exam

These have been largely covered above.
• Know the algorithms. Following them precisely will secure a pass.
• Keep it simple and organised.
• If in doubt, think back to the beginning.

• In such scenarios, the exam will often position you as the team leader and ask you to allocate tasks rather than expect you to do everything yourself.

• Chest compressions should **not** be interrupted for anything except rhythm analysis and delivery of the shock. Chest compressions must continue even during charging of the defibrillator.

• During the 2 minutes of chest compressions, it is important to address the following:

  • Secure a definitive airway

    • This would normally be the job of the anaesthetist, who would intubate the patient with an endotracheal tube.

    • However, one does not need specialist skills to insert a laryngeal mask airway (LMA), which literally slides along the palate to the throat. Although an LMA does not protect the airway from aspiration, it provides a more secure airway that allows continuous, uninterrupted chest compressions.

  • Obtain intravenous access.

  • Send off basic bloods and a blood gas:

    • Blood gas analysis (even a venous sample) allows a quick analysis of key facts, for example potassium level, haemoglobin, etc.

• Check the good placement and adherence of the defibrillation paddles to the chest wall.

• Check adequacy of the chest compressions:

  • One should be able to palpate a central pulse if a chest compression is adequate.

  • It is important to rotate this role frequently between team members. Fatigue is a key cause of inadequate chest compression.

• Think of each of the reversible causes of the arrest:

  • Take measures to address them if they may have contributed; for example, start insulin/dextrose if hyperkalaemia is suspected, give fluids for hypovolaemia, warm the patient if they are hypothermic, etc.

• **Practice** makes perfect!

• It is often helpful to ask your resuscitation officers about any doubts or queries, and possibly help you work through some simulation sessions. Most resuscitation officers are friendly, approachable and very keen to teach.

70 Completing a death certificate

Task (5 minutes): Read the two clinical cases given to you by the examiner and then use these to fill out death certificates for the corresponding patients.

Checklist	CP	MP	F
Fills out 'name of the deceased'			
Fills out 'date of death as stated to me' in words and correctly fills out 'age' in numbers			
Correctly fills out 'last seen alive' line in words			
Correctly fills in line 1A			
Correctly fills in line 1B			
Correctly fills in line 1C			
Correctly fills in line 2			
Correctly fills in time interval between onset of illness written on lines 1A, 1B, 1C and 2 and death			
Writes in full without using abbreviations			
Does not use modes of death or 'failure'			
Identifies whether the death may have been contributed to by the deceased patient's occupation			
Ensures handwriting is legible			
Signs and dates certificate			
Correctly answers whether this death needs to be reported to the coroner			

On questioning, is able to identify cases that would need to be referred to the coroner:			
• Death within 24 hours of admission to hospital			
• Unknown cause of death			
• No doctor has seen the patient within 14 days of death			
• Death in prison			
• Death that is suspicious or related to violent causes			
• Sudden/unexpected death			
• Death during surgery or before recovery from anaesthetic			
• Accidental death			
• Death related to occupation			
• Death that may be the result from neglect			
On questioning, is able to state the criteria that must be fulfilled to be able to complete a valid death certificate:			
• Must be a registered medical practitioner			
• Must have seen the patient within the last 14 days			

Hints and tips for the exam

This is a very commonly tested finals OSCE station. Note that you will probably be required to fill out death certificates for at least two separate clinical scenarios in a 5-minute OSCE station, so you should practise pacing yourself accordingly in your study groups.

You are unlikely to get much practice at this task during any of your clinical attachments, so the best way to practise is by photocopying blank death certificates and setting each other example scenarios to complete within 5 minutes. Another option is to find out whether it would be possible for you to visit the bereavement office at your teaching hospital and spend a couple of hours going through some clinical histories and corresponding death certificates. In addition, you should memorise the criteria for referral to the coroner and the conditions that must be fulfilled before you can complete a death certificate.

Listed below are three example OSCE scenarios to get you started:

1. Mrs Winters is a 95-year-old lady who was admitted 7 days ago with a complete anterior circulation infarct. She deteriorated after admission and developed an aspiration pneumonia 2 days ago. *Escherichia coli* was isolated from a sputum sample. She was treated with antibiotics but subsequently went into cardiac arrest and was not resuscitated as she had a DNAR order. She had not been in good health for the previous 2 years and had a history of diabetes and Alzheimer's disease.

- 1A: Aspiration pneumonia caused by *E. coli*
- 1B: Complete anterior circulation territory cerebrovascular accident (**not** stroke)
- 1C: [BLANK]
- 2: Diabetes mellitus, Alzheimer's disease

2. Mrs Jones is 68-year-old lady with a history of multiple myeloma. She was admitted under the haematology team for an exchange transfusion. Five days into her hospital stay, she died from a pulmonary embolism. She is also known to have suffered from three miscarriages in the past, which were found to be secondary to antiphospholipid syndrome.

- 1A: Pulmonary embolism (**not** PE)
- 1B: [BLANK]
- 1C: [BLANK]
- 2: Antiphospholipid syndrome and multiple myeloma. (NB. Antiphospholipid syndrome and all malignancies contribute towards a procoagulant state)

3. Mr Smith is a 65-year-old man who was admitted 10 days ago with an anteroseptal STEMI. He was recovering on the ward but developed sudden shortness of breath and passed away from pulmonary oedema secondary to acute heart failure. He had a past medical history of angina, diabetes and hypercholesterolaemia.

- 1A: Acute pulmonary oedema (NB. **not** acute heart failure)
- 1B: Anteroseptal ST elevation myocardial infarction (**not** MI)
- 1C: Ischaemic heart disease
- 2: Hypercholesterolaemia, diabetes mellitus

Index

OSCEs for Medical Finals, First Edition. Hamed Khan, Iqbal Khan, Akhil Gupta, Nazmul Hussain, and Sathiji Nageshwaran.
© 2013 John Wiley & Sons, Ltd. Published 2013 by John Wiley & Sons, Ltd.

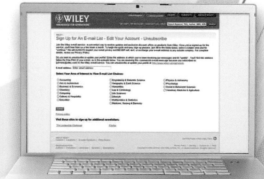
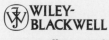

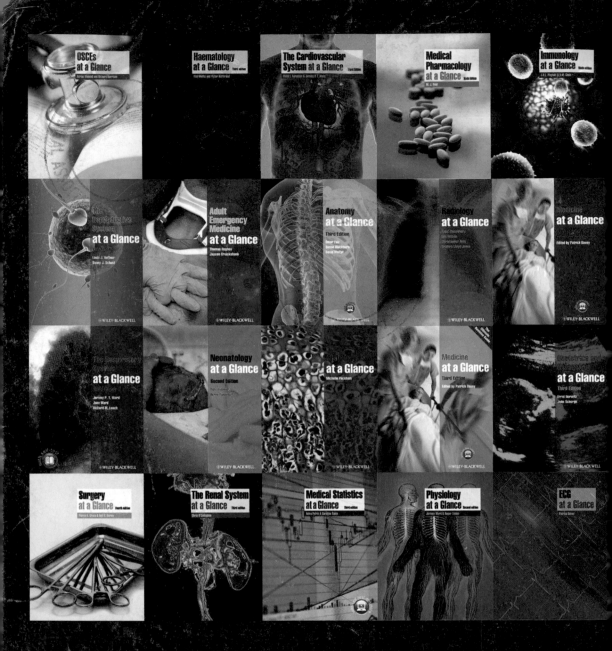

The at a Glance series

Popular double-page spread format › Coverage of core knowledge
Full-colour throughout › Self-assessment to test your knowledge › Expert authors

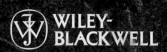